GAYELORD HAUSER'S
TREASURY OF SECRETS

Gayelord Hauser's Treasury of Secrets

By GAYELORD HAUSER

New York
Farrar, Straus and Company

Contents

Preface

A boy lay dying in a hospital in Chicago. He had undergone many operations and countless injections, and still his tubercular hip refused to heal. Finally the doctors decided: "Send this boy home. There is nothing more we can do for him."

So the unhappy boy was sent back home to die in the serenity of the Swiss mountains. There a miracle happened. One morning the boy was having his usual breakfast of coffee, rolls, and marmalade, when an old man, a family friend who had spent his life as a missionary, said to him, "If you keep on eating such dead foods, you certainly will die. Only living foods can make a living body."

"What are living foods?" asked the boy.

The gentle old man described them: "Fresh young growing things, especially green and yellow garden vegetables, saturated with earthy elements; lemons, oranges, and other tree fruits, full of sunshine and living juices." The old man knew nothing about proteins, vitamins, minerals, and the many other nutrients discovered since. But the sick boy listened thoughtfully. And from that day on, he began to eat enormous amounts of fresh living foods. And wonder of wonders, the hip that had defied all sorts of treatment, now, slowly but surely, healed. Through this amazing recovery, I discovered for the first time what fresh food can do. Yes, food saved my life—for I was that boy.

This is how, more than forty years ago, I decided to make food, diet, and nutrition my lifework.

I work hard. I spend long hours writing books. For many months of the year I lecture all over the United States, England, Germany, and France. And I am still hale, hearty, happy, and full of the enjoyment of life.

After all these years of seeing countless thousands of people eat their way to new-found health and vitality, I am more deeply convinced than ever that good nutrition can reduce human suffering and misery. And what is yet to be accomplished dwarfs everything we have so far achieved!

In the early Twenties I learned a bitter lesson. I realized then, for the first time, what Plato meant when he said: "Woe unto him who teaches a new theory and tries to change people's habits." I was called every name in the book by the *Fressers* who couldn't give up their "smashed" potatoes, greasy gravies, and devil's cakes —they were proud of their jowls and their paunches and even their gout. They wore them like badges of wealth and affluence. But the fiercest and most vicious attacks came from rather high places. Especially bitter were the manufacturers of foods I condemned then, as I do to this day: empty white flour, empty white sugar, denuded breakfast cereals, those processed cake mixes, the saturated greases and fats known as shortening. All are robbed of their life-giving nutrients: the vitamins, minerals, enzymes, and many elements that are still nature's secrets.

That's what the old man in Switzerland, with his God-given knowledge, meant when he gave me my all-important first lesson, a million dollar secret I pass on to you: Fresh food, the fresher the better—and it alone—contains all the living elements. Fresh food should be the basis of every meal we eat if we wish to stay young and vital. It is a secret I want to share with the millions of sad, sick people the world over: *Only living food can build a living body*. Every one of our daily meals should give our bodies living food: the freshest milk, cheese, and eggs; lean meat, fish, liver and other organ meats; and always the freshest green and yellow fruits and vegetables, served as huge salads or as fresh juices or espressos.

People from all over the world travel to Zurich, Switzerland, to take such a *Frisch Kost* diet at the Bircher-Benner Sanatorium; hundreds of these patients who were given up by their physicians have found new health. Yet the diet is such a simple one. It consists entirely of such living foods as green salads, fresh vegetables, vegetable juices, milk, and their famous fresh Bircher Apple Muesli. For many years I knew the beloved physician Dr. Bircher-Benner. I listened to many of his lectures (given at six o'clock in the morning). Fresh food had also saved his life, and fresh food was his favorite subject. He often spoke of "sun-cooked food," especially green leaves which are saturated with sun energy and therefore have the most potent health-giving properties.

The Hunza People Know the Secret

Twenty-five thousand people called the Hunzas are living today in a little isolated region of Pakistan. They never heard of sun energy, vitamins, or enzymes in food. They simply accept nature's gifts. They till their soil, they sow their precious seed, and they wait for the harvest. These people have no refrigerators. Their simple food consists of fresh vegetables, fruits, goat milk and meat, and whole grains. All comes fresh from the land, directly into their cooking houses. And as Dr. McCarrison, of London, who lived among the Hunza people, said: "They know no sickness. The women are small and beautiful, and the men are tall and tough. The only work for a doctor is to help them with fractures or other accidents." Isn't it good to know, in this day of synthetics, calorie charts, and TV dinners, that there still are healthy people on this earth who live simple, happy lives, close to nature and far away from delicatessen stores?

I realize that we cannot all live today like these lucky people of Hunza Land. But these healthy men and women are living proof that fresh, simple food is superior to our sophisticated, over-refined empty foods.

A Long Life for Our Foods or for Ourselves?

Dr. E. V. McCollum, of the famous Johns Hopkins Hospital, expressed the whole thing in a few words when he said: "Eat only food that decays or spoils easily, but eat it before it does."

How many foods did you eat today that spoil easily? Too many foods in our pantries keep indefinitely; they have been emptied, peeled, pickled, chemicalized, and embalmed for a long shelf life. Manufacturers, of course, want a long shelf life for their products. But you and I want a long life for ourselves!

Happily, our government is making stricter laws forbidding the use of harmful chemicals. The cranberry scare started many people to thinking. Scientists and other intelligent people everywhere now agree that we need more wholesome, natural foods, preferably grown in fertile soil and without artificial sprays. Such foods are already being produced on a large scale in England, Germany, and Switzerland. In Japan, where they do not have the abundance that we enjoy in the United States, researchers are trying to modernize the Japanese people's eating habits. Milk has been introduced into the spare Japanese diet, with noteworthy success. Already there are signs that the Japanese have stronger legs and are growing taller.

Fortunately, the soybean and soybean milk, cheese, and the golden oils are still mainstays in Japan. Europeans are always amazed to see so few overweight Japanese. Japan has the lowest death rate from heart and circulatory diseases; and how interesting it is that the Japanese consume only 8 percent of their calories in fat—and that fat is unsaturated vegetable oil extracted from the soybean. According to Dr. Philip S. Chen, professor of chemistry and author of the splendid book, *Soy Beans for Health, Longevity and Economy,* the soybean is rich in lecithin, which seems to be most helpful in keeping cholesterol moving through the body instead of allowing it to become deposited in the arteries. Dr. Chen definitely feels that the humble soybean and its products, and particularly the lecithin in it, are of tremendous value to those with heart and circulatory difficulties.

Prosperity Has Perils Too

In West Germany, where great prosperity is also responsible for great trouble, eating rich and refined foods has become the favorite indoor sport. Bulging waistlines are back—and with them, the same old metabolic diseases: gout and gall bladder and digestive troubles, which had disappeared during the lean years. German doctors wonder what this will lead to. Many now recommend drastic juice and tea fasting. The two most famous sanatoriums are under the direction of the Drs. Buchinger, father and son, both physicians. I have been a guest in Bad Pyrmont and in Uberlingen am Bodensee. Both of these beautiful places are constantly filled. They specialize in the fasting cure with outstanding success, especially in cases of rheumatism, digestive diseases, and obesity. You will learn later on about my personal experiences in these sanatoriums.

Since German physicians discovered that overweight patients prefer the short juice fasts to the long, drawn-out low-calorie diets, ten more such diet sanatoriums have sprung up. Now the idea has spread to England. Who knows? It may even spread to the United States. If some modern young doctor were to establish such a sanatorium, it would prove a blessing, especially for the grossly overweight. However, no one should ever undertake a prolonged fruit or vegetable juice fast without the supervision of a physician trained in that special field.

One of Germany's distinguished physician-nutritionists is Dr. Werner Kollath, author of many books on nutrition. His whole philosophy can be condensed into one single sentence: "Let things be natural, as natural as possible." In other words, Mother Nature knows best; let your diet consist of natural, fresh things. Dr. Kollath asks his patients to eat only fresh foods—even to grind their own grains—to get all of the living elements. There is a special Kollath Breakfast Mixture, very much like the Bircher Apple Muesli (page 411) which Dr. Bircher-Benner originated for the sturdy Swiss to eat instead of empty cereals.

The good work of Sir Arbuthnot Lane, that grand old man under whose auspices I lectured in England, is still going on. Sir Arbuthnot, a great surgeon, for many years observed in the operating room the damage that bad eating habits did to the liver, heart, kidneys, and digestive organs. He organized the New Health Society to teach the English people to eat in the modern manner—less of the rich suet puddings, starches, and sweets, and more of the good proteins and fresh things.

Even in Russia, where life is unbelievably difficult, and unthinkable for free people, I found tremendous interest in better nutrition. There are posters everywhere that tell people to eat fresh food, to gather herbs, to take vitamins—especially vitamin C, for which they especially cultivate rose hips. According to our standards, food in Russia is poor and terribly monotonous; but it is much more earthy and natural. They forbid the use of chemicals in or on foodstuffs. I assure you they are desperately trying to be tops in nutrition.

The Russians Ask Embarrassing Questions

Interviewing some of the Russian nutritionists was embarrassing at times. One asked bluntly: "Why have you so many sick people in your rich country? Why have you more deaths from atherosclerosis and heart attacks than any other country in the world? Why do you not teach people to use more sunflower oil? We are doubling our output; we order our small farmers to plant the big-kernel variety along the roads or wherever else there is a bit of unused ground."

I could not deny that we in the United States have the highest death rate from heart disease, for statistics prove it. But I did say proudly that we have not only sunflower oil, but we also have safflower, peanut, corn, sesame, and olive oils galore, and more and more people are using them. I did not want to say that many of our people are spoiled or indifferent to the modern way of eating because I know what he would have said: We *make* our people eat what is best for them. You see, they have dictatorship in all phases of life. We're lucky, we free people who can choose with our own free will.

But I could not help thinking what Paul de Kruif wrote a few years ago in his book, *The Hunger Fighters*: There is hidden hunger that lets folks starve to death while they're eating plenty. In our own rich, lovely land we suffer from too many over-refined, empty foods; we starve for the living elements, the vitamins, minerals, and enzymes, and the many as-yet-undiscovered elements found in fresh food.

Our Physician Researchers Find the Answers

Dr. E. H. Ahrens first alerted Americans to the dangers of eating heavy cholesterol foods. From Dr. J. M. Beveridge, Professor of Biochemistry at Queens University in Ontario, Canada, came the happy discovery that the unsaturated fatty acids of our golden vegetable oils are helpful in reducing high cholesterol levels. (Dr. Beveridge used corn oil in his experiments.)

For a while, nutritionists and dietitians everywhere had recommended low-fat diets to reduce their patients' cholesterol. This worked in some cases; but many patients could not get their cholesterol levels down with low-fat foods. Then another important discovery came from the Donner Laboratory of the University of Berkeley in California. An experiment, under the direction of Dr. J. W. Gofman, demonstrated that blood cholesterol levels would rise even on a low-fat diet when the carbohydrates (starches and sweets) were increased.

At Harvard University School of Public Health, a research team specifically studied the relationship between cholesterol and a diet high in white sugar and found that diets high in refined sugar cause an increase in cholesterol. And Dr. G. Cheney, of the

Department of Medicine at Stanford University in California, announced that so simple a food as fresh cabbage juice would heal ulcers. He later identified the healing factor as vitamin U.

I was delighted that at least one fresh vegetable juice had official recognition as a potent healer; I knew from personal experience that fresh carrot juice had helped me to get well. As you probably know, I am most enthusiastic about fresh "living" juices, not just cabbage juice (which is unfortunately the least tasty), but also carrot juice, celery juice, and apple juice, singly or mixed; these contain vitamins, minerals, enzymes, and other still unidentified "living" substances. Since I introduced the drink-your-vegetables idea in America, several excellent books have been written about the "blood of the plant," a natural and quick way to increase the whole family's well-being.

Dr. Tom Douglas Spies, when he received the Distinguished Service Award from the American Medical Association in 1959, told the doctors, among other things: "All disease is caused by chemicals, and all disease can be cured by chemicals. All the chemicals used by the body, except for the oxygen we breathe and the water we drink, are taken in through food." Dr. Tom, as they lovingly called him at the Hillman Hospital in Birmingham, Alabama, rescued thousands of those poor hill people (I never saw poorer and more miserable people in my life), and his secret was a diet rich in fresh foods, high-potency vitamins, high-potency food yeast, and peanut butter. Dr. Tom, who did so much for the science of nutrition and to help the lowliest of poor and sick, unfortunately died much too soon. This was a great personal loss to me, for he was the only one who stuck by me when I was attacked so ferociously for recommending such foods as yeast, wheat germ, yogurt, and blackstrap molasses. "Why all the fuss?" asked Tom Spies. "We've been eating blackstrap molasses down here for years, and it's a darned good food."

Are We So Healthy?

I know there are many Americans who still laugh at the idea of eating natural wholesome food: Some even claim that we are the healthiest and best-fed nation in the world. Nothing could be further from the truth. The report which that Russian nutritionist thrust under my nose was correct: We do have the highest death rate from atherosclerosis and heart attacks. It also pointed out that Americans consume 40 percent of their calories in saturated fats, compared with the 8 percent consumed by the slender Japanese, who use chiefly vegetable oils. And if we are so well-fed and healthy, why did our President tell a nation-wide television audience, on December 5, 1961: "To get two men today, the United States Army must call seven men. Of the five rejected, three are turned down for physical reasons and two for mental disabilities . . . and the rejection rate is increasing each year."

I find it a tragedy that our young people should have such a miserable record at a time when we know more about building healthy bodies than ever before. We know today what foods and elements are essential for building health and vitality, what foods are the best sources of each vitamin and mineral, how fatigue can be prevented, how most sickness can be warded off, and how to live longer—in short, how to build a good body that houses an alert mind.

Fortunately, food research is now going on in all parts of the world. But what good is all our research if it is not used and applied in that unsung laboratory and center of the home—the kitchen? There the wise homemaker can apply all the million dollar secrets discovered by scientists of many lands. A wise homemaker—and I meet thousands of them—knows that the well-being of her whole family is largely in her two hands. Her menus can make or mar her husband's success as a good father and provider. They can build the health and good looks of her growing youngsters. What she selects for her market basket can vitally affect both the physiological and phychological health of her loved ones, as individuals and as a family. Her whole happiness in marriage may be in direct ratio to what she knows about modern nutrition and how to apply her knowledge.

And here, I believe, is where I come in. In schools and clinics, in laboratories and sanatoriums, I have asked thousands of questions, made tests, and always offered myself as an experimental guinea pig to demonstrate my conviction that with good nutrition comes a good life. I have always taken great pride in interpreting the complicated and confusing technical language of the latest scientific discoveries into plain everyday speech so that everyone could understand and apply them. I wrote a book about good food and good health, and how it affects our happiness and *joie de vivre*, called *Be Happier, Be Healthier*. Later I wrote a book for the harassed overweighters, *The New Guide to Intelligent Reducing*, with a few fundamental reducing secrets and no gimmicks. It quickly became a best-seller and was translated into French, German, Swedish, and Italian. When many requests came from England and France I finally wrote *Mangez Pour Etre Belle*, or *Eat and Grow Beautiful*, giving the ladies their heart's desire—showing them how a cosmetic diet creates an inner vitality and the kind of beauty that does not come off at night. This book created a sensation in France.

But my most popular book, written to appeal to both men and women, was *Look Younger, Live Longer*. That did it. Almost overnight I became a hero. With it came offers for radio and television; King Features Syndicate serialized the book in every large city; the *Saturday Evening Post* and many other magazines did feature stories about me and my Wonder Foods; and the *Reader's Digest* did a condensation. *Look Younger, Live Longer* has been translated into 27 languages.

I learned an important lesson during those hectic days. Wherever I went, little people, big people, all people, had one thing in common: They were hungry. They were not particularly interested in me, nor were they hungry for more food. They were hungry for more life, for better health, for younger bodies and keener minds. And only because I could satisfy this hunger and teach them the secret of eating for health, good looks, and high vitality, did they become my devoted friends and followers. My Town Hall lectures are now filled to overflowing whenever I appear, whether in New York, London, Berlin, or Paris. One of the great joys of my full life is the countless letters I receive (in many languages) telling me how people have been able to transform their lives from mediocrity into a state of positive health and vitality.

Occasionally some people with serious medical problems ask for my help. These people I always advise to find a local physician, preferably one who knows and applies modern nutrition. Sick people should always be under a doctor's care. Then, I tell them, when they are well, they should make every effort to apply the secrets of modern nutrition to prevent future troubles.

Nothing, I believe, pays higher dividends in health and happiness than knowing how to apply modern nutrition—not for a day or a week, but for a lifetime. I hope you will let me be your guide to this splendid investment in yourself.

Two years ago my publishers asked me to build another book, putting together a selection of the most important materials from my books and nutrition classes, and telling all the new and exciting things happening in the world of nutrition—a sort of *Treasury* of all my million dollar secrets. I hesitated, thinking it would not be possible to get so much into one book. But with much writing, and rewriting, and pruning, trying to get the work of many years down to my most essential teachings, I hope I have succeeded in making this book the most helpful one in your library—a book that will answer most of the thousand and one questions I am constantly asked.

Some years ago a noble and very rich maharaja came to see me in Paris. He was a troubled man: He could not sleep. Through our mutual friend, Lady Mendl, I learned that His Highness had spent a fortune for every kind of treatment; but still he could not sleep. With the cooperation of the Maharaja's personal physician, we put His Highness on a high-vitality diet, high in protein and extra high in calcium and all the B vitamins. The frightened man had been tense from head to foot, and he needed to learn to relax. This was difficult at first, but he was most cooperative. Within just two weeks, this troubled man slept peacefully. His tense expression was gone and his whole attitude toward life changed. He was a most gracious and grateful man. I shall always remember his parting words: "Mere money cannot pay for your priceless secrets. I would not take a million dollars for what you taught me."

Those million dollar secrets are all in this book. I know that if you apply them faithfully, they can bring to you and your family, as they have to so many others, a new vitality and a joy in living worth many times a maharaja's millions and his treasure of jewels.

For even the greatest wealth is worthless without health, and joy in living is more precious than rubies.

GAYELORD HAUSER

Springtime, 1963
19 Union Square West
New York 3, New York

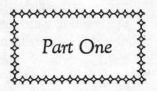

Part One

LOOK YOUNGER, LIVE LONGER

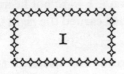

Passport to a New Way of Life

The book you hold in your hands is no ordinary book. You are holding a passport to a new way of living. You are not just beginning to read. You are beginning a new adventure, a journey of discovery.

Like any journey, this one requires a certain amount of courage at the outset. Courage to do new things, think in new ways, entertain new ideas, some of which may surprise and startle you. Like any journey, too, this one requires at the outset a certain amount of confidence and a sense of excitement. Confidence in the guide and in the value of the goal. Excitement at the prospect of setting forth into unfamiliar territory, of testing your own ability to grasp new concepts and accept new points of view, some of which may seem not only unfamiliar but unorthodox.

However, I promise you that like any adventure undertaken with courage, confidence, and excitement, this one will reward you richly from beginning to end, every step of the way.

Before we start, you should know who I am, since I am to be your guide on this journey. I am a doctor, not of medicine but of natural science. I have taken my inspiration from the teachings of Hippocrates, Paracelsus, Father Kneipp, Hindhede, Bircher-Benner, and other great teachers of ancient, medieval, and modern times. The word *doctor* comes originally from the word *docere* meaning "to teach." Even if I were not licensed to practice a healing art, I would feel that I had earned the right to this title.

You and Me and a Longer Life

I have three special qualifications for teaching people how to live longer. One is my own great relish for living. There was a time, many years ago, when I had a supposedly incurable disease and hope for me was given up. Perhaps I relish life more because at that time I had to fight for it. At any rate, I find it very good and very satisfying to be alive. Each year on May 17 I celebrate my birthday; I like to receive the good wishes of my friends and the good thoughts of my students. But I refuse to get older. I celebrate each birthday not just as the end of another good and satisfying year of life but as the beginning of a new year of exciting work, travel, and accomplishment.

My second qualification for teaching people how to live longer is my great relish for people. Perhaps the fact that I grew up in a large family (I am the ninth of ten children) has something to do with this.

As a dietitian, nutritionist, lecturer, and writer, I travel constantly, all over the United States and Europe. Wherever I go, I meet more and more people. Many of these are People—spelled with a capital P. Many of these are my good friends. They include royalty, society leaders, stage and screen stars, statesmen, business executives, sportsmen, writers, philosophers, doctors, artists, scientists, teachers, and preachers.

I meet people in large and small cities, on trains, ocean liners, and air liners. I meet them at Hollywood parties, in drawing rooms in New York, London, Paris, and Rome. I meet them in the learned circles of Vienna and Copenhagen and in the crowds that gather around my lecture platform all the way from Boston, Massachusetts, to Seattle, Washington.

Also, I meet people in another place—on the shelves of the nearest library, wherever I happen to be—for my appetite for reading books by and about people is almost as great as my appetite for knowing the people themselves. Many of these library-shelf people also are People. Many of these, also, are my good friends.

My third qualification for teaching people how to live longer is my own great relish for longevity. I have always devoured every-thing bearing upon the subject of longevity—in the fields of nutri-tion, endocrinology, surgery, biology, biochemistry, osteopathy, naprapathy, chiropractic naturopathy, psychiatry, philosophy, phys-ical culture—wherever I could find it.

I have visited many of the famous watering places in Europe and the United States, and tested their special diets and regimes. I have visited doctors in their offices and sanatoriums, research scientists in their laboratories, and many health resorts and beauty-farms. I have assembled rooms full of books and filing cabinets full of pamphlets, reprints, and clippings dealing with my favorite subject. I have inquired into and experimented with or speculated upon everything I could find that anyone has said, thought, written, discovered, developed, invented, promised, prophesied, or dreamed of, that had to do with living a long life.

Why?

Well, I myself would like to live for a long time. I would like to live for at least one hundred years.

Would you?

I know what you are thinking. You are thinking, "This man is mad. Suppose I can live to be one hundred. Who wants to hang onto life—frail, dried-up, useless—just for the sake of proving that it can be done?"

Who, indeed? Not I. You are thinking in old terms. I have told you that this book is an adventure into new ways of thinking.

Do you want to live one hundred years if, at the age of one hundred:

> Your body will not be wracked with aches and pains?
> Your face will not look like a dried-up apple?
> You can still be of definite use in the world?

Then come along with me.

In this book, this journey that we are taking together, I will teach you how to eat not merely to satisfy hunger, but to eat for health, good looks, youth, vitality, the joy of living. I will show you that you are not old at forty, fifty, sixty, seventy. That you need not be old at eighty, ninety—shall I go on?

Certainly I shall. I have friends and students who have passed seventy, eighty, ninety, and one hundred without getting old. I shall talk about them in this book. You will meet some of them and share their secrets.

You will learn how to nourish your entire body. You will learn how to eat so that your own blood stream will contain all the vital elements for nourishing the inside of your body, your arteries, glands, colon, bones, connective tissues. So that, whatever your age, you will *feel* young.

You will learn how to eat, also, so that your own blood stream will contain all the vital elements for nourishing the outside of your body, your muscles, skin, hair, teeth, eyes, complexion. So that, whatever your age, you will *look* young.

And you will learn how to eat so that your own blood stream will contain all the vital elements for full, energetic enjoyment of living, for nourishing your mind, heart, spirit, your total personality. So that, whatever your age, you will *be* young.

Forget your age. It does not matter. This is what matters: are you alive? Do you want to stay alive until you are one hundred or more years old? Do you consider the possibility that you may live to be one hundred an exciting idea? A challenge? An opportunity? A great adventure?

Then come along with me.

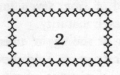

2

Forget Your Age

Now, put this book down for a moment. Say to yourself, "I—this person sitting here in this chair—I can live to be one hundred years old." Say it aloud. Listen to your words. Repeat them.

This idea is new to you. It is a new kind of thinking. Take your time with it. Accept the idea of living to be one hundred. In imagination, extend your life forward, far into the future. Figure out what the calendar year will be when you are one hundred. Think what the world will probably be like, what new, interesting, unheard-of things probably will be happening. Say to yourself, "I shall be alive then. I can be alive in the year ——."

Accept those years. They are yours. This is not wishful thinking or idle daydreaming. It is simple acceptance of scientific fact. Science has increased your life span beyond your wildest expectations.

You can live one hundred years. This means that whatever your present age is, you are young.

Suppose you are forty. Heretofore you have been saying to yourself, "I am *forty.*"

But now that you have been told that you will live to be one hundred, you are saying to yourself, "I am *only* forty."

It is not possible, at this time, for us to place a limit on the age to which man may aspire, if he is assured of a life reasonably free from tensions, and is fed an ideal diet rich in every vital necessity. It has been stated by certain scientists that living creatures may well attain a life period of from seven to fourteen times as long as the time required to reach maturity.

Man attains maturity at the age of twenty; therefore he might live one hundred and forty years. Said the Russian Dr. Alexander A. Bogomolets: "A man of sixty or seventy is still young. He has lived only half his natural life. Old age can be treated just as any other illness because what we are accustomed to regard as normal old age is actually an abnormal, premature phenomenon."

Scientists have proved that the spark of life can be prolonged indefinitely. The Russian professor Kuliabko removed a human heart, from a soldier killed in battle, and restored its action twenty-four hours after it had ceased beating. Another scientist, Briu-khonenko, restored life in dead dogs by artificially renewing their blood circulation. *The stuff of which we are made is potentially immortal.* Many scientists have demonstrated this, notably Dr. Alexis Carrel who experimented with a piece of heart tissue cut from a chicken and put into an ideal nutritive medium. This piece of chicken heart lived on, as long as the "broth" in which the tissue lived contained all the necessary nutrients and the waste products were eliminated.

But to live long without growing old—how can that be done? From the dawn of recorded history, mankind has sought the fountain of youth.

You are as young as your glands, some scientists have said. The French scientist, Charles Edouard Brown-Séquard, believed that the secret of youthfulness lay in intravenous injections of extracts of animal testicles. Steinach, in Vienna, hoped that tying off the spermatic cord would flood an aging man's entire body with sex hormones and make him forget the calendar. Voronoff, in Paris, transplanted the sex glands of monkeys into male and female patients in the quest for rejuvenation. Following the same quest, American biochemists harked back to Brown-Séquard and developed testosterone, which has helped some and disappointed many.

You are as young as your colon, other scientists have said, notably the bacteriologist Metchnikoff. He believed that the body is prematurely aged by toxins released by the decomposition of food in the bowels. His secret of youthfulness was to wage war on the bacilli producing the toxins in the colon by marshaling against them armies of the beneficent bacilli contained in acidophilus buttermilk and yogurt.

Said the Canadian Dr. William Osler: You are as young as your arteries.

Said Bogomolets: You are as young as your connective tissues. Bogomolets made world-wide headlines by perfecting A.C.S. (anti-reticular cytotoxic serum) and stating that with regular injections of A.C.S., plus reasonable care, we can all live to be one hundred and forty.

Says the French Dr. Saint-Pierre in his book *Prolonger La Vie*: You are as young as your blood. In Paris today, people in search of rejuvenation are flocking to Dr. Saint-Pierre who, out of fresh young human blood, makes a serum and injects it into the bodies of older men and women; and in Switzerland Dr. Niehans injects fresh cells (*Frisch Zellen*) of unborn animals, usually lambs or calves, into the tired and aging. His method has attracted world-wide attention. I will discuss this treatment more fully later on.

But I believe that the answer lies not just in the glands, the colon, the arteries, the connective tissues, the blood, or in any *one* part of the body, but in the whole body.

Steinach himself realized that. He once said to me, "I have opened *one* door to the palace of truth. No doubt there are a hundred corridors I have overlooked, a hundred doors that others luckier than I will enter."

I belive that I am one of those lucky ones.

I believe that you are as young as you *look, feel, think, hope, believe, and act*. And I believe that the way you look, feel, think, hope, believe, and act depends on three things:

An adventurous young spirit
Good food
A strong vibrant body

In short, I believe that *you are as young as your diet*.

The world over, scientists studying the extension of life are finding more and more evidence that the fountain of youth is *good nutrition*. Dr. Henry C. Sherman of Columbia University is considered one of the world's outstanding authorities on nutrition. In a lecture given before the New York Academy of Medicine, Dr. Sherman stated that, given the right selection of foods, human life can be greatly extended. Furthermore, says Dr. Sherman, the later years can be lived in much fuller measure of usefulness.

What is meant by good nutrition? First, it is adequate nutrition, giving the individual cells of the body not only the quantity but also the quality of nourishment they require. Second, it is balanced nutrition, supplying the body cells with vital nutrients in the proper proportion. Scientists are unanimous in agreeing that overnutrition, through excess calories stored as fat, contributes materially to physical deterioration and the aging process.

As a simplified, perhaps crude, illustration, think of your body as a motor car. It is made of protein, inside and out. Arteries, glands, colon, connective tissue; muscles, skin, bones, hair, teeth, eyes: all contain protein and are maintained and rebuilt with protein. Fats and carbohydrates are your body's oil and gasoline; they are burned together to produce energy. Vitamins and minerals are its spark plugs, essential to the utilization of food and its assimilation into the blood stream.

It is a marvelously sturdy motor car, this body of yours—marvelous in its ability to maintain and rebuild itself. Given care, consideration, and respect, it will function smoothly, on and on. Provided that none of its important organs have been allowed to break down, it can and will heal and regenerate itself at any age. It cannot be neglected or abused. It must be fed and cared for faithfully. When it does not hit on all cylinders, it must be examined by an expert mechanic who can not only find out what is wrong but also detect hidden weaknesses, forestall serious breakdowns. Even when it is functioning adequately it should have regular over-all checkups, preferably always at the same "machine shop" where its history is known and its special characteristics and needs are understood.

Headed by the Mayo Brothers in Rochester, Minnesota, and Johns Hopkins Hospital in Baltimore, Maryland, human "machine shops" are springing up all over America. Wonderful clinics are staffed with topnotch physicians and equipped with the most superb diagnostic facilities in the world—equipment which private doctors could not possibly afford. Doctors at such clinics look for specific symptoms; but more than that, they consider the individual as a whole—his body, his mind, his special circumstances and problems. They are interested, these expert "body mechanics," in the over-all picture. Their aim is to arrest deterioration and more, to forestall such deterioration, prevent it.

One by one, the so-called infectious diseases are being controlled. Heart disease, hardening of the arteries, arthritis, strokes, high blood pressure—all are giving ground to science. I am convinced that with our growing knowledge of prevention, plus the immense progress the science of nutrition is making, America is leading the world into a new era, a Look Younger, Live Longer Era.

"Your body may seem much the same to you as it was a year ago, plus or minus a few pounds or inches, but . . . in a single year, 98 percent of the old atoms will be replaced by the new atoms which we take into our bodies from the air we breathe, the food we eat, and the water we drink."

Dr. Paul G. Aebersold
Head of the Atomic Energy Commission
Washington, D. C.

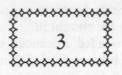

3

Vital Foods for Longer Life

Age is a physiological and psychological matter; it has no relation to the calendar. Examination of men and women over one hundred years of age at some of our famous clinics revealed that they had four outstanding qualities:

> Strong digestive juices
> A slow, rhythmic heartbeat
> Good elimination
> Happy dispositions

Let me introduce to you one of the happiest people I have ever known. I first met her twenty years ago. She had worked with Wallace Beery, Sonya Henie, Charles Laughton, Don Ameche, Bette Davis, James Stewart, and a dozen others, but I did not know that. To me she was one of the hundreds of people who had crowded into a large auditorium in Los Angeles to hear me lecture.

I had never seen her before but I recognized her at once. She was one of my People. I knew by the way she sat—erect and disciplined, her shining white head resting proudly on straight shoulders. I knew by her face—strong as well as sweet, revealing inner beauty as well as beauty of line and feature.

She was a Person, no question about it. After my lecture, I saw her among the crowd gathering around the platform to meet me. We shook hands, and then I realized that she was an actress, too.

"Tell me," she said, her eyes sparkling with humor, her trained, resonant voice carrying clearly. In mock despair she put her hands on her stomach, which was perhaps not quite so flat as it might have been. "Tell me—*what* am I going to do about this *jelly belly?*"

Of course she brought the house down.

Adeline de Walt Reynolds was then eighty-two. At the age of sixty-five, she told me, having raised four children and helped raise a raft of grandchildren, she had decided to go to college. At sixty-nine, she was graduated from the University of California. Then Hollywood discovered her and the new star "Grandma Reynolds" was born. At the age of eighty-two, with thirteen years of stardom behind her, she saw no limit to the years of stardom ahead of her. *If* she could get rid of her "jelly belly."

That was not difficult. With a lifelong habit of regular exercise, a natural talent for relaxation, and the drive that comes from sheer zest for living, she had long since made of her body a well-trained, responsive instrument. Her basic dietary habits already were good; I advised only such changes as would make sure that her diet contained many, many of the good proteins needed to rebuild tissue more firmly and strengthen the natural "muscular corset" which has been given to all of us to protect the abdomen, the most vital and vulnerable region of the body. I added brewers' yeast, yogurt, and cottage cheese to her diet and taught her the one exercise which I consider indispensable—the Stomach Lift. She bought herself two Yoga Slant boards—one a plain board, the other with a motor attached which mildly rocked her to sleep after a hard day's work at the studio. (I shall have more to say about the Stomach Lift and about Yoga Slant boards later.)

Six months passed. I lectured again in Los Angeles. Again Grandma Reynolds was in the audience. She was at my elbow the minute my lecture was over.

Her head was prouder than ever; her eyes were full of excitement and delight. She had just begun work on a new picture, she told me. It was the best role she had had yet. She was starring with Bing Crosby in *Going My Way*.

The "jelly belly"?

Neither of us even mentioned it. Grandma Reynolds was as flat across the midriff as I am.

At the ripe young age of 96, Grandma was still starring on television. What was her secret for long life, good health, and happiness? She herself could not have told you. She had a strong constitution, she had always loved life and believed in living each day to the full. She did not know her own secret. She had never analyzed it. But her secret was that all of her life she followed *instinctively* the basic principles of the Look Younger, Live Longer program.

Long ago I discovered that my friends and students who are youthful at seventy, eighty, and ninety had many of the same principles and beliefs that I had. The difference was that, while I had arrived at my principles and beliefs through study, research, and experiment, they had arrived at theirs intuitively. It had been their lifelong habit to eat a balanced diet, keep their bodies in topnotch condition, and maintain a cheerful, positive attitude of mind. I found that they knew without being told that it is better to undereat than to overeat, that they had been given, apparently by the good fairies who presided over their cradles, a supreme gift—the gift for complete body relaxation.

I have checked this evidence over and over again.

Another outstanding example of its soundness: a good friend of mine who lived to be 106—Hiram R. Gale, a veteran of the Civil War.

I met him more than twenty years ago in Seattle. In full uniform, complete with medals and decorations, this grand old soldier stood long in line at the reception which followed a lecture I gave there. He was erect, buoyant, with bright blue eyes and rosy skin.

"I wanted to shake your hand," he said. "I listened to every word you said. Not that I needed telling. Been doing everything you talk about as far back as I can remember."

A "natural" Hauser student all his life, Hiram Gale was a literal follower of my regime. As a result, Hiram Gale in his second century was exceptionally healthy, happy, and ambitious. His big ambition—to be Commander-in-Chief of the G.A.R.—was fulfilled in 1945–46.

What you eat between the ages of 40 and 60 largely determines how you feel, look, and think at 70 and 80. Now is the time to take stock of yourself. Now is the time to discard myths of "age," and concentrate on agelessness. Now is the time to discard careless habits and swing into the Look Younger, Live Longer way of life.

The body can be rebuilt at any age. Well and wisely fed, the body and all its organs are capable of reaching a greater age than most of us ever before dared hope for.

ENJOY YOUR FOOD

It was stated recently in one of the medical journals that 75 percent of the senior half of our population suffers from malnutrition. Studies reveal that most people over sixty suffer from a number of nutritional deficiencies. My own personal observation corroborates these facts; rarely do I find, among the thousands of people—rich and poor—who come to me for advice, a person midway in life who could not profit by improved nutrition.

Many things may contribute to this needless "running down" of life. With years of food for food's sake, the appetite becomes dull. With lessening of appetite, interest in preparing and eating good foods lessens. Perhaps mealtime is lonely. Poor teeth may make chewing difficult; one may consider eating a tedious task to be finished as quickly and easily as possible, without thought of its life-giving potential.

Food is made for man. By all means, let us enjoy it. I believe in eating all kinds of good food, either fresh or cooked (never overcooked) in infinite variety. I believe in spiking meats and sauces with herbs and fragrant spices, much as the French people do. I believe that everyone should not only consider a large, crisp salad as an important part of the main meal but also *eat it as the first course of the meal, when appetite is keenest.* Fruit should become the favorite dessert, either fresh or stewed in the modern manner with honey. (See Lady Mendl's *compote des fruits* on page 513).

Food makes amazing contributions to health. Consider this with every mouthful you eat, for many of the vital food factors are hard to get, and you cannot afford to miss any opportunity. The secret of longevity largely lies in eating intelligently. Learn to like foods that are health-giving. This becomes easy as you learn about food values and also the values of vitamins and minerals. It becomes exciting to feel yourself a kitchen chemist rather than a kitchen slave.

Looking back over all these years I have studied and taught nutrition, I realize that one of the most important factors is the *satisfaction center.* Certainly eating should be a pleasure. But too many people—especially people who are not happy—try to use rich, fattening foods as a substitute for other pleasures. And often these foods are eaten absent-mindedly or bolted hurriedly, with a minimum of satisfaction. If you will choose wholesome, natural foods, eat them slowly, chewing them twice as long as you now do, you will then feed your satisfaction center. You will eat half as much and enjoy it many times more. Then you can throw away your calorie charts, throw away your diets, and never again overeat. You can keep your slim, healthy, attractive body for the rest of your long life.

WHY BOTHER TO EAT INTELLIGENTLY?

Students sometimes ask, "Why must we be everlastingly intelligent about diet? Our forefathers knew nothing of vitamins, minerals, amino acids, and the rest. They ate without thought of balanced diet and food values and maintained a high degree of health. Why must we bother always to eat in what you call the modern manner?"

The answer is: You must eat in the modern manner because you live in the modern age.

Going back far enough, the probabilities are that our forefathers enjoyed considerable adequacy of diet. Sugar itself was at a premium and certainly white sugar was not a poor man's food; white flour was unheard of. Cold-storage fruits and vegetables were unknown. Processed, oversterilized, and highly refined foods were not articles of commerce. Soils were richer in humus, vitamins, and minerals, thus producing foods richer in vital factors. Foods went from the fields to the tables more quickly. There was no need to count calories.

No calories were derived from synthetic pick-up beverages and pops such as are popular today and which consist mainly of empty sugar and synthetic flavors.

Ever since we learned to refine and "preserve" food, deficiencies began suddenly to develop. What science has accomplished in combating disease is nearly offset by the outrages done to our food by the processors. Only a small percent of foods in our super-duper markets contain the good nutrients that our forefathers enjoyed in their simple home-cooked meals. Today, when over-refined foods are the rule rather than the exception, we should rely primarily on the finest fresh foods available and supplement the diet with the wonder foods (page 33) and the best vitamin concentrates available.

The sound combination of medical and nutritional sciences will promote the longevity of the individual—true longevity, the addition of years at the end of life's span. I am not talking of impersonal averages, based on statistics, but of the long lives that every one of you may live. To bring this ideal about, the layman, the individual man in the street, must be conscious of the need for adequate, well-balanced nutrition. He must have a sound background knowledge of the needs of nutrition, and he must exercise care in the selection of the food he eats. Until such knowledge has become general, we shall never know man's potentiality in longevity. It is not a bother, or even a duty; it is an act of self-preservation.

It is my belief that, because man long has been adapted to foods as produced in nature, he should eat *natural* foods. (See also page 23.) I advocate the use of whole-grain flour and cereals instead of refined products, even the so-called "enriched" variety. For by means of what is termed "enrichment," they put back only a fraction of what has been taken out. In the lost portion are vital nutritive factors that, in the earlier days of nutritional science, were brushed off with the expression that "their need in human nutrition has not been established." Today we are constantly learning more and more about how important these factors are. I am willing to learn from broad practical experience, and I shall always give reasonable processing the benefit of the doubt. If at times it fails, at other times it is valid; if I make a mistake in my judgment, it will always be on the side of conservatism and safety.

I hope to see the day when everyone, especially growing children and persons over forty, will eat intelligently, consuming foods adequate to their bodily needs for vital factors. Undereating is better than overeating, for surplus fat is an enemy of health. But overeating of vital factors never hurt anyone. I believe in a reasonable abundance of proteins, vitamins, and minerals. Mastication, particularly in older people, and also digestion and absorption, are not always perfect. A reasonable oversupply of the essential factors to compensate in such cases is much to be desired.

I believe that a well-fed body is the best defense against the many tensions of modern living. There is a great need for the practice of moderation—in the use of spirituous liquors, smoking, and quest of physical excitement. When the body is well nourished, when no cravings of the tissues produce a physiological unrest, then and only then do I believe that man has attained a state in which he can more easily realize moderation, under the social, economic, and political pressures of the day.

How Much Shall I Eat?

That is a question that I am frequently confronted with. First, we *will* eat to satisfy our energy requirements. I emphasize "will" because simple physical hunger demands it. Moreover, unless we supplied our energy requirements reasonably well, we would lose so much weight that our bodies would become emaciated. It is too bad that we do not also have a mechanism that tells us about the hidden hunger of the cells for vital nutritive factors. However, we are endowed with intelligence and we are supposed to use it.

We cannot use our brains if we have no knowledge. How can you, my reader, use your intelligence in regard to eating if you are told little, if anything, about the specialized knowledge of modern nutritional science? It is the purpose of books such as this to bring you that knowledge, in a form that you will understand and that will so impress you that you will want to be guided by it, even to the extent of making a very special effort.

Food for energy is measured in calories, and the term *calorie* is simply a unit of energy. Physical hunger—not to be confused with emotional cravings for food, sometimes caused by frustrations and tensions—generally is a good guide to the amount of food we need for energy; certainly, to the person who is at all observant, experience, together with honest hunger, is an ample guide to how much to eat.

The insistent inquirer often asks this question: "Is there no simple guide that can be followed to ensure a good supply of each vital factor? I am told that I need some thousands of units of vitamin A, a few milligrams of vitamin B₁—and a different number for each vitamin. How can I remember them all? It is all very confusing.

Why did they not devise their units so that every factor works out to the same number?" What could be a more logical request—and it can be answered!

All we have to do is to forget units and milligrams, and call the quantity of each vital factor we require 100 percent. In this way the needed amount is reduced to the same figure for every factor.

It is my philosophy, born of years of experience and my long study of nutrition, that generous allowances of the vital food factors make a definite contribution to health and longevity. I grant that the necessary quantity of some of the vitamins and minerals, particularly some B vitamins, is conditioned by energy requirements. However, to reduce general dietary considerations to the finest distinctions is both tedious and unnecessary, and, moreover, it discourages the busy person whose table is not set with a slide rule along with a knife and fork!

Just remember that the wholesome, natural foods give much greater appetite satisfaction and are therefore your best guardians against overeating.

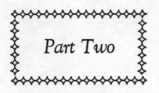

Part Two

YOU ARE WHAT YOU EAT

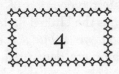

4

Eat Natural, Wholesome Foods

When I first taught and lectured before Town Hall groups, I was delighted by the general good looks of these audiences. They were women of culture, intelligence, and wealth, who knew a great deal about art, literature, music, economics, and politics, and even something about nuclear physics. But they knew so little about food. How could I tell? Long before they began asking questions on the subject it was woefully apparent as I looked out across row after row of women about one-third of whom were overweight.

Well, they were there to learn about food—and I was there to teach them. They followed my lecture intently, faces lighting up as I explained how within thirty to sixty days they could, if they truly desired to do so, change their lives and become their vital selves again, with better skin and shiny hair. Most important, that it could be done sensibly and enjoyably without grim do-or-die dieting or mad calorie counting.

One of the reasons why we have more overweighters in America than in any other country is because we have more food and more money to spend for it. But the thought I want to impress upon the minds of all intelligent people is that, nutritionally, man has been asking for trouble ever since he began tampering with the quality of Nature's foodstuffs. It is my opinion, based upon observation and experience in nutrition for more than forty years, that the country which produces the most denatured, artificial, over-refined foods will have the greatest proportion of overweighters—and that country, I am sorry to say, is the United States of America.

Practically all the food we *habitually* eat has been tampered with. Our bountiful grains are denatured in the milling process, vitamins and minerals removed, and the bleached-out remainder is processed into soft, fluffy white breads that would be laughed at in Europe. Sugar is refined, bleached, and processed. Most fats and oils are over-refined and hydrogenated to negative value. Fruits and vegetables frequently are sprayed with poisonous insecticides. (I hope that Rachel Carson's wonderful book *Silent Spring* will help to remove these poisonous sprays and chemicalized foodstuffs from our markets.) And then, in our kitchens, chefs and housewives habitually overcook, overpeel, overlook and throw away many valuable food elements.

Of course I know that life can no longer be lived as naturally and as simply as in our forefathers' day, but even in our overcivilized age there is much we can do to protect ourselves, nutritionally. If we are to keep our bodies slim and fit and wholly alive, we must have more wholesome food—food that is 100 percent nourishment, as Nature intended it to be. It can be had in lean meats, short-cooked tender vegetables, crisp and tasty green salads, ripe fruits, fruit and vegetable juices, natural sugar with all its vitamins and minerals, and breads that still contain the "staff of life" nutrients of the original grain. It cannot be had in devitalized foodstuffs that are overcooked and over-refined, or in soda pops and colas.

I have had to get accustomed to ridicule during the past forty years because I constantly insist upon naturally nutritious foods. It is tough going at times, and it may take another forty years before it is generally realized that one of the reasons we have so many sick and overweight Americans is that so many of our foods are relatively foodless. If it seems shocking to you, may I remind you that President Kennedy, during Physical Fitness Week, said: "In order to get two healthy young men for the armed forces, we now have to call seven." And these are *our* young men, remember.

The late Dr. William Howard Hay influenced the eating habits of Americans and Europeans through his writings and nutrition classes. Some years ago, when the first big revolt against foodless foods swept America, I spent an evening talking nutrition with Dr. Hay. It was interesting to hear him definitely blame the refinement of our food for the increase in obesity and heart trouble and many other diseases. Imagine my pleasure when this famous doctor said to me, "Hauser, I am impressed by your personal story of how you ate yourself from sickness to health. I like your gospel of 'living foods.' If people were given natural foods their appetites would be natural; they would not constantly overeat and there would be no need for us to teach them. Stick to this gospel. You are young and will see many changes; you can have great influence. Never weaken in your conviction that natural food is best for man's health and happiness."

I have never weakened. I believe that "We are what we eat." I look forward to the day when smart Americans will demand more naturally nourishing foods, and I hope and believe that when that time comes our great industrialists and food processors will ungrudgingly supply it.

Meanwhile, we thinking people can find many complete and unrefined foods available, and supplement them with extra vitamins and minerals. Such good, wholesome fare nourishes and satisfies so that you cannot overeat and will not want to.

Good meals—nourishing meals—mean much more than a certain quota of calories; they mean balanced proportions of proteins, carbohydrates, fats, vitamins, and minerals. You'll find them in the foods recommended in this book. Let me show you, now and forever, how well you may eat, how many good foods you may enjoy, and how you can maintain your health and good looks.

Proteins, carbohydrates, and fats are the BIG THREE. In order to eat well, of course, you need the "hidden" food elements—the vitamins, the minerals, and the many as yet undiscovered food factors. The last word in nutrition has not yet been spoken, but this we do know: that most people do not get an excess of proteins, vitamins, and minerals. They overeat on starches, sugars, and hard fats. Here, then, is what every homemaker should know about the foods she selects and prepares for the family table.

Proteins—Body Builders, Repairers, and Youthifiers

Proteins are of first importance for growth, development, and maintenance of life. They are "protective foods." They satisfy hunger; they stick to the ribs, nourish, and keep the body young and elastic.

In addition to building and repairing body tissue, protein is used in making hemoglobin, the iron-containing substance of the red blood corpuscles. Hormones are made of proteins. All of the enzymes in the body, which aid in the production of energy, the digestion of foods, the building of new tissue, and the tearing down of worn-out tissue, are made of protein. Proteins in the blood are responsible for the collection of urine and waste from the tissues. Proteins also help prevent the blood and tissues from becoming either too acid or too alkaline. They are important in making possible the clotting of the blood. Proteins even form substances known as *antibodies,* which combine with and render harmless the bacteria, bacterial toxins, and other foreign materials that act as poisons in the blood. When proteins are not supplied to carry on these many functions, the body is susceptible to sickness and even premature death.

For overweighters who want to cut down the size of their bodies and rebuild them closer to the heart's desire, ample amounts of first-class proteins are a *must.* Remember that they prevent hunger and they prevent the body from going soft and flabby. All too often we see people who have reduced their weight by drastic diet and insufficient protein foods, looking old, haggard, and wrinkled in consequence.

Keep in mind that when protein foods form the basis of a reducing plan, the body is helped to metabolically *subtract* the stored-up fats and carbohydrates.

Protein is an "active" nutrient, busily employed in repairing the daily wear and tear. Nutritionists agree that every man and woman should have, daily, about one gram of first-class protein for each two pounds of body weight. (This means your real weight, not overweight; the right weight for a person of your height, bone structure, and sex. See the chart on page 388 if you are not certain, or let your doctor help you.) A woman weighing 120 pounds should have 60 grams of protein a day; a man weighing 150 pounds should have 75. Many people ignore this important point, and without sufficient proteins they feel weak, tired, and irritable, and their best plans go overboard. Also, protein foods are not the lowest in cost—and this cost factor is one of the reasons why I introduced the "life saving" proteins of powdered skim milk, brewers' yeast, soya flour, and wheat germ, which are excellent fortifiers for those who cannot afford the more expensive forms of protein foods.

Irrespective of cost, the first-class proteins are found in eggs, cheese, milk, yogurt; the glandular meats such as liver, kidney, heart, brain, sweetbreads; and of course, the roasts, chops, steaks, poultry, and fish. But glandular meats take first place because they are richest in essential vitamins and minerals as well. Among vegetables, only a few contain first-class proteins; they are soybeans, nuts, some seeds, and fresh wheat germ. Second-class proteins are found in dried beans, lentils, corn, rye, and gelatin.

From long experience I have found that meals including both animal and vegetable proteins are the best insurance of a firm and healthy body. Here, then, is a check list of good protein foods. May I suggest that you check your protein intake for the last twenty-four hours? You may be surprised.

Fresh Meats and Fowl	Amount	Grams Protein
beef, lean	1 serving*	20
chicken	1 serving	23
ham	1 serving	20
heart, beef	1 serving	19
kidney, lamb	1 serving	18
lamb chop	1 medium	14
liver, calf	1 serving	21
meat, average lean	1 serving	20
sausage, bologna	5 slices	12
steak	1 serving	21
turkey	1 serving	22

Fresh Dairy products		
cheese, American	2 × 1 × 1 inches	14
cottage	3 tablespoons	10
cream	1½ tablespoons	0.6
cream soups	¾ cup	4
egg	1 large	8
milk, whole	1 quart	34
powdered skim	½ cup, level	20
skim	1 quart	34
yogurt	1 cup	9

* The average serving is usually considered to be about ¼ pound of meat.

Fresh Fish and Seafood	Amount	Grams Protein
clams	6	14
fish, average	1 serving	21
oysters	7 medium	12
salmon, canned	⅓ cup	11
shrimp	6 medium	8
tuna	⅓ cup	12

Nuts		
almonds	10 medium	6
peanuts	2 tablespoons	8
peanut butter	2 tablespoons	9
pecans	10 large	3
walnuts	½ cup	8

Vegetables		
beans, lima (green)	½ cup	6
navy	½ cup	6
beans, soya, dry	½ cup	36
soya grits	½ cup	25
soya flour	1 cup	40
corn, fresh or canned	⅓ cup	3
lentils	½ cup	10
peas, dried & cooked	½ cup	6
fresh	½ cup	5
potato, white	1 medium	3
sweet	1 medium	3
yeast, brewers'	1 level tablespoon	8

Grain products		
barley, whole, cooked	½ cup	8
bread, whole wheat	1 slice	3
buckwheat, whole (dark)	⅓ cup	5
oatmeal, cooked	½ cup	3
rice, brown or white	¾ cup	3
shredded wheat	1 biscuit	3
spaghetti	¾ cup	3
wheat germ	½ cup	14

The average serving of many vegetables contains only 1 gram of protein. This amount is so small and the protein so inferior that it is best not to consider it.

Fortify Your Meals with Extra Protein

1. Make your own Hi-Vi milk. Mix one cup of powdered skim milk with one quart of fresh skim milk. Believe it or not, you have about 70 grams of protein—practically a whole day's supply of first-class protein in a single bottle. Keep this in the refrigerator and use any time during the day.
2. Add one or more tablespoonfuls of food yeast to all stews and gravies.
3. Add half a cup of fresh wheat germ to meat loaves and hamburgers, and sprinkle wheat germ over cereals.
4. Use yogurt in place of sour cream.
5. Learn to use soya flour and soya grits in your cooking and baking. Two tablespoons can be added to your favorite recipe for waffles and biscuits. Remember, just one cup of soya flour gives you 40 grams of good protein.

QUICK-ENERGY FOODS—THE CARBOHYDRATES

The chief function of carbohydrates in nutrition is to provide energy for the body and for muscular exertion, and to assist in the digestion and assimilation of other foods. In moderation, they are indispensable to the metabolic processes. Taken in excessive quantities, such as gorging oneself with sweets, pastries, and starchy foods, the carbohydrates cannot be used up by the body and are only stored as fat where you least want them—in the double chin, potbelly, and buttocks. Carbohydrates, as they are broken down by the body, eventually form pyruvic acid, which not only inhibits the disposal of body fat but is actually converted into more fat. It can safely be said that most people overeat on overprocessed empty carbohydrates.

Another minus factor of excessive carbohydrate intake, recently reported, is that it causes B vitamin deficiency. In an effort to burn up the unnecessary carbohydrates, the body uses extra B vitamins—which are rarely sufficient for other metabolic needs. The vast consumption of white sugar, which is a chemically-pure sucrose without vitamin content, is the No. 1 vitamin-depleting factor in the American diet.

The best carbohydrates, with all their important vitamins and other nutrients intact, are found chiefly in whole-grain flours and cereals, fresh fruits, fresh vegetables and their juices. Nutritionists suggest about one gram of carbohydrate daily for each three pounds of your body weight. This means about 40 grams for the 120-pound woman and 50 grams for the 150-pound man. I strongly urge you to do away with your white-sugar bowl and in its place get one of those drip-cut honey jars, especially if you have to feed a large family. Honey is one of our finest natural sweets, containing its own vitamins and minerals; whereas, white sugar contains no vitamins, no minerals, no real nourishment.

Actually, you never need to worry about not getting enough sugar. You may be surprised to know how many other sources of sugar there are. Practically every mouthful of fruit and vegetables you eat contains sugar. All breads, cereals, dried beans, and other starchy vegetables are changed to sugar in the process of digestion. Even meat and liver contain some starch which is changed into sugar—and listen to this: about 10 percent of the fats you eat yield glycerin, when digested, and this in turn becomes sugar. In fact, about 65 percent of the food you put into your body is turned to sugar.

Yes, you can get your full quota of sugar without your beloved sugar bowl, and I can promise you that your craving for sweets will become less and less as you eat more natural foods. If you crave sweets, you can satisfy that hunger with honey, molasses, sweet fruits, or fruit drinks.

Here is a list of the wholesome carbohydrates you can use with good conscience:

YOUR BEST CARBOHYDRATES

Wheat, rye, barley	Short-cooked vegetables
Brown rice	Fresh vegetable juices
Whole-grain breads	Fresh fruits
Whole-grain cereals	Fresh fruit juices

YOUR BEST SWEETS, IF YOU NEED THEM

Honey, unheated	Brown sugar, natural
Unsulphured molasses	Dried fruit, unsulphured
Maple sugar	Carob powder, in place of chocolate

BEST FATS—FOR SUSTAINED ENERGY AND SMALLER WAISTLINES

Fat is used as a source of sustained energy, as heat insulation under the skin, as a padding for the framework, to round out the contours of the body, and prevent excessive fat deposits around the middle. Fat foods supply more than twice the number of calories available from the same amount of protein or carbohydrate. Meals containing some fat have greater "staying power" because fat is more slowly digested and absorbed than all other foodstuffs. This aspect is an important point for those wishing to reduce; it means that the stomach feels full and contented for a longer time.

When liquid vegetable fats are used in normal amounts—never less than 2 tablespoonfuls a day (even on reducing diets)—they are completely and easily digested. Unfortunately, with our increased prosperity, Americans instead of using 25 percent fat in their daily meals, today consume from 40 to 50 percent of their calories in hard fats. No wonder Carl Sandburg, our beloved poet, said: "We are dripping in fat." The unsuspecting public doesn't know that so many of our foods such as crackers, cakes, and cookies are often saturated with the wrong kind of fat.

I believe two events, more than anything else, made the civilized world sit up and take notice: (1) Dr. Bronte Stewart's experiments in 1956. When he gave his patients oil instead of animal fat, he actually brought about a rapid decrease in their blood cholesterol. (2) President Eisenhower's heart attack. This brought the danger of excess animal fat in the diet to the attention of the general public. The arguments still continue, and probably always will; but the fact remains that the hard animal fats can and do create high cholesterol content in the blood, whereas the liquid golden vegetable oils do not. In fact, our golden oils even help to lower high cholesterol levels and thus already have been a godsend to millions.

All animal fats, including cream, butter, lard, and all meat fat, are frequently guilty of contributing to overweight, hardening of the arteries, heart trouble, gallstones, and many other diseases. There are those who say that tension and stress and strain can also create excessive amounts of cholesterol. No doubt that is also true, but diet can be much more easily controlled than one's emotions.

All vegetable oils contain the unsaturated fatty acids—especially linoleic acid, which is so important not only for good health, but also for good looks. A German chemist, in his experiments with animals, proved that when he deprived his animals of linoleic acid their skin became very dry and scaly and the hair became dry and thin. As soon as the important linoleic acid was returned to the diet, the skin and hair again became normal.

Last, and most important, the golden vegetable oils, with their rich supply of unsaturated fatty acids, actually stimulate (via the pituitary) the burning of stored fat. Thus you never need to be afraid of these oils—they are not weight adders; instead, they even help to burn up excessive fat deposits. Golden oils have become more and more important for reducers. Whole books have been written about them.

Here is your choice of golden oils, with their approximate percentages of valuable linoleic acid.

Safflower	70	Sesame	41
Poppyseed	62	Avocado	39
Sunflower	57	Peanut	25
Soybean	53	Flaxseed	20
Corn	53	Sardine	15
Wheat germ	50	Olive	10
Cottonseed	50		

Sunbutter

Many who object to the taste of the new oil margarines on the market like the delightful combination of highly unsaturated sunflower oil and fresh butter. Here you have both the health benefits of sunflower oil, with its valuable unsaturated fatty acids, plus the excellent taste and vitamins of fresh dairy butter. My cook in Sicily first made a combination of one pound of fresh butter with one cup of olive oil. It is delicious. Of course, Sicilians love the strong olive oil flavor. However, sunflower oil is cheaper. For an all-around delightful buttery combination, on toast or sandwiches and over cooked vegetables, use butter mixed with one of the milder oils; cold-pressed sunflower oil makes the best-tasting combination. It is most important, when using oils, that they be absolutely fresh.

Sunflower oil stays fresh much longer than safflower oil and is ideal for our sunbutter:

Sunbutter

1 pound fresh dairy butter
1 cup sunflower oil
  season to taste

Place fresh butter in bowl and whip until soft and smooth. Gradually add sunflower oil, and mix thoroughly. When blended, put mixture in square butter dish or small cake pan and place in refrigerator until hard enough to be cut into squares or pats.

For variety, spike mixture with vegetable salt, your favorite herbs, or fresh garlic. Keep refrigerated at all times.

Food cooked with sunbutter will delight a gourmet!

THOSE WONDER FOODS

There are certain foods I call "wonder foods." I have often been criticized for using this term, but still I continue to use it. I believe that it says exactly what I mean, and it is as appropriate as the term "wonder drugs." These wonder foods are so full of such concentrated goodness—and they are so inexpensive and always available—that they are indeed wonderful.

They provide excellent quantities of many of the hard-to-get B vitamins; or they are rich in easily digested protein—and ease of digestion is of great importance, especially in the second half of life. They also provide generous quantities of calcium and iron, two minerals that become more and more difficult to obtain from ordinary foods. These wonder foods also can easily be eaten every day without becoming tiresome, and they can be mixed with other foods to add valuable nutritive factors. I talk a great deal about them, for I am convinced that if they are used generously they will so improve the nutritive quality of the diet that your health is bound to be benefited. Wonder foods can also help you to look younger and live longer.

Brewers' Yeast

This wonder food has been found to contain 17 different vitamins, including all of the B family; 16 amino acids; and 14 minerals, including the "trace" minerals, held to be essential. It also contains 36 percent protein (sirloin steak, not counting the bone, may contain as little as 23 percent protein). Brewers' yeast contains only 1 percent fat, whereas sirloin steak contains 22 percent!

The calorie requirement of the average woman is about 2,000 per day. One tablespoonful of brewers' yeast adds up to only one-hundredth of this calorie requirement, but it provides over one-third of my generous daily allowance of vitamin B_1 (thiamine) and very nearly one-fifth each of the vitamin B_2 (riboflavin) and niacin allowances. Put in another way, on the basis of its calorie contribution, it contributes 354 times as much vitamin B_1, 160 times as much vitamin B_2, 176 times as much niacin, and 91 times as much iron!

Remember, the amount of brewers' yeast we are talking about is just *one tablespoonful*—8 grams, only 22 calories! Think how easy it is to add to your B vitamins and iron, to be sure that you get a true abundance, simply by stirring a tablespoonful of brewers' yeast in a glass of tomato juice, fruit juice, or buttermilk, by sprinkling it over your salad or your whole-grain cereal.

The figures given here are derived from ordinary brewers' yeast. Specially cultured strains, sometimes referred to as food yeast, are even richer in B vitamins. When you purchase brewers' yeast, examine the label carefully. Always, it should give you in 8 grams (a little over one-fourth ounce) not less than 0.78 milligram of vitamin B_1; 0.44 milligram of vitamin B_2; and 2.9 milligrams of niacin. Do not be confused if the label states the quantity in micrograms. There are 1,000 micrograms in one milligram; therefore, 0.78 milligram would be 780 micrograms. If you encounter micrograms and want to transpose them into milligrams, just move three places to the left and place a decimal point. The food yeasts, which are richer in vitamins than ordinary brewers' yeast, cost only a very little more and are cheaper in the long run because they give you more vitamins. Moreover, they are more convenient to store, as you need a smaller quantity. If you do not care for the flavor of ordinary brewers' yeast, you can obtain it in a pleasantly flavored form.

I use the terms *brewers' yeast* and *food yeast* because these indicate a palatable form of yeast. Many kinds of yeast are produced, primarily for baking, that have an unpleasant, bitter taste. If you have trouble finding brewers' yeast, any diet and health food shop has it on hand. Under no circumstances should you ever eat fresh yeast which is used in baking.

Powdered Skim Milk

Powdered skim milk has many properties that cause me to classify it as a wonder food. First and foremost, it gives you protein of high biologic quality, practically free from fat, and in combination with rich quantities of calcium and riboflavin (vitamin B_2). Moreover, its vital nutritive factors are in a form readily available to the body and easily digested. Of secondary importance is its convenient physical form; being a dry powder it can be kept on hand in the pantry at all times. It is well to store it in an air-tight container, preferably a metal one with a screw-on closure provided with a rubber liner. This will exclude the moisture of the air and light, prevent the product from "staling" or becoming lumpy, and also preserve its riboflavin content.

Add powdered skim milk (also called nonfat milk solids) to fresh milk, sauces, soups, custards, waffles, muffins, and all breads; no change of recipe is necessary. It is also delicious whipped into potatoes.

A nourishing beverage for everyone—youngsters and oldsters alike—can be made by mixing one-half cup of powdered skim milk into a quart of whole or skimmed fluid milk. If whole milk is used, the calories are increased by only 17 percent, whereas the vital food factors are increased by the following percentages: protein, 62.3; calcium, 62.5; iron, 50; vitamin B_1, 60; vitamin B_2, 100; niacin, 63.

Yogurt

Yogurt is an important wonder food because it is an excellent source of easily assimilated, high-quality protein and contributes significant quantities of calcium and riboflavin to the diet. Yogurt fills a need that has long existed—that of a luncheon dish or a between-meal or bedtime snack. So many people eat what I call "foodless foods" at such times—devil's cakes, pastries, cinnamon toast made with white bread lavishly sprinkled with white sugar. A taste for yogurt is acquired quickly; you will become fonder and fonder of it as time goes on. It is a good hunger satisfier and, most important of all, contributes much-needed vital food factors with every mouthful. A cup of yogurt, fortified with powdered skim milk provides only about 7 percent of the calories for a 2,000 calorie a day diet; at the same time it provides, in terms of my generous daily allowances, protein, 17.5 percent; calcium, 50 percent; and vitamin B_2, 30 percent.

Yogurt and the acidophilus cultured milks have undergone many ups and downs in popularity. They have been advocated for everything from "that tired feeling" to typhoid fever. My interest in yogurt is wholly concerned with *nutrition*, and from a nutritional point of view it is tops.

Bulgarians are credited with retaining vigor, vitality, and the characteristics of youth to an extremely advanced age; their longevity is traditional. Yogurt and certain cultured milks constitute a major item of diet for the Bulgarian peasant. To state that all of these virtues stem solely from the consumption of yogurt is to treat the subject most superficially; climate, heredity, and other factors must be considered. But clearly the Bulgarians have established the nutritional excellency of yogurt. That, and that alone, first attracted me to yogurt and caused me to investigate and study it. Its superior nutritive qualities caused me to recommend it to my students, and my faith in it has been justified in every respect. The extent to which the bacteria present in yogurt may reach the colon is to me of passing interest only. They are "friendly" and helpful bacteria, active in the synthesis of certain B vitamins, and the acid they produce from milk sugar tends to suppress the activities of pathogenic and putrefactive types of organisms. If yogurt eaters receive these benefits in any measure at all, they are just that much ahead.

While excellent yogurt can be purchased in dairy and food stores, the homemade variety is far less expensive and can be made with inexpensive skim milk. The recipe for my favorite yogurt appears on page 536.

Yogurt can be eaten plain, seasoned with chives or other herbs, served with fresh or canned fruits, or made into a sundae with maple syrup, honey, or molasses. Real yogurt connoisseurs prefer it plain! I'm indeed sorry that many dairies now sell "jazzed up" yogurt, loaded with white sugar and glucose preserves. Buy it plain or—better still—make your own.

World's Best Cereal—Fresh Wheat Germ

Fresh wheat germ is worth its weight in gold. It takes its place on my list of wonder foods as an outstanding source of vitamin B_1. One-half cup provides about three and one-half times my generous daily allowance of this so-important vitamin. Moreover, on the basis of the calories it contributes, it is richer in protein and provides nearly three times as much iron. It substantially exceeds the calories in vitamin B_2 and niacin.

Fresh wheat germ should be sprinkled over hot or cold cereals. Excellent hot cakes, waffles, muffins, and breads can be prepared by substituting from one-half to one cup of wheat germ for an equivalent quantity of flour. If you own an electric liquefier-blender, you can make delicious drinks with a pint of any fruit juice, a small section of banana, and half a cup of wheat germ.

Wheat germ also contains vitamin E. Man, over centuries of time, became adapted to the consumption of whole cereal grains, including the germ. He cannot now lightly drop the germ from his diet. Many modern processes of refining natural foods have led to a number of dietary deficiencies, some of them dramatically clear cut, others more subtle and difficult to identify.

If at all possible, do get the fresh wheat germ. If you live near a mill that produces it, by all means buy it directly. If not, you will find it on sale at your local health shop. Not only is the fresh wheat germ better for you, but it will cost about half as much as the processed toasted wheat germ. Stored in a tight can or jar in a cool place, it will keep its freshness for a month. And above all, avoid the "processed" wheat germ that has other ingredients added—especially foodless white sugar. The best of all wheat germ is made in France. There the Moulin de Paris exposes the freshly milled wheat germ to the rays of a powerful ultraviolet lamp, which adds sweetness and brings out the natural flavor of the "heart of the wheat." On page 498 you will find a recipe for making your own honeyed wheat germ.

Unsulphured Molasses

For many years I have advocated the use of blackstrap molasses because it is an unusually rich source of iron and the B vitamins. The late Dr. Tom Spies, of Hillman Hospital in Birmingham, Alabama, first told me of the wonders he performed with it. It has long been an important staple in the diets of many Southerners in the United States. However, because of its unusual taste, it invokes in most people a strong *yes* or *no*—and, unfortunately, more often *no* than *yes*. So, if you are one of those who say *no* to blackstrap molasses, use instead the darkest molasses you can find—but do be sure it's unsulphured.

Molasses is an excellent source of nutritionally available iron. On the basis of a 2,000 calorie per day diet, it provides seven times as much iron as it does calories. Moreover, it is the best source of natural sugar, and it also provides significant quantities of thiamine and riboflavin.

I list it as a wonder food primarily for its rich iron content. It lends itself in dozens of ways to the preparation of foods; added to muffins, waffles, spiced cookies, and the like, it enriches them significantly with much-needed iron. Milk is poor in iron, yet the growing youngster requires three or four glasses a day; a tablespoonful of molasses stirred into each glass turns an iron-poor food into an iron-rich one, providing from 50 to 75 percent of the daily iron allowance. Used in place of table syrups, which for the most part are nascent sugar solutions, its nutritional superiority is undoubted.

Six-Course Dinner Growing on One Tree

When I first wrote about the fabulous avocado in the Gaylord Hauser *Newsletter,* thousands of my students asked for more details and more recipes. So let me tell you more about this special wonder food.

Mother Nature put many of her best ingredients into this fruit-vegetable that grows on a tree. In each avocado are combined the proteins of meat, the fat of butter (unsaturated, as an extra bonus), the vitamins and minerals of vegetables, and the flavor of nuts. Thus you might say that the avocado is a complete meal from soup to nuts—plus several other pleasant surprises.

The avocado (or alligator pear) is a semitropical plant, originally grown in South America, Mexico, the West Indies, and Hawaii. Now it is also grown in southern California and Florida.

California produces avocados from November to June, and Florida avocados are available during the rest of the year. This means that there is a good supply of avocados throughout the year. (It was my pleasure to introduce this wonder food to Italians, and I now have several trees in my garden in Sicily.)

The avocado, like the olive, is an acquired taste, and it took time for it to become popular. However, it has now captured the public taste, and demands for it have increased tremendously. It is estimated that between California and Florida, the crops are close to a hundred million pounds!

The protein content of the avocado is the equal of many kinds of meat; when fully ripe, it contains little starch and practically no sugar. It offers generous quantities of calcium, magnesium, potassium, sodium, copper, phosphates, manganese, and iron. It is loaded with vitamins A, B₁, B₂ and C, and has some vitamins D and E.

About one-fourth of the avocado consists of fat or oil—10,000,000 pounds of this oil were produced last year. What makes avocado oil so valuable is its high percentage of polyunsaturated fatty acids. This oil gives the avocado its mellow texture and nutlike flavor. The Mexicans call the soft green pulp "butter growing on trees"; and they spread it generously on their tortillas. A very ripe, soft avocado, mashed with a few drops of lemon juice and spiked with herbs, makes an utterly delicious dressing over fruit and vegetable salads. Because the vegetable oils are easily burned by the body, even overweighters can enjoy this "butter growing on trees."

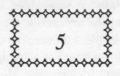

5

More Vitamins for Longer Life

Dr. H. C. Sherman, in his longevity experiments at Columbia University, pointed out again and again that not fewer, but more, vitamins are necessary for a long and healthy life. He insisted that the ideal intake of vitamins should be four times the maintenance amount, and by that he meant optimum amounts—as I suggest to all my students.

Today the eating habits in the United States are, unfortunately, no longer those of our forefathers who lived on simple earthy fare. It is a fact that today 80 percent of the foods available to us have been meddled with to prevent them from spoiling and a great deal of our important nutrients are lost. For this and many other reasons, intelligent people the world over have learned to fortify and supplement their diets with extra vitamins and minerals. In the next few pages I shall list the foods and nutrients that help to fortify and supplement the average American diet. Do not hesitate to use extra vitamin concentrates, but *not* at the expense of the good basic foods—these must always come first. But to be sure there is no possible deficiency in your daily meals, I suggest you use the best vitamin-mineral concentrates that money can buy.

VITAMIN A

Dr. Sherman particularly stresses an abundance of vitamins A and C, together with the B vitamins. First we shall deal with vitamin A. In the interest of a longer and healthier life, your daily diet should provide you with one hundred percent of my generous allowance. Should your diet provide two hundred percent daily, and even frequently go higher, it would be all to the good. The table below gives you the best sources of vitamin A. The values given are generally for cooked foods, unless the foods are commonly eaten raw, as fruit.

FOODS FOR VITAMIN A

Rich Sources	Serving	Units
* Liver, calf	3 Ounces	19,130
Dandelion greens	1 Cup	27,310
Spinach	1 Cup	21,200
Carrots, diced	1 Cup	18,130
Turnip greens	1 Cup	15,370
Collards	1 Cup	14,500
Squash, Hubbard	1 Cup	12,690
Sweet potato	1 Med.	11,410
Beet greens	1 Cup	10,790
Mustard greens	1 Cup	10,050
Kale	1 Cup	9,220
Pumpkin	1 Cup	7,750
Cantaloupe	½ Med.	6,190
Broccoli	1 Cup	5,100

Good Sources		
Apricots	3 Whole fruit	2,990
* Kidney, lamb	3 Ounces	980
Tomato	1 Med.	1,640
Cheese, Cheddar	2″ × 1″ × 1″	740
Peas, green	1 Cup	1,150
* Egg	One	550
* Butter	1 Tbsp.	460
Peach, fresh	One	880
Beans, green	1 Cup	830
Asparagus	6 stalks	760
Corn, yellow	1 Med. ear	500

* These foods contain actual vitamin A, which is about twice as effective in the body as carotene (pro-vitamin A), provided by foods not marked with an asterisk.

Here's how to fortify your daily meals with more vitamin A:

1. A cup of finely chopped carrots added to your green salad bowl gives you an added 13,000 units of vitamin A.
2. A piece of inexpensive lamb liver, about 4 ounces, ground up with your meat loaf or hamburger, fortifies it with about 57,000 units of vitamin A.
3. Adding just one cup of finely chopped spinach, turnip tops, or parsley to stews or soups fortifies them with thousands of additional units of vitamin A.
4. Use an egg yolk for thickening gravies instead of pasty white flour. Each egg yolk gives you an additional 500 units of vitamin A.
5. The richest of all sources of vitamin A is fish-liver oils, which doctors and dietitians recommend for extra fortification. Small capsules contain as much as 25,000 units. They are nonfattening and no longer have an unpleasant fishy taste.

Those Important B Vitamins

The B vitamins represent an extensive family; its many members play a wide variety of roles in the economy of the body. The maintenance requirements of the three best-known members of the family —thiamine (B_1), riboflavin (B_2), and niacin—are well established and agreed upon by the authorities. Maintenance requirements suffice only to protect the body against deficiency diseases, and should not be confused with the requirements for buoyant health and longevity. My generous daily allowance of these three B vitamins significantly exceeds the maintenance requirement.

FOODS FOR
THIAMINE, RIBOFLAVIN, AND NIACIN

Food	Serving	B_1 Thiamine mgs.	%	B_2 Riboflavin mgs.	%	Niacin mgs.	%
Brewers' yeast	1 Tbsp.	.78	39	.44	17.6	2.9	19.3
Peas, split, raw	½ Cup	.76	38	.28	11.1	3.15	21.0
Wheat germ	½ Cup	.7	35	.27	10.8	1.6	10.6
Soybean flour, low-fat	½ Cup	.55	27.5	.18	7.2	1.45	9.7
Heart, beef, raw	3 Ounces	.5	25	.75	30.0	6.6	44.0
Flour, whole-wheat	½ Cup	.33	16.5	.07	2.8	2.6	17.3
Rice, brown, raw	½ Cup	.33	16.5	.05	2.0	4.8	32.0
Kidney, beef	3 Ounces	.32	16.0	2.16	87.0	5.5	36.0
Flour, white, enriched	½ Cup	.24	12.0	.145	5.8	1.9	12.6
Skim milk, dried	½ Cup	.21	10.5	1.175	47.0	0.7	4.65
Liver, calf	3 Ounces	.18	9.0	2.65	106.0	13.7	93.0
Liver, beef	2 Ounces	.15	7.5	2.25	90.0	8.4	56.0
Lamb, leg	3 Ounces	.12	6.0	.21	8.4	4.4	29.4

Oatmeal	½ Cup	.11	5.5	.025	1.0	0.4	2.66
Peanuts	¼ Cup	.105	5.25	.05	2.0	6.0	40.0
Turkey	4 Ounces	.1	5.0	.16	6.4	9.1	60.0
Turnip greens	1 Cup	.09	4.5	.59	23.5	1.0	6.7
Chicken	4 Ounces	.09	4.5	.18	7.2	9.1	60.0
Bacon, med. fat	2 Slices	.08	4.0	.05	2.0	0.8	5.3
Kale	1 Cup	.08	4.0	.25	10.0	1.9	12.6
Peanut butter	¼ Cup	.08	4.0	.08	3.2	10.4	69.5
Bread, whole-wheat	1 ½" Sl.	.07	3.5	.03	1.2	.7	4.65
Molasses	1 Tbsp.	.06	3.0	.05	2.0	.4	2.66
Beef, sirloin	3 Ounces	.06	3.0	.16	6.4	4.1	27.4
Rice, converted	½ Cup	.05	2.5	.01	0.4	.95	6.3
Egg	1 Medium	.05	2.5	.14	5.7	—	—
Salmon, red	3 Ounces	.03	1.5	.14	5.7	6.2	41.4
Cheese, Cheddar	1 Pc. 2" x 1" x 1"	.02	1.0	.24	9.6	—	—

Here's how to fortify your meals with the Vitamin B Family foods:

1. Sprinkle fresh wheat germ or corn germ over green salads, over hot or cold cereals; also add one tablespoonful to every cup of flour in all your baking.
2. Use fresh wheat germ in place of bread crumbs to coat fish or veal chops.
3. Eat several glasses of yogurt a day, and use it in place of sour cream.
4. Add a tablespoon of food yeast to all gravies, stews, and tomato juice.
5. Have broiled liver at least twice a week. The less-expensive beef or lamb liver is just as rich as calf liver.
6. Use molasses for sweetening instead of white sugar.
7. If you eat in restaurants all the time, it is wise to take a concentrate of vitamin B Complex.

You can see from the table above that these three vitamins are much harder to get, for example, than vitamins A and C. The B vitamins are present in foods in much smaller amounts than vitamins A and C. No single food will provide 100 percent of a generous requirement of *thiamine* in an ordinary serving. Of the twenty-eight foods listed, only five provide between 25 and 39 percent, and eighteen of the twenty-eight foods provide less than 10 percent per serving. For *riboflavin*, only three foods, all of which are organ meats, provide between 87 and 106 percent. One-half cup of skim milk provides 47 percent, and another food, also an organ meat, provides 30 percent. All the rest provide less than 25 percent, with the majority falling below 10 percent. *Niacin* is a little more richly distributed; however, no single food provides 100 percent per serving, and only one as much as 90 percent.

To render the table as informative as possible, the values for the three B vitamins are given in milligrams and in percentages of my generous allowance. The table is compiled in descending order of the percent of thiamine present, as adequate quantities of thiamine are the most difficult to obtain of the three.

THE LESSER-KNOWN B VITAMINS

The lesser-known B vitamins, even after they were discovered and isolated (and in most cases synthesized) labored for a long time under the legend: "their need in human nutrition is not yet established." That appears on the label of all vitamin concentrates containing these lesser-known B vitamins. As the legend is misunderstood by many people, a discussion of it here may be informative and of considerable interest.

It is required by law to place the above statement about nutrition on the label of all products containing the lesser-known B vitamins, if the claim is made that they are present. The purpose of the law is to protect the public against imposition, and is laudable in every respect, since the law was made at a time when there were virtually no data to indicate that such vitamins were needed by humans. You see, in general, these vitamins display a subtle and diffused effect in the body. A gross deficiency of thiamine, for example, causes the disease beriberi; the symptoms are unmistakable, and, on the administration of adequate quantities of thiamine, promptly start to disappear. The lesser-known B vitamins, however, do not appear to be associated with such clear-cut deficiency states. For example, choline and inositol, either separately or in combination, have recently been found to play a role in preventing and relieving atherosclerosis, or "fatty" hardening of the arteries (page 188). However, as the condition involved is slow in developing, requiring a good portion of a lifetime, the shortage of these vitamins does not display its effect so quickly or dramatically as a shortage of thiamine or niacin.

Recent research has led some leading nutritional authorities to make recommendations as to the desirable quantity of certain lesser-known B vitamins in the diet. As expressed by these authorities: ". . . in some cases where there *may* be no nutritional requirement under normal circumstances, it is nevertheless suggested that a level of these vitamins be provided in the diet as a precaution, in view of our lack of knowledge regarding the subject."

Pyridoxine-Vitamin B₆

Vitamin B₆ is an important factor in the use of protein by the body. Also, it stimulates the production of antibodies, which should be present in the blood to help protect against the invasion of bacteria. In many nervous conditions it has proved to be of definite help. Authorities recommend 1.5 milligrams per day.

FOODS FOR PYRIDOXINE—B₆

Food	Serving	Percent per Serving
Beef liver	4 Ounces	60
Bananas	1 Med.	27
Beans, lima, dry	1 Cup	26
Sweet potato	1 Med.	26
Cabbage, cooked	1 Cup	24
Chicken, broiled	8 Ounces	20
Cabbage, raw shredded	1 Cup	19
Brewers' yeast	1 heaping Tbsp.	18
Lettuce	½ Head	11
Irish potato, baked	1 Med.	11
Spinach, cooked	1 Cup	10
Turnips, diced, cooked	1 Cup	9
Beef heart, cooked	3 Ounces	9
Halibut	1 Pc. 4″ × 3″ × ½″	7
Veal cutlet, no bone	3 Ounces	7
Peanuts, roasted	¼ Cup	7
Beef, round steak, no bone	4 Ounces	6
Green peas	1 Cup	5
Cantaloupe	½ Large	4
Dark molasses	1 Tbsp.	4
Apple	1 Average	4
Wheat germ	1 Tbsp.	2
Cauliflower, cooked	1 Cup	2
Cheddar cheese	1 1″ Cube	1
Whole milk	1 Cup	1
Egg	1 Med.	1

Pantothenic Acid

This B vitamin has been shown to stabilize the adrenal glands, and in this way is thought to help keep the natural color of our hair. Also, it has been shown to be an important nutrient for the nervous system. Recommended daily requirement, about 10 milligrams.

FOODS FOR PANTOTHENIC ACID

Food	Serving	Percent per Serving
Beef liver	4 Ounces	58
Broccoli	1 Cup	21
Chicken, broiled	8 Ounces	12 to 20
Mushrooms	10	17
Beef heart, lean	3 Ounces	17
Whole wheat	1 Cup	15
Beef brains	3 Ounces	15
Wheat bran	1 Cup	14
Wheat germ	1 Cup	13
Egg	1	13
Oysters	1 Cup, 13–19 med.	12
Sweet potato	1 Med.	11
Cauliflower, cooked	1 Cup	11
Soybeans, dry	¼ Cup	10
Green peas	1 Cup	9 to 16
Cauliflower buds, raw	1 Cup	9
Roasted peanuts	¼ Cup	9
Orange	1 Med.	8
Lima beans, dry, cooked	1 Cup	7
Whole milk	1 Cup	7
Salmon	½ Cup	6 to 11
Leg of lamb	3 Ounces	5
Rolled oats, cooked	1 Cup	5
Ham, smoked	4 Ounces	4 to 7
Irish potato	1 Med.	4 to 6
Cheddar cheese	1 1" Cube	1 to 3
Whole-wheat bread	1 Slice ½"	1
Veal cutlet	3 Ounces	1 to 2
Bacon, broiled	4 Slices	1 to 3

Inositol

The effect of this B vitamin, together with another B vitamin, choline, is that of protecting against fatty hardening of the arteries. Authorities recommend one gram per day.

FOODS FOR INOSITOL

Food	Serving	Percent per Serving
Orange	1 Large	49
Wheat germ	1 Cup	48
Grapefruit	½ Med.	40
Watermelon	1/16 Melon 16″ × 10″	30
Peas, green	1 Cup	26
Beef heart, lean	3 Ounces	22
Cantaloupe	½ Med.	22
Whole wheat	1 Cup	20
Peas, dry	⅓ Cup	20
Beef brains	3 Ounces	17
Lima beans, dry	1 Cup	15
Cabbage, cooked	1 Cup	13
Lettuce	½ Head, Med.	12
Cauliflower, cooked	1 Cup	11
Peaches, frozen	4 Ounces	11
Chicken, broiled	½ Bird, 8 oz.	11
Oysters, raw	1 Cup (13-19 med.)	10
Onions, dry	1 Med.	10
Cauliflower buds, raw diced	1 Cup	9
Cabbage, raw, shredded	1 Cup	9
Strawberries	1 Cup	9
Sweet potato, baked	1 Med.	8
Tomato, raw	1 Med.	7
Roasted peanuts	¼ Cup	6
Turnips, diced	1 Cup	6
Beef liver	4 Ounces	6
Cornmeal, white	1 Cup	5
Leg of lamb	3 Ounces	5
Raisins	¼ Cup	5
Spinach	1 Cup	5
Banana	1 Med.	4
Whole milk	1 Cup	4
Ham	4 Ounces	3 to 6
Apple	1 Med.	3
Veal cutlet	3 Ounces	3
Irish potato	1 Med.	3
Carrots	1 Med.	2
Halibut	1 Pc. 4″ × 3″ × ½″	2
Mushrooms	10 Large	2
Salmon	½ Cup	2

Food	Serving	Percent per Serving
Egg	1 Med.	2
Whole-wheat bread	1 Slice ½"	1
Beef, round steak	4 Ounces	1
Cheddar cheese	1 1" Cube	1

Biotin

Man is less likely to be deficient of this B vitamin than any of the others, for it is made in appreciable amounts in the intestinal tract. It is essential to certain enzymes of the body fluids. Only very little is needed, about 0.15 to 0.3 milligrams per day.

FOODS FOR BIOTIN

Food	Serving	Percent per Serving
Beef liver	4 Ounces	75
Chicken, broiled	8 Ounces	15
Oysters	1 Cup (13–19 med.)	14
Cauliflower, cooked	1 Cup	14
Cauliflower, raw, diced buds	1 Cup	11
Mushrooms	10 Med.	11
Peanuts, roasted	¼ Cup	10
Whole milk	1 Cup	8
Egg	1 Med.	8
Peas, dry	⅓ Cup	7
Lima beans, dry	1 Cup	6
Corn	1 Ear, Med.	5
Grapefruit	½ Med.	5
Strawberries	1 Cup	4
Whole wheat	1 Cup	4
Banana	1 Med.	3
Salmon	½ Cup	3
Onions, dry	1 Med.	3
Spinach	1 Cup	2
Peas, green	1 Cup	2
Tomatoes	1 Med.	2
Bacon	4 Slices	1
Molasses	1 Tbsp.	1
Carrots	1 Med.	0.7
Halibut	1 Pc. 4" × 3" × ½"	0.7

Folic Acid

This is an important B vitamin, essential to the proper formation of red blood and also to the growth of the cells. The quantity required is not large, about 0.2 milligrams daily.

FOODS FOR FOLIC ACID

Food	Serving	Percent per Serving
Salmon	½ Cup	427
Watermelon	1/16 Melon 16″ × 10″	356
Oysters	1 Cup (13–19 med.)	288
Spinach	1 Cup	222
Lima beans, dry, cooked	1 Cup	150
Chicken, broiled	8 Ounces	136 to 282
Cantaloupe	½ 5″ dia.	218
Whole wheat	1 Cup	114
Asparagus, cut spears	1 Cup	106
Wheat germ	1 Cup	95 to 112
Orange	1 Large	97
Broccoli	1 Cup	75
Irish potato	1 Med.	68
Banana	1 Med.	64
Beef liver	4 Ounces	56
Kale	1 Cup	50 to 55
Peanuts, roasted	¼ Cup	50
Mushrooms	10 Med.	49
Parsley, chopped	1 Cup	47
Green string beans	1 Cup	45
Veal cutlets	3 Ounces	39 to 72
Leaf lettuce	½ Head, Med.	38 to 46
Beets, diced	1 Cup	35
Endive, French	2 Stalks, Med.	35
Ham	4 Ounces	33 to 68
Cauliflower	1 Cup	26
Carrot	1 Med.	24
Radish	8 Small	22 to 26
Cauliflower buds, raw, diced	1 Cup	22
Egg	1 Med.	21
Beet greens	1 Cup	18
Peas, green	1 Cup	17
Beans, wax	1 Cup	16
Tomato	1 Med.	10
Whole-wheat bread	1 Slice ½″	8
Cheddar cheese	1 1″ Cube	4

Choline

The two B vitamins choline and inositol cooperate to prevent fatty hardening of the arteries, and to protect the liver and kidneys. The exact amount of choline required daily has not been established for man, but foods rich in choline should be used frequently in the diet.

FOODS FOR CHOLINE

Food	Serving	Milligrams per Serving
Beef liver	4 Ounces	790
Spinach	1 Cup	425
Beans, string	1 Cup	425
Cabbage, cooked	1 Cup	420
Kidney, lamb	3 Ounces	306
Egg yolk	From 1 egg	289
Wheat germ	1 Cup	272
Cabbage, raw, shredded	1 Cup	250
Asparagus, cut tips	1 Cup	227
Rolled oats, cooked	1 Cup	222
Beans, soy	¼ Cup	185
Turnip, diced	1 Cup	126
Whole wheat	1 Cup	108
Beef	4 Ounces	101
Irish potato	1 Med.	99
Dried skim milk	½ Cup	96
Lamb	3 Ounces	94
Liver sausage	1 Slice 3¼″ × ¼″	73
Peanuts, roasted	¼ Cup	60
Carrots, raw	1 Med.	48
Sweet potato	1 Med.	42
Corn on the cob	1 Med.	37
Whole milk	1 Cup	31
Bologna	1 Pc. 2⅛″ dia. × ½″	30
Cheddar cheese	1 Ounce	14
Beets, diced	1 Cup	13
Pecans, halves	¼ Cup	11
Butter	1 Tbsp.	8

VITAMIN C—ASCORBIC ACID

Dr. H. C. Sherman stresses the value of vitamin C in the retention of youthful characteristics, and in lengthening the span of life—to add more youthful years.

There is no reason why anyone should fail to get an abundant supply of this very important vitamin from the diet. The generous use of citrus fruits and green leafy vegetables is all that is required—but do use them generously.

In the table which follows, the rich and good food sources are listed.

FOODS FOR ASCORBIC ACID (VITAMIN C)

Food	Serving	Milligrams
Rose hip powder	100 Grams	500*
Orange juice	1 Cup	122
Broccoli	1 Cup	111
Grapefruit juice	1 Cup	99
Strawberries	1 Cup	89
Turnip greens	1 Cup	87
Collards	1 Cup	84
Pepper, green	1 Med.	77
Mustard greens	1 Cup	63
Brussels sprouts	1 Cup	61
Cantaloupe	½ Med.	59
Kale	1 Cup	56
Spinach	1 Cup	54
Cabbage, cooked	1 Cup	53
Cabbage, raw, shredded	1 Cup	50
Asparagus, cut spears	1 Cup	40
Tomato juice	1 Cup	38
Tomato	1 Med.	35
Cauliflower	1 Cup	34
Pineapple, fresh, diced	1 Cup	33
Liver, calf	3 Ounces	30
Chard, leaves only	1 Cup	30
Dandelion greens	1 Cup	29
Sweet potato	1 Med.	28
Tangerine	1 Med.	25
Lima beans, immature	1 Cup	24
Peas, green	1 Cup	24
Beet greens	1 Cup	22
Liver, beef	2 Ounces	18
Endive	1 Cup	18
Beans, green	1 Cup	18

* Sometimes even more, depending on variety.

Here's how to fortify meals with extra vitamin C:

1. Have citrus fruit cups often, either as appetizers or for dessert. (Eating the fruit is preferable to drinking the juice for reducers. The pulp helps to prevent that hungry feeling.)
2. Add to salad dressing the juice of one lemon.
3. Sprinkle lemon juice and vegetable salt on all flat-tasting vegetables.
4. Drink at least one glass of fresh vegetable juice a day.
5. Fortify tomato juice with a tablespoon of lemon juice and spike with herbs.
6. Add a half a cup of chopped dark-green parsley to your stews, salads, dressings, hamburgers, mashed potatoes. Tastes wonderful; the vitamin C is free.
7. Serve pink rose-hip tea with your meals as they do in Switzerland. And serve rose-hip jam for breakfast, or use high-potency rose-hip tablets. (Those coming from the cold Scandinavian countries are the most potent.)

Grow Your Own Vitamin Roses

Roses delight us with their subtle fragrance and beautiful colors. But I believe the real secret of the rose, which so few people know, is the red seed, the hip, a treasurehouse of life-giving vitamin C. In Northern Europe, where oranges and lemons are very expensive, many housewives have learned to grow their own inexpensive vitamin C. Some rose hips contain twenty times as much of this important vitamin as citrus fruit, and the wild Scandinavian varieties are even richer. Rose hips are easily grown, and the most nutritious variety can now be bought in the United States. The *Rosa Rugosa* bushes grow the large, meaty variety and can be used for jam, syrup, marmalade, and a delightful beverage—the pink rose hip tea, which is the great favorite at the famous Bircher-Benner Sanatorium in Switzerland. Even if you have only a small plot, plant some "vitamin roses," as the Russians call them. (Stern Nurseries in Geneva, New York, ship them all over the United States.)

Rose-Hip Marmalade: The ruby red seed of the rose makes an excellent marmalade. If you have been to Switzerland or Sweden you have probably enjoyed it for breakfast. Simply soak the cleaned rose hips for two hours in plain cold water; then let boil for 2 hours, and strain. Measure the puree, and add 1 cup of brown sugar to each cup of rose-hip puree. Let boil down to thick consistency, pour into sterilized glasses, and seal.

VITAMIN D

Certain misunderstandings are current regarding vitamin D, to the effect that it is not needed by adults. Nothing could be further from the fact, and after forty it assumes an increased importance. There is need for an abundance of calcium all through life; and as we get older, for a variety of reasons, we do not absorb calcium as efficiently as we should. However, if vitamin D is present in the body in adequate amounts, the absorption of calcium is promoted.

Almost no common foods contain vitamin D in significant amounts. The quantity present in butter, which is consumed daily in relatively small amounts, is so small that butter is out of consideration as a dietary source of vitamin D. Fortified or irradiated whole milk provides 102 units of vitamin D per eight full ounces (a cup, or drinking glass brimming full); thus four glasses, or a quart, would have to be consumed daily to meet requirements. Because of the fat in whole milk, this quantity amounts to 664 calories, which few adults can afford to use up solely on milk. Vitamin D is not present in skim milk or buttermilk.

Eggs vary in vitamin D content according to the diet of the hens. An egg will vary between 25 and 65 units. Clearly, eggs cannot be relied upon as the sole source of vitamin D in the body. Four ounces a day of tuna fish or Atlantic herring would provide adequate vitamin D, and four ounces per day of mackerel or canned salmon would go a long way toward supplying it; but, manifestly, the daily consumption of these fish is impractical, not to say monotonously impossible.

Vitamin D is produced in the skin through the exposure of the body to sunshine or direct skyshine (reflected sunlight from the blue sky).

An adult reasonably exposed to sunlight, in amounts sufficient to produce a reasonable tan every season, doubtless has sufficient vitamin D produced in the skin. However, persons who do not, or for any reason cannot, obtain adequate exposure to sunshine would do well to fortify their diet with fish-liver oil concentrates of vitamin D. The daily requirement for maintenance is set at 400 units, but after the age of 40, up to 1000 units per day would be much better.

Here's how to fortify your meals with extra vitamin D:

1. Simply put your golden oil in the bright sunshine and irradiate it. This is how my cook in Sicily does it. She pours the oil in a flat tin pan, not more than one half inch deep; then she puts the pan into the noonday sunlight for at least two hours. After that she pours this sun-drenched vitaminized oil into dark bottles. This is the humble forerunner of the scientific irradiation process patented by the University of Wisconsin.
2. Golden orange, lemon, and grapefruit peelings also contain some vitamin D because the oil in the peel is constantly exposed to the sun. So instead of wasting this citrus peel, chop it and use it as often as possible in baking and cooking. It is delicious in stewed fruit.

VITAMIN E

No other vitamin has ever provoked such controversy as vitamin E. It appears to act as a regulator of the metabolism of the nucleus of the cells. It is reported to help prevent abortion; authorities disagree as to the amount of vitamin E required, but a teaspoon of wheat germ oil a day is often recommended.

A serious deficiency of vitamin E in the diet of the male leads to degeneration of the germinal epithelium; there is a tendency toward muscular wasting, an increased demand for oxygen by the tissues, and an improper use of phosphorus. The Doctors Shute, of Canada, have done extensive research with vitamin E in relation to heart trouble; thousands of people, including myself, have benefited by their work. For the last year I have taken 200 units of vitamin E with my other concentrates, with the result that after my last examination the doctor found my heart to be that of a young man. The Doctors Shute do not approve of self-medication; they insist on adjusting the proper dosage for each individual, as they did for me. You may wish to discuss this with your doctor. You can read all about the Shute experiments in their book, *Your Heart and Vitamin E* (Devin-Adair, New York).

The principal dietary sources of vitamin E are given in the following table.

FOODS FOR VITAMIN E

Food	Serving	Milligrams
Wheat germ oil	1 Tbsp.	45.0
Corn oil	1 Tbsp.	35.0
Soy oil	1 Tbsp.	13 to 17
Cottonseed oil	1 Tbsp.	11 to 13
Meats (average)	4 Ounces	9.0
Kale	1 Cup	8.0
Corn	1 Med. ear	6.0
Wheat germ	¼ Cup	4.6
Peanut oil	1 Tbsp.	3.7 to 4
Spinach	1 Cup	2.55
Carrots, diced	1 Cup	2.1
Whole-wheat flour	½ Cup	0.72 to 2.24
Brussels sprouts	1 Cup	1.87
Egg	1 Med.	1.5
Celery	3 Inner stalks	1.0
Oatmeal	1 Cup	0.5
Parsley	4 Med. sprigs	0.35

Here's how to fortify your meals with the important vitamin E: Add a tablespoonful of wheat germ oil to any of the golden oils and use as salad dressing. Eat all cereals (hot or cold) "a la mode," by sprinkling a heaping tablespoon of fresh wheat germ over them. You can also buy high vitamin E concentrates in capsule form.

Vitamin F

This possibly unexpected letter in your alphabet of vitamins stands for those essential unsaturated fatty acids which we talk so much about. It is a grave mistake to eliminate these even when on a reducing diet. They are essential to arterial and organic functions, the control of cholesterol level in the blood, and body warmth. Meat fats and the hardened or hydrogenated fats in solid shortenings should be replaced by the golden vegetable oils, which contain the unsaturated fatty acids, especially linoleic acid.

Foods richest in vitamin F: All the natural golden vegetable oils. Use them generously in salad dressings and for general cooking purposes.

VITAMIN K

This vitamin is essential to normal ability for the blood to clot. The daily need is very small. One or two milligrams per day is sufficient for normal nutrition. Larger amounts, from foods, are in no way harmful. The Japanese claim that the large amount of sea greens in their diet give them extra quantities of vitamin K.

FOODS FOR VITAMIN K

Food	Serving	Percent per Serving
Spinach, cooked	1 Cup	814
Cabbage, cooked	1 Cup	534
Cauliflower, cooked	1 Cup	384
Cabbage, raw, shredded	1 Cup	320
Cauliflower, raw, diced	1 Cup	320
Tomato, raw	1 Med.	60
Peas, green, cooked	1 Cup	48
Carrots	1 Med.	5

MINERALS FOR MAXIMUM NUTRITION

Your body requires many minerals for maximum nutrition and high vitality. Minerals help to maintain in the body the amount of water necessary to the life processes. They keep blood and tissue fluid from becoming either too acid or too alkaline. They help draw chemical substances into and out of the cells. They influence the secretion of glands. They help set up conditions responsible for the irritability and contractility of muscle and tissue. And they are important in sending messages through the nervous system.

Calcium and Phosphorus

Calcium and phosphorus are necessary for maximum vigor. They are largely used in the body to give hardness to the teeth and bones. Although 99 percent of the calcium in the body is found in the bones and teeth, the remaining 1 percent plays an important role in regulating certain physiological functions. Calcium aids in the transmission of nerve messages, and helps the nerves to be steady and relaxed. Conversely, a calcium-deficient person is inclined to be grouchy and irritable, and to have a feeling of tenseness and uneasiness that quickly results in fatigue. Serving calcium-rich foods increases the efficiency, peace, and happiness of your family. A lack of calcium also may prevent a person from sleeping soundly. Needless dollars are spent each year for sleeping powders and tablets that could be replaced by calcium-rich foods.

Muscular cramps may also result from a lack of calcium. And abdominal cramps during menstruation are often caused by a decrease in blood calcium. This period is frequently accompanied by nervousness, headaches, mental depression, and other symptoms of calcium deficiency. An extra supply of calcium and vitamin D will usually cause these symptoms to disappear.

Calcium is also necessary for the clotting of blood; and a lack can lead to hemorrhage following the extraction of teeth or an accident, or during an operation. In treating hemorrhaging of any type, calcium—and vitamin D, necessary for the efficient absorption of calcium into the blood—should be given.

The best sources of calcium are milk, powdered skim milk, buttermilk, and yogurt. (Very fine bone flour or tablets are recommended for "milk haters.") Various types of cheese may be good or poor sources of calcium, depending on the way they are made. If the milk has been soured to develop flavor in the cheese, some calcium is lost. Commercial cottage cheese, for example, often contains little calcium; but if it is prepared at home it is an excellent source. (See page 534.)

Calcium and phosphorus are used by the body in chemical combination with each other; one without the other is of little value. Good sources of phosphorus are meats, dairy products, all foods made from whole grains, and many vegetables. Phosphorus is used to build and maintain bones and teeth. It is also a part of each of the billions of cells in the body, and is a constituent of all glandular secretions and all body fluids.

Vitamin D is necessary for the efficient use of calcium and phosphorus. It helps in their absorption into the blood and in depositing them in the bones and teeth. Most people get no more than 100 units of vitamin D daily, although about 1,000 units seems nearer the requirement. It is little wonder that people are nervous and tired, suffer from insomnia, and must resort to sleeping tablets.

Regardless of the amount of calcium and phosphorus in the diet, calcium and phosphorus are excreted daily in the urine and feces. If you are not getting enough of these minerals to supply the nerves, muscles, and body fluids, they are taken from the bones and teeth. On the other hand, if you receive an excess of calcium and phosphorus, the excess will be excreted.

Phosphorus is so readily available in many foods there is little danger of deficiency. Calcium, however, is more difficult to obtain. It can be furnished by one quart of milk, whole or skim, buttermilk, or yogurt. No other foods supply the amount of calcium needed daily.

As a correction for nervousness, and before operations of any kind, some doctors now recommend concentrated calcium such as dicalcium phosphate blended with very fine bone flour and fortified with vitamin D. Since calcium dissolves only in acids, it should be taken on an empty stomach, before meals or between meals, and preferably in or with citrus juice. Usually about a fourth of a teaspoonful of powdered dicalcium phosphate or two to four tablets daily are sufficient. Small amounts, taken frequently, can be absorbed more completely than a larger amount taken at one time.

Foods richest in calcium:

Powdered skim milk	Molasses
Fresh milk	Almonds
Buttermilk	Sesame seeds
Yogurt	Turnip greens
Cottage cheese	Broccoli

Also in concentrates: very fine bone flour, dicalcium phosphate, plus vitamin D in tablet form.

Rich Red Blood Needs Foods Rich in Iron

Iron is necessary to enable the blood to carry oxygen throughout the body; and it is also of great value in helping to remove carbon dioxide from the tissues. The number of red corpuscles in the blood varies widely with various people, depending on their health. In addition to red corpuscles, each blood cell must contain a normal amount of hemoglobin, which actually carries the oxygen to every cell in the body.

Anemia is a condition in which the body fails to produce either enough red corpuscles or enough hemoglobin. Both abnormalities may exist at once. In this case, sufficient oxygen cannot be carried to the cells throughout the body, nor can carbon dioxide be completely removed. As a result, the anemic person is tired, listless, and lacking in endurance. He cannot think clearly or quickly.

The most common cause of anemia is a lack of iron in the diet. Iron is used more efficiently by the body in building blood if a trace of copper is present. Fortunately copper and iron occur together in several foods. The richest sources are liver, wheat germ, food yeast, and turnip greens. The greatest single cause of anemia in America may be the discarding of iron in the refining of breadstuffs and empty white sugar; that is why I insist on the use of whole grains and natural sugars such as honey and dark molasses.

Only about 50 percent of the iron in foods is freed during digestion to pass into the blood. The other 50 percent is lost in the feces. Thus, even though the diet may contain iron, if it does not reach the blood and bone marrow, anemia can exist. The quantity of iron in foods is less important than the actual amount that can be used by the body.

Fruits are not especially rich in iron, but most of the iron they do contain reaches the blood stream. Apricots are particularly valuable for correcting anemia. The iron in peanuts, celery, and carrots is well absorbed, as is that from molasses. Meats are rich sources of iron, especially liver and heart. Soybeans and eggs are also rich in easily assimilable iron.

Iron is dissolved only in acid, and unless it is dissolved it cannot pass through the intestinal walls. Normally the hydrochloric acid produced by a healthy stomach dissolves iron; but in many persons, especially those lacking the vitamins of the B family and those addicted to taking soda and alkalizers, sufficient acid is not present, and the end result is the same as if no iron were supplied by the diet.

It is by no means easy to plan a diet that supplies adequate iron. Average servings of the foods listed below furnish approximately the following amounts of iron, given in milligrams:

FOODS FOR IRON

Food	Serving	Milligrams
Turnip greens	½ Cup	9
Liver	Average serving	8
Wheat germ	½ Cup	8
Yeast, brewers'	1 Tbsp.	8
Molasses, dark	1 Tbsp.	5
Beet tops	½ Cup	4
Kidney	Average serving	4
Wheat bran	½ Cup	4
Dates, dried	4	4
Spinach	½ Cup	4
Apricots	4 Halves	3
Eggs	2	3
Prunes	4	3
Chard	½ Cup	3
Dandelion greens	½ Cup	3
Raisins	⅔ Cup	3
Muscle meat, fish, or fowl	Average serving	3
Nuts	½ Cup	3
Banana	1 Large	2
Whole-wheat bread	1 Slice	1

There are many iron salts on the market, such as ferrous mucate and ferrous chloride, which are put up in tablets. These are inexpensive and are of great value in curing or preventing anemia. However, the tablets should not be used as an excuse for bad food habits. Deficiencies of protein, iodine, and calcium, and of vitamins A, C, and those of the B family, particularly of vitamins B_6, B_{12}, folic acid, choline, and niacin, can also lead to anemia and tiredness.

Iodine Is Important

Iodine forms part of the active substance thyroxine, produced by two small thyroid glands located on either side of the windpipe. The iodine-containing thyroxine not only has a powerful effect on physical and mental development, but gives the body its normal verve, its urge for work and play. A lack of iodine causes a corresponding lack of thyroxine and results in decreased stamina and vitality.

A partial lack of iodine may cause goiter, an enlargement of the thyroid gland. This enlargement is an attempt by the body to overcome the iodine lack by developing a larger amount of tissue to produce thyroxine and to use more efficiently the small amount of iodine available. In this case, the production of thyroxine is usually normal. Aside from the slight fullness and perhaps a mild pressure in the neck, there may be no other body changes. Goiter is a danger signal, pointing to possible trouble ahead. If it is at all suspected, consult your physician.

Another disease caused by too little iodine is called exophthalmic, or toxic, goiter. It appears to occur in people whose thyroid glands are already weakened because of lack of iodine. In this disease, too much thyroxine is produced and the body engine races. The heart beats too rapidly. The patient loses weight, is extremely nervous, and suffers from heat; the eyes often become prominent and somewhat protruding. This type of goiter should be supervised by your physician, who will probably prescribe large amounts of iodine.

In no other condition is diet so important as in exophthalmic goiter. All vitamins and all minerals must be given in larger than usual amounts. The need is particularly increased because the body is working at such a high speed that all requirements are much greater.

The amount of iodine in foods grown in this country varies widely; almost no food is a reliable source. The exceptions are ocean fish and seafoods, which are excellent sources. Many of my students use an iodized vegetable salt, which contains iodine from sea vegetables. It is a convenient way to get a small amount of iodine daily.

Many authorities believe that no salt should be sold except the kind that has iodine in it. Yet, although iodized salt has been on the market for over a quarter of a century, only about 15 percent of the people use it. It is difficult to understand such indifference to health.

Foods richest in iodine:

Fish	Iodized vegetable salt
Shellfish	Sea water
Sea vegetables	

Also in concentrates: sea greens made from sea vegetables; one single tablet contains the daily iodine ration.

You Need Potassium

Even a partial deficiency of potassium leads to nervousness, constipation, gas distention, and sleeplessness. The heart beats slowly and irregularly, and the heart muscles become damaged. Potassium is also necessary for the normal contraction of all muscles. The green leafy vegetables and their juices are excellent sources of potassium, as well as other minerals.

While whole-grain breads and cereals and molasses are extremely rich in potassium, three-fourths of this mineral is lost in refining grains; and white sugar contains none. In refining foods, practically all of the minerals are lost. A diet high in refined foods can cause a deficiency of a number of minerals.

You Need More Sodium and Chlorine in Hot Weather

Sodium and chlorine are of tremendous importance in the body. Chlorine is used in the stomach to form hydrochloric acid, which is necessary for normal digestion of protein and the absorption of minerals into the blood. Many foods contain sodium and chlorine; and, of course, salt contains both of these minerals. Excessive amounts of salt are not needed, but it should never be entirely omitted except on the recommendation of your physician.

A healthy person who eats a reasonably varied diet runs little risk of a deficiency of sodium and chlorine. In extremely hot weather, however, particularly if the air is dry, so much salt can be lost through perspiration that death may result. In milder cases, a lack of sodium and chlorine can cause heat cramps or heat stroke. This condition is common among people who work in furnace rooms, in mines, or in any surroundings where the temperature is unusually high. Heat stroke is accompanied by nausea, dizziness, general exhaustion, and muscular cramps in the legs, back, and abdomen. People working under conditions of extreme heat should always be supplied with salt tablets.

Hot-weather fatigue is largely due to the loss of salt through perspiration. During very hot weather, keep on hand a supply of salty foods such as peanuts, popcorn, pretzels, or soybeans. At least one well-salted food should be served with each meal. In addition, the person who perspires freely and must work in the heat is wise to add a pinch of vegetable salt to each glass of water—actually, it makes a pleasant drink.

Don't Miss Out on Trace Minerals

We do not know everything about trace minerals, but some of them are extremely important to our health and well being. For example, when magnesium is omitted from the diet of experimental animals, their hearts beat with extreme rapidity, their blood vessels expand, and low blood pressure results; the animals are extremely irritable, and slight noises may cause them to go into convulsions.

The blood of some people suffering from extreme irritability has been found to be low in *magnesium*. It is possible that extreme irritability and even some types of mental disturbance may be connected with lack of magnesium. People who consume over-refined foods and neglect to eat green vegetables could easily become deficient in this mineral.

Aluminum is found in various parts of the human body. Whether its presence is necessary to health has not yet been determined.

Zinc is present in human tissues, especially in the thyroid and the sex glands. It is one of the constituents of insulin, which is necessary for the normal utilization of sugar. Liver and milk are good sources of zinc; people who avoid these foods might be deficient in this mineral.

Cobalt is also found in small amounts in most of the organs of the human body. It is a part of vitamin B_{12}. It appears to be related to the development of red corpuscles. In persistent anemia, doctors recommend cobalt, iron, and copper with beneficial results. Liver of all kinds appears to be the best source of cobalt, iron, and copper.

Manganese is also necessary to human health, but its exact action is little understood. Manganese is found in green leaves and whole-grain breads and cereals.

Several other trace minerals seem to be essential to health. For example, *tin* is found in many human tissues, especially in the liver, brain, and thyroid gland. Relatively large amounts of *arsenic* are found in the liver; the concentration in the blood varies with glandular activity. *Bromine*, like arsenic, is best known as a drug and a poison; yet it is always in human blood. *Mercury* is found in the human liver; *nickel* is concentrated in the pancreas; *silver* occurs in the blood, liver, sex glands, heart, spleen, kidneys, and especially the thyroid and tonsils. However, the functions of these minerals are not well known.

Although a great deal is still to be learned about the exact role of trace minerals in human nutrition, they are undoubtedly of importance. Leafy vegetables, organ meats, and whole-grain breads and cereals should always be included in the diet to fulfill our needs in this respect. Since many of our minerals are washed into the oceans, thousands of people have learned to fortify their diets with sea vegetation and sea greens. These are extremely rich in so many of the trace elements.

THOSE IMPORTANT AMINO ACIDS

Amino acid molecules are small and contain from ten to thirty-five atoms! It took about one hundred years of research for this momentous discovery—a discovery as vital for the *good* of man as the atomic bomb can be for the destruction of man. Another great victory of this hundred-year research is the discovery that only eight of the twenty-odd amino acids are necessary for health and longer life. The others can be manufactured by the body. And now, before you wonder what this is all about, let me say that all protein foods are made up from amino acids. So it is for a very good scientific reason that I recommend larger amounts of first-class protein, rich in essential amino acids, such as milk, lean meats, eggs, yeast, and the unappreciated soybean. The names of the eight essential amino acids may sound strange, but in years to come you will hear a great deal about them, so let me introduce you to:

Lysine	Phenylalanine
Leucine	Threonine
Isoleucine	Methionine
Tryptophan	Valine

Don't be confused by these strange-sounding names; just remember that all of these are obtained in first-class proteins. Also remember that you have to have enough protein foods each and every day. The average man should eat not less than 70 grams of protein, the average woman not less than 60 grams, each and every day. This is the most expensive item, especially for people with large families. For that reason, I recommend the fortification of ordinary foods with dried skim milk, an inexpensive source of good protein, as well as brewers' yeast, wheat germ, and soya products. Before or after surgery, in burns and ulcers, your doctor will recommend extra amounts of first-class proteins, which contain all of those eight atomic amino acids. See page 27 for a list of the best protein foods. Use it to check your protein intake until you have formed the habit of eating not less than 60 to 70 grams a day for the rest of your life.

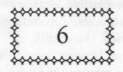

High Vitality Meal Planning

If we relied on our *natural* appetites, we would never make a mistake in eating. In the brain there is a built-in regulator for thirst, hunger, appetite; and when the body needs a certain kind of food, that built-in regulator creates the appetite for that particular food.

Perhaps you have heard of a famous experiment that was made years ago with a group of healthy toddlers, still young enough to follow their natural unspoiled appetites. Every day, at every meal, these babies were set down before a table loaded with all kinds of simple, natural foods, and they were allowed to eat what they wished—and somehow, they selected the foods which they needed.

Yes, nature would regulate our eating for us, if we would only allow her to do so. To get you started, come along with me and see how easy it is to arrange your meals so that you feel nourished and vital all day long.

Your breakfast is your vitality determinator for the day. I say this over and over again. Whether you will begin your day tired or glowing with energy is no longer a matter of guesswork. It is simple arithmetic.

When your blood sugar is at 90, you are comfortable. At 80, you are slowing down. At 70 you are hungry and your lassitude becomes fatigue. At 65 you are craving for sweets and your insides are grumbling, and if the level continues to drop you may suffer headache, weakness, wobbliness, heart palpitations, mental confusion, nausea, and worse. And your nerves, which feed only on the sugar supply in your blood, suffer first and most from this needless starvation!

Now let us see what happens when you begin your day with your habitual breakfast. It is about twelve hours since your last meal, and the average level of blood sugar after twelve hours of fasting is between 90 and 95. In a famous study which was reported some years ago by the United States Department of Agriculture, two hundred volunteers ate various kinds of breakfasts, from black coffee alone or "coffee-and" to a heavy breakfast of juice, oatmeal with sugar and cream, bacon, toast with butter and jam, coffee with sugar and cream.

With only coffee, the blood sugar went steadily down during the morning, and the volunteers became more and more irritable, nervous, headachy, and exhausted.

PROTEIN BREAKFAST PREVENTS LETDOWN

But for those who had taken a first-class protein with their breakfast, either eggs or fortified milk (page 29), the blood sugar rose to a vigorous 120 and remained at that level through the morning hours.

Here is the most remarkable part of this remarkable story: All through the day, no matter what those volunteers ate, those who had eaten a breakfast without protein continued to have low blood sugar, with all its miseries. And those who had taken good protein with their breakfast enjoyed high blood sugar, high vitality, high efficiency, and high spirits all day long.

Now, do you understand why I say that breakfast is your vitality determinator for the day? As for your looks, when you are irritable, nervous, fatigued, how do you imagine you look? Your mirror has shown you, many times. When your blood sugar falls, everything falls—including the muscles in your face!

Now I know what you will say—I have heard it so many times: "But I *can't* eat such a big breakfast!" My answer to you is, you *will be able* to eat it, and enjoy it too. Begin by eating a bit less the night before, and in just a few days your natural morning hunger will return.

Do you realize what upside-down people we have become? We give our bodies the biggest load of food at night, before going to sleep, exactly when we need it least. And then we cheat ourselves at breakfast, the meal with which we begin the day's working and living, just when we need food most and when calories can be worked off easiest.

Another argument I hear, especially from people who rush off to work each day, is "But I haven't got the time!" My answer is that it takes only five minutes to boil an egg and toast a piece of good bread, which with coffee and fresh fruit makes an adequate breakfast. And it takes only another five or ten minutes to eat it and put the dishes in the sink. Isn't it worth getting up fifteen minutes earlier to function all morning in your most efficient way?

For small eaters, I offer this suggestion: If you really find it impossible to manage a substantial breakfast each day, then make sure to have a midmorning vitality booster that will keep your blood sugar at high level—not an empty deceptive snack like coffee or cola and a doughnut, but a fortified milk drink, a bit of bread and cheese, a sweet fruit with a handful of nuts or a handful of sunflower seeds, which you can keep at the office.

Blueprint for High Vitality Breakfasts

First: Unsweetened fruit juice or whole fruit, preferably fresh

Second: Large helping of protein, not less than 20 grams

Third: Helping of whole-grain bread, gluten bread, or whole-grain cereal

Fourth: For enjoyment and more protein, have one or two cups of Swiss coffee (hot coffee with foaming hot milk, half and half, with honey, if you must have sweetening).

Now let us set a buffet on a big long table so you can see the tremendous variety to choose from. I have listed the most popular breakfast dishes; you need not have ham and eggs every day of the week. They are a fine protein dish, but actually we need variety. The English people like fish, South Americans eat steaks, the Swiss people enjoy their famous cheese. These are all first-class breakfast proteins. If your pocketbook does not permit these proteins, then at least eat a whole-grain cereal, hot or cold, and fortify it with one or two tablespoons of wheat germ and lots of fortified skim milk. I urge you to try different kinds of breakfasts. Soon we will be traveling in space and I predict that concentrated protein breakfasts will become a must for all strenuous tasks. I suggest you start now. See how lucky you are; in this land of variety you can have a different breakfast for every day in the month.

I recommend average helpings of most foods and large portions of protein dishes. Animal proteins are best; fresh and dried milk, lean cottage cheese, and dried chipped beef are also extremely high in first-class protein. Use them generously to get your protein quota of 20 to 30 grams in every meal. (See page 27.)

Breads and cereals are disappointingly low in protein unless you fortify them with gluten flour, soya flour, powdered milk, or food yeast. But we *need* one good helping of carbohydrate to help keep energy and spirits high all day long.

I also urge you to learn to enjoy Swiss coffee in place of the health-destroying, heavily sugared and creamed beverage. Swiss coffee for breakfast is much to be preferred to black coffee; the milk adds extra protein, plus milk sugar for extra morning energy. Some manufacturer could make a fortune by mixing instant coffee with dry milk powder. All we would have to do then is stir in hot water.

Fresh Things First

Each morning make a fresh beginning. Take my words literally, and make a fresh beginning with each meal. By this I mean: begin each meal with something fresh whenever you can.

Those of us who for many years have begun each meal with a fresh fruit or vegetable have always believed we were following the latest dictates of scientific nutrition—and so we were. But the truth of the matter is that, even without the aid of modern science, the wise Greeks practiced this rule 400 years before the birth of Christ. More than 2,000 years ago, the Greek physician Diocles Carystos wrote, "Eat your raw fresh foods first of all and follow with cooked food as your second course, and let fruit be the end of your meal."

In California and Florida and the sunny Mediterranean lands of Europe it has long been a custom to begin a meal with something fresh, melon or fruit cup, or the crisp raw vegetables of French hors d'oeuvres and Italian antipasto. The lively fragrance and flavor refresh the taste buds, start the digestive juices, and set the body's wonderful chemistry going for the rest of the meal.

German Scientist Tells Us Why

We know all this scientifically today. One of the great scientists of the last century, Dr. Rudolf Virchow, discovered and proved that there are physiological reasons for eating fresh foods at the *beginning* of a meal. He observed that cooked food called up a great increase of white blood corpuscles in the blood, the same reaction that the body makes to disease germs and bacteria. This is the wonderful defense system of the body, the "immune reaction" that protects us against disease. But it was Virchow's astonishing discovery that the body makes this same defense against processed foods! Then he found that when he fed his patients fresh, unprocessed food *first*, this rise in white blood corpuscles did not occur. Even more important, his patients *then* could eat their cooked meal without causing this irritating reaction of the blood.

I believe I am the first American nutritionist to apply Virchow's discovery. In Europe, Dr. Bircher-Benner of Zurich and Dr. Werner Kollath of Hanover for many years have prescribed fresh fruits or vegetables at the beginning of breakfast, lunch, and dinner.

The fresh color and flavor will set the "appetite juice" flowing. And I have discovered other wonderful advantages to this agreeable custom.

Fresh things, eaten at the beginning of the meal when appetite is keenest, satisfy that first sharp hunger and prevent overeating.

Your salad, with its mildly acid dressing, also stimulates all the digestive processes and contributes bulk to encourage those muscular intestinal walls that might otherwise become lazy. Then too, crisp fresh salads are our best vehicles to get valuable golden oils into our daily menus, and now we have more and more proof that the golden vegetable oils with their valuable unsaturated fatty acids help to burn up ugly fat deposits in the body. They help Adam to keep his cholesterol level down; and for Eve, golden vegetable oils moisturize the inside and outside of her skin—permanently, not just temporarily as cosmetics do.

Thus your fresh beginning for each meal serves health, good looks, and a slim waistline, as well as appetite and the pleasure of eating.

Make Lunch Time Salad Time

To save time and a lot of dishwashing, I have devised what I call a meal in just one bowl—tempting, compact, not too expensive, and above all nourishing enough to keep energy at a high level all through the afternoon.

I am convinced that the eating of heavy and greasy luncheons causes much afternoon tiredness and mental letdown, which leads to short tempers and four o'clock letdowns, and costs Big Business millions. You can prevent this by forming the salad-lunch habit.

Whether you order this salad at your favorite restaurant or are lucky enough to have it at home, here are its essentials:

For a base, cut up the freshest, greenest, crispiest vegetables (at least a cupful); add to this a good portion, not less than twenty grams, of your favorite stick-to-the-ribs protein food (see list, page 27); and toss it all together with a golden oil dressing of your choice (page 481).

On beautyfarms, salads like this are served in great bowls with a choice of half a dozen different kinds of dressing. The salad itself can be different every day, with the endless variety of delicious fresh things we have to choose from all the year round. And there need never be monotony in the dressing with the many golden oils providing their different nuances of taste. I urge you to try them all, individually and in combination. Mix these oils, two or three different kinds in one dressing, the less expensive to extend the more costly ones, and by all means add a little of a good grade of olive oil. Olive oil is not rich in the polyunsaturated acids, but it is extremely rich in the mono-unsaturated acids (82%), it is far richer in flavor than any of the other oils, and it gives an elegance to salads that no other oil can.

Good oils deserve good vinegars, and again we have a wealth of them to choose from. Shun the white synthetic kind, which contributes neither goodness nor flavor but only an edge sharp as a knife. It is just as easy to use cider vinegar, with its mellowness of ripe apples; or if you have a French or Italian taste, flavorsome wine vinegar (but use it more sparingly). A salad must never have an outright acid or sour taste; sheer sourness is so strong and dominating that it kills all other flavors. It is best to follow the classic French proportions of two-thirds oil and one-third vinegar.

Add Spice and Sparkle

For fresher and more exciting-tasting dressings use both lemon juice, rich in vitamin C, and vinegar; I know some excellent cooks who sprinkle a few drops of lemon juice over all salads, no matter what dressing they use. And to give their salads of all kinds a bit of mystery and to soften any sharpness in the dressing, they use their imagination and spike them with various flavors—vegetable salt, salad herbs, or something unexpected like a drop or two of honey, wonderful when fruits are in the salad. You can be a true gourmet and make your own delicately flavored herb vinegar, as is done in thousands of French homes. They really add new spice and sparkle to your salads, which should be eaten with gusto and not just because they're good for you.

Learn to Use Golden Oils

No matter what you may have heard or read, take my word for it that vegetable oils are necessary at all times, even when you are reducing or weight-watching. The excess of hard animal fats and the many hydrogenated pure white and highly tooted inert fats in the diets of millions of Americans has given a bad name to all fats, including the oils that are so necessary to keep the body fires burning bright and the skin and hair beautiful.

It is true that the health and vitality-giving values are destroyed when manufacturers shoot hydrogen into otherwise good oils so that they can stand in warehouses and on market shelves for a long time without spoiling. But why should you pay that hidden price in health? I believe that much of the excess fat which thirty million Americans carry around their waists is in part due to these fats. The human body is not equipped to metabolize such quantities of inert fats, so they are deposited where circulation is slowest—around the middle!

But with the fresh, unsaturated, liquid oils it is quite a different story. They are untreated by heat, especially if you take pains to buy them at a diet and health shop, and so they have not lost their abundance of the essential fatty acids, especially linoleic acid, and most of the antioxidants. Liquid oils are easier for the body to burn; they are not deposited as excess fat unless you are overeating generally.

So whether you are keeping your ideal weight or reducing, have not less than two tablespoons of your favorite oil a day, *every* day, in some form; use it in cooking, in plain salad dressing, or in your own delicious homemade mayonnaise. Real mayonnaise, made with unheated fresh oil, a fresh egg yolk, and a dash of vinegar, is a splendid food. The oil furnishes your body with the fatty acids; the fresh egg yolk contributes important lecithin and vitamin A; and the vinegar adds flavor and speeds digestion. Many of my students now make their own mayonnaise, not only for salads but also for a spread on bread when doctors have forbidden butter.

Blueprint for High Vitality Luncheons

First: A fresh start with any and all fresh green salad vegetables, broken up or chopped, the more the merrier (at least a cup).

Second: Your favorite salad protein, at least 20 grams, never less than half a cup. Have lean cottage cheese, shredded meat, eggs, or fish. Toss the salad with a golden oil dressing or mayonnaise.

Third: A carbohydrate for prolonged energy. A muffin, a slice of protein, rye, or whole-wheat bread, lightly buttered or with mayonnaise.

Fourth: For enjoyment and stimulation, a glass of milk, yogurt, buttermilk, or your favorite beverage. No white sugar, please, or you'll have a letdown.

PROTEINS FOR YOUR SALAD BOWL

Cottage cheese	Conch
Chicken	Tuna

Cheddar cheese   Eggs, hard-cooked
Lean ham   Leftover meat
Tongue   Soybean
Lobster   Gelatin meat or fish (aspic)
Shrimp   Fruits and nuts

MIDAFTERNOON VITALITY LIFT

One of my most difficult Hollywood assignments was to keep the glamor girls from looking wilted by midafternoon. Making motion pictures is the cruelest, most strenuous kind of work; after a few hours of repetitious "takes" in stuffy air, under hot Klieg lights, even the brightest of stars began to droop, and the sharpest of all eyes, the movie camera, caught every listless line.

Once at the Hal Roach studio my task was to sustain the gorgeousness of twelve showgirls who really deserved the word *gorgeous*; the picture was *The All-American Coed*, and Frances Langford was its lovely star. Lady Mendl was my guest in Beverly Hills at the time, and since she was interested in all phases of the theatre I took her along to see how drooping glamor girls can be revived without benzedrine and other pep pills. I knew it would be inspiring to the girls, too, to see how an internationally famous hostess kept her glamor and vitality undimmed even at the age of eighty. All went well through lunch and after, until in midafternoon those long-stemmed American beauties began to fade visibly.

My answer was to set up a beauty bar, the first in Hollywood. At three o'clock sharp the cameras stopped turning, and all those beautiful girls came to the bar to replenish their beauty. For fifteen minutes, in their gold and silver lamé gowns, they sipped my booster cocktails and nibbled at the proteins laid out for them on platters.

They had their choice of these cocktails: orange juice with fresh egg yolk beaten into it; fortified skim milk flavored with orange-blossom honey; chilled yogurt fortified with dark molasses; and Lady Mendl's own favorite, which I call my Hi-Vi Booster, cool glasses of lushly red tomato espresso, spiked with one or two heaping teaspoons of celery-flavored food yeast and a teaspoon of lemon juice. On the platters were the more solid Hi-Vi beauty treats: crisp whole-wheat crackers with cubes of cheese; nonhydrogenated peanut butter; avocado slices spiked with vegetable salt, spices, and lime juice; and that ever-wonderful, ever-popular standby, Hi-Vi cottage cheese with parsley, chives, basil, and all the fresh herbs we could find in the Farmer's Market.

After a few days of our beauty bar refreshment, the girls and the director saw the difference. More important, the day's run of film showed the girls as fresh-looking and their dancing as crisp in the afternoon as it had been in the morning.

DINNER TIME IS RELAXING TIME

All over this great land, dinner time is homecoming time, the end of the working day and the beginning of evening leisure; in many homes it is the one time when families can sit down together to a meal and eat in an atmosphere of peace and relaxation. The man of the house needs a chance to unwind before sitting down to dinner. The American cocktail before dinner can be a relaxing custom, but it is too often misunderstood and abused. I am sorry to see people pickle their stomachs with martinis, killing their natural appetites and all sense of taste of food. It is then that most people tend to overeat, not knowing *what* they are eating and getting no pleasure from savoring their food.

Intelligent people need not be slaves to strong cocktails simply because that is the custom. Occasionally, why not try nature's own cocktail, a tall glass of cool vegetable espresso, spiked with fragrant garden herbs and spices, or that old standby—a cool glass of tomato juice, vitalized with a spoonful of good-tasting brewers' yeast and a few drops of fresh lemon juice.

After a busy and perhaps a tense day, such a drink does wonderful things. It helps to unwind taut nerves; it quickly erases fatigue with its high content of natural sugars; most important, it raises the blood sugar level to the point where you will have no wish to overeat.

Every dinner should be nutritious, light, and lean; about twenty to thirty grams of good protein in lean meat, fish, or fowl, with a green short-cooked vegetable, an occasional baked potato or kasha or brown rice, and always a crisp salad with golden oil dressing. For pleasure and digestion, there is a bowl of fresh fruit or honey-sweetened compote, occasionally an open-face fruit pie, a custard, or a tangy cheese.

Blueprint for High Vitality Dinners

Your choice of appetizers:
Fruit cup
Green salad
Finger salad
Vegetable espresso
Hot or cold jellied broth occasionally

Your choice of protein dishes:
Lean meat
Liver
Lean fish
Nut loaf
Lean cheese
Eggs
Soybeans

Your choice:
Short-cooked vegetables
Light-hearted baked potato
Kasha
Rice

Your choice of delightful desserts:
Fresh fruit of the season
Honey compote
Gelatin with fruit
Custard
Open-face fruit pie
Cheese
Yogurt
Plus your favorite beverage

RECIPES AND MENUS TO GUIDE YOU

Sound nutrition demands that all the important nutrients for the entire body be eaten every day. There follow some menus to guide you. If you like them, use them; or if you prefer, make up your own. Eating, as we have learned, should be fun and not regimented. I thoroughly agree with Dr. Margaret Mead when she says: "The present phase of American 'dieting' and 'slimming,' counting *calories*, has something of the same pathetic rigidity that accompanied early bottle feeding. Eventually bottle feeding was modified according to the needs of 'self-demand' or 'self-regulation.'"

It is this self-regulation we must strive for so that we can once and forever say goodbye to all diets, including those of Gayelord Hauser. For the present, all I ask of you is to remember that we cut down on all unfriendly hard fats, we eat fewer starches and sugars, but we eat more proteins and we include as many fresh fruits, vegetables, and unprocessed foods as possible.

I have said very little about the few "skinnies," those lucky ones who would like to gain weight. They can follow the same principle, perhaps eat smaller meals and between meals enjoy the rich milk shakes made with very ripe bananas. A French physician says that with greatly underweight people it is not so much a question of eating more as it is a matter of learning to *relax* so that they assimilate their food better. His recommendation is to relax ten minutes before meals and five minutes after meals. This certainly is a simple procedure, and I suggest that you underweighters eat in the modern manner and apply the French doctor's advice. (See also page 427, "How to Gain Weight.")

Since breakfast to a very great measure determines how we feel and look throughout the day, let me give you a few sample menus. I ask you only to have a protein-rich breakfast for ten days. If you do not like the proteins in my breakfast menus, select those that you like better. If you do not feel and look much better after these ten days, then go back to your limp and empty "coffee-and" combinations.

Since protein foods are the most expensive of all foods, I suggest again, that you with small budgets obtain a large part of your proteins from the inexpensive Hi-Vi lean milk, cottage cheese, or homemade cream cheese. Good bread—wheat germ or soya or whole wheat—can add another three to five grams of protein to your most important meal.

MILLION-DOLLAR EYE-OPENER

If you are a slow riser, easily irritated or just naturally mean in the morning, this eye-opener can help you to get going, make you more amiable and attractive. The minute you get out of bed, drink a small glass of your favorite fruit juice. It must be naturally sweet, never sugared, orange juice, pineapple juice, apple juice, or papaya juice. The natural sugar in any unsweetened fruit juice, taken on an empty stomach, performs the magic. It raises your blood sugar level quickly and makes everything, including you, look more rosy at the breakfast table.

Between-Meal Vitality Boosters Unlimited

There is exciting evidence coming from a famous nutrition laboratory that "nibbling" animals, who eat throughout the day, keep their vitality at a higher level than when given three squares a day. So do not hesitate to nibble one of the between-meal vitality boosters should you feel hungry or have a sense of letdown. If you enjoy a coffee break, drink Swiss coffee (half hot coffee and half hot foaming milk). Remember it's the protein, and the protein alone, which gives a sustained lift, and the thrifty Swiss have known for years that their Swiss coffee sticks to the ribs.

Quick Hi-Vi Milk (Hot or Cold)

Put four tablespoons of instant dry milk into a glass of fresh skim milk. Waistline watchers can flavor this with a bit of instant coffee powder, vanilla, nutmeg, or cinnamon. Those with normal waistlines can add a bit of honey, molasses, caruba (carob) powder, or frozen fruit juice. Or you can put 1 cup of dry milk into a quart of fresh milk and keep it in the refrigerator. This is a wonderful standby for busy mothers.

Hi-Vi Booster Par Excellence

Beat two or three teaspoons of good-tasting brewers' yeast into a glass of chilled tomato juice, spike with a slice of lemon and a pinch of vegetable salt.

Hi-Vi Chocolaty Drink (Hot or Cold)

Stir one tablespoon of caruba powder into a glass of skim milk. If necessary, sweeten with a bit of honey. Real chocolate prevents the calcium in milk from being assimilated and is especially undesirable for youngsters.

Hi-Vi Eat and Run Drink

Stir one fresh egg yolk into a glass of fresh orange juice; half a teaspoon of honey gives added taste and very quick energy.

Hi-Vi Swiss Broth

Mix one tablespoon of instant skim milk powder, one teaspoon food yeast, half teaspoon of dried herbs (savory, parsley, dill, tarragon, etc.). Stir into a cup of hot skim milk or tomato juice and spike with vegetable salt. This instant Swiss broth is already available in health and diet shops.

Hi-Vi Bomb

Into one cup of skim milk, stir one teaspoon *each* of golden honey, dark molasses, good-tasting food yeast, and caruba powder. Can be taken hot or cold for a quick burst of vitality.

Hi-Vi Golden Drink

A favorite on beautyfarms and with children. Mix half a cup of fresh cold milk with half a cup of freshly made carrot juice. Undernourished, finicky eaters thrive on this delicious combination.

Tranquilizing Nite Cap

Mix one tablespoon of dry skim milk powder into a cup of hot skim milk and flavor with a teaspoon of honey or molasses. Sip slowly. For more tranquilizing calcium and vitamin D, some nutritionists now recommend two calcium tablets to be taken with the hot milk drink instead of habit-forming sleeping tablets.

Hi-Vi Egg Snack

Fresh hard-cooked eggs, when eaten very slowly, can sustain a high level of vitality. Contrary to popular opinion, they are not hard to digest. Keep them in the refrigerator. Before eating, spike them with herbs and a bit of vegetable salt. Hard-cooked eggs are especially valuable for reducers.

Hi-Vi Yogurt

Lean yogurt is extremely valuable. It supplies hard-working bacteria, useful acids, and easily digested protein. A cup of plain yogurt, or yogurt spiked with honey, molasses, or frozen fruit concentrate, makes an ideal between-meal boost.

Hi-Vi Cheese Spread

Two or three tablespoons of cottage or yogurt cream cheese mixed with chives, parsley, or green onions, spiked with herbs and vegetable salt, served with a slice of whole-wheat or gluten toast, is excellent for those wishing a more solid between-meal or bedtime snack.

Let these samples help you. There is really no limit to the delightful between-meal vitality boosters you can make. Let your imagination guide you.

Now, hold up your right hand and swear that, henceforth, you will not insult your body with empty coffee breaks, colas, pops, or other white-sugar concoctions which give you a swift lift and then a kick in the pants and drop you to an all-time low!

HIGH VITALITY BREAKFASTS, LUNCHEONS, AND DINNERS

HIGH VITALITY VITAMIN RITUAL

So that there is no possible chance for any of the many known nutrients to be missing in your daily meals, it is wise to take your vitamin and mineral concentrates with your breakfast and be fortified for the day ahead. Let your doctor recommend the supplement best suited to your needs.

BREAKFAST: Fruit juice
                    Scrambled eggs
                    1 portion lean ham
                    1 slice whole-wheat or gluten toast,
                    lightly buttered

	Choice of beverage: coffee, tea, or milk Preferably Swiss coffee: half hot coffee and half hot foaming milk
MIDMORNING:	If hungry: your choice of between-meal vitality boosters
LUNCHEON:	Salad bowl: cottage cheese on bed of dark green lettuce Golden oil dressing 1 slice whole-wheat bread, buttered lightly Fresh or honeyed fruit, if desired Choice of beverage: mint tea, English tea, papaya tea, coffee, milk, or yogurt
MIDAFTERNOON:	If hungry: your choice of between-meal vitality boosters
DINNER:	Mixed salad Golden oil dressing Large lean hamburger, tenderized Steamed zucchini Apple Snow or baked apple Choice of beverage: demitasse, milk, or tea
BEFORE RETIRING:	If hungry: Treat yourself to a between-meal snack or a hot tranquilizing nite cap

---

HIGH VITALITY VITAMIN RITUAL

So that there is no possible chance for any of the many known nutrients to be missing in your daily meals, it is wise to take your vitamin and mineral concentrates with your breakfast and be fortified for the day ahead. Let your doctor recommend the supplement best suited to your needs.

BREAKFAST:	Half grapefruit Your favorite hot or cold cereal a la mode

(Serve all cereals a la mode: topped with 2 tbsp. wheat germ, 1 tsp. honey)
Serve with half-cup Hi-Vi milk
3 slices crisp lean bacon
Choice of beverage: coffee, tea, or milk
Preferably Swiss coffee: half hot coffee and half hot foaming milk

MIDMORNING: If hungry: your choice of between-meal vitality boosters

LUNCHEON: Salad bowl: half-cup shrimp on bed of green leaves
Golden oil dressing
One wheat-germ muffin, buttered lightly
Fresh or honeyed fruit, if desired
Choice of beverage: mint tea, English tea, papaya tea, coffee, milk, or yogurt

MIDAFTERNOON: If hungry: your choice of between-meal vitality boosters

DINNER: Red apple and red cabbage salad
Your favorite golden oil dressing
Lean pot roast
Short-cooked beets
Kasha
Fresh or stewed fruit
Choice of beverage: demitasse, milk, or tea

BEFORE RETIRING: If hungry: Treat yourself to a between-meal snack or a hot tranquilizing nite cap

HIGH VITALITY VITAMIN RITUAL

So that there is no possible chance for any of the many known nutrients to be missing in your daily meals, it is wise to take your vitamin and mineral concentrates with your breakfast and be fortified for the day ahead. Let your doctor recommend the supplement best suited to your needs.

BREAKFAST:
Applesauce, sprinkled with 1 tbsp. wheat germ and 1 tsp. honey
Chipped beef, simmered in Hi-Vi lean milk
Served on whole-wheat toast
Choice of beverage: coffee, tea, or milk
Preferably Swiss coffee: half hot coffee and half hot foaming milk

MIDMORNING:
If hungry: your choice of between-meal vitality boosters

LUNCHEON:
Salad bowl: shredded Swiss cheese on bed of watercress and lettuce
Golden oil dressing
1 slice rye bread, buttered lightly
Fresh or honeyed fruit, if desired
Choice of beverage: mint tea, English tea, papaya tea, coffee, milk, or yogurt

MIDAFTERNOON:
If hungry: your choice of between-meal vitality boosters

DINNER:
Raw tender spinach salad
Golden oil dressing
Tender broiled liver
Baked onions with oregano
Broiled grapefruit
Choice of beverage: demitasse, milk, or tea

BEFORE RETIRING: If hungry: Treat yourself to a between-meal snack or a hot tranquilizing nite cap

---

HIGH VITALITY VITAMIN RITUAL

So that there is no possible chance for any of the many known nutrients to be missing in your daily meals, it is wise to take your vitamin and mineral concentrates with your breakfast and be fortified for the day ahead. Let your doctor recommend the supplement best suited to your needs.

BREAKFAST: Large slice of melon or berries
Your favorite hot or cold cereal a la mode (Serve all cereals a la mode: topped with 2 tbsp. wheat germ, 1 tsp. honey)
Serve with half-cup Hi-Vi milk
Choice of beverage: coffee, tea, or milk
Preferably Swiss coffee: half hot coffee and half hot foaming milk

MIDMORNING: If hungry: your choice of between-meal vitality boosters

LUNCHEON: Salad bowl: chunks of tuna fish or chicken on bed of lettuce and celery
Your favorite golden oil dressing
One slice gluten toast, lightly buttered
Fresh or honeyed fruit, if desired
Choice of beverage: mint tea, English tea, papaya tea, coffee, milk, or yogurt

MIDAFTERNOON: If hungry: your choice of between-meal vitality boosters

DINNER: Carrot and pineapple salad
Golden mayonnaise dressing
Lean broiled steak

Braised celery
Light-hearted baked potato
Fruit compote, Lady Mendl
Choice of beverage: demitasse, milk, or tea

BEFORE RETIRING: If hungry: Treat yourself to a between-meal snack or a hot tranquilizing nite cap

---

HIGH VITALITY VITAMIN RITUAL

So that there is no possible chance for any of the many known nutrients to be missing in your daily meals, it is wise to take your vitamin and mineral concentrates with your breakfast and be fortified for the day ahead. Let your doctor recommend the supplement best suited to your needs.

BREAKFAST: Pineapple juice
Finnan haddie, poached in Hi-Vi milk
One slice old-fashioned rye toast, buttered lightly
Choice of beverage: coffee, tea, or milk
Preferably Swiss coffee: half hot coffee and half hot foaming milk

MIDMORNING: If hungry: your choice of between-meal vitality boosters

LUNCHEON: Salad bowl: chopped hard-cooked eggs on bed of dark green lettuce
Golden oil dressing
One whole-wheat muffin, lightly buttered
Fresh or honeyed fruit, if desired
Choice of beverage: mint tea, English tea, papaya tea, coffee, milk, or yogurt

MIDAFTERNOON: If hungry: your choice of between-meal vitality boosters

DINNER: Celery-carrot espresso
                       Grilled halibut
                       String beans with slivered almonds
                       Fresh fruit gelatin
                       Choice of beverage: demitasse, milk, or
                       tea

BEFORE RETIRING: If hungry: Treat yourself to a between-
                       meal snack or a hot tranquilizing nite
                       cap

HIGH VITALITY VITAMIN RITUAL

So that there is no possible chance for any of the many known nutrients to be missing in your daily meals, it is wise to take your vitamin and mineral concentrates with your breakfast and be fortified for the day ahead. Let your doctor recommend the supplement best suited to your needs.

BREAKFAST: Sliced orange
                       Soft-cooked eggs, spiked with herb salt
                       Two slices lean Canadian bacon
                       One soya muffin, or slice whole-wheat
                       toast, buttered lightly
                       Choice of beverage: coffee, tea, or milk
                       Preferably Swiss coffee: half hot cof-
                       fee and half hot foaming milk

MIDMORNING: If hungry: your choice of between-meal
                       vitality boosters

LUNCHEON: Salad bowl: lean fish or meat salad on
                       bed of crisp greens
                       Golden oil dressing
                       One slice El Molino or rye bread, but-
                       tered lightly
                       Fresh or honeyed fruit, if desired
                       Choice of beverage: mint tea, English
                       tea, papaya tea, coffee, milk, or yogurt

MIDAFTERNOON: If hungry: your choice of between-meal vitality boosters

DINNER: Avocado and grapefruit salad
Golden fruit dressing
Roast herbed chicken
Short-cooked shredded cauliflower
Peas with fresh mint
Honey ice cream
Choice of beverage: demitasse, milk, or tea

BEFORE RETIRING: If hungry: Treat yourself to a between-meal snack or a hot tranquilizing nite cap

---

HIGH VITALITY VITAMIN RITUAL

So that there is no possible chance for any of the many known nutrients to be missing in your daily meals, it is wise to take your vitamin and mineral concentrates with your breakfast and be fortified for the day ahead. Let your doctor recommend the supplement best suited to your needs.

BREAKFAST: Fresh berries, sprinkled with honey
Cottage cheese pancakes, with maple syrup or honey
Three slices lean crisp bacon
Choice of beverage: coffee, tea, or milk
Preferably Swiss coffee: half hot coffee and half hot foaming milk

MIDMORNING: If hungry: your choice of between-meal vitality boosters

LUNCHEON: Salad bowl: Waldorf salad on bed of tender lettuce
Yogurt dressing
One square cornbread Carrotte, lightly buttered

	Choice of beverage: mint tea, English tea, papaya tea, coffee, milk, or yogurt
MIDAFTERNOON:	If hungry:your choice of between-meal vitality boosters
DINNER:	Summer soup, Persian style *or* Watercress and nasturtium salad Golden oil dressing Chicken curry Indienne Fluffy brown rice Fresh pineapple or melon Choice of beverage: demitasse, milk, or tea
BEFORE RETIRING:	If hungry: Treat yourself to a between-meal snack or a hot tranquilizing nite cap

Summing up

I repeat, you do not need to follow these menus; you may not like the arrangement or you may not always have the recommended foods in your pantry. But for keeping vitality high all day long, promise yourself to eat a protein breakfast. Use no white sugar whatsoever. Should you be hungry between meals, do have one of the vitality boosters. Enjoy a big salad luncheon, and eat a leisurely, lean, protein dinner. For a good night's sleep, treat yourself to that tranquilizing calcium-rich nite cap. Remember that hot milk drinks, sipped slowly at bedtime, are by far the best sleep inducers. The warm drink in your stomach coaxes the blood away from the overactive brain—calcium is the great tranquilizer-relaxer—and before you know it, you're in the arms of Morpheus. The next morning, tension and tiredness are a thing of the past; and you face the new day with courage and confidence.

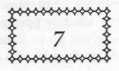

7

Eating Should Be Fun

I shall never forget the favorite maxim of my favorite teacher, Ragnar Berg, the Swedish nutritionist: "There must be pleasure in eating." The pleasure principle is essential in the biological scheme of things; or as Dr. Iago Gladstone says it, "Life is not logical; it is biological."

Please, never think or speak of nutritious food as being "good for you" or let the family table be approached as though it were a prescription counter. Let's revive the great art of dining—but with nutritionally sound meals.

Ladies, don't be satisfied with the old-fashioned compliment, "She sets a good table." And don't be satisfied merely with setting before your family the freshest, best, and most nourishing foods available. Make your table attractive, with immaculate linen, silver, and chinaware. Plan interesting color combinations in foods; have hot dishes hot and cold dishes cold. Above all, set an unhurried, pleasant atmosphere, and a new, slower tempo of family eating and living, especially at the end of the day.

This is important: Never eat when you are emotionally upset or overtired. Lie down before dinner, if possible (this is a perfect time for fifteen minutes on the Yoga Slant). Perhaps the rest of your family will follow your example. Half an hour or so before dinner, your whole family (I hope) enjoys a refreshing fruit or vegetable juice cocktail, the natural appetite normalizer that is now part of your daily living. (See page 505.) I hope that you make this cocktail time a leisurely get-together to which you all look forward, from which you go to dinner looking and feeling relaxed. I hope you indulge in a lot of conversational nonsense. Nonsense is the best thing I know to keep family machinery well oiled.

Eating slowly and chewing well helps make smaller amounts of food more satisfying. Also, take your time about beginning to eat. Did you grow up in a family where grace was said before meals? I did, and it gives me a sense of inner peace to recall it—the big round table presided over by our parents and surrounded by ravenous, growing children; the moment's pause, before wading into our food, to say "Thank you." How I would like to see this fine old custom generally reinstated!

However you do it—with candles, soft music, good conversation —your aim is to create the peaceful "homey" atmosphere in which families forget their worries and individual differences—in which good fellowship is as plentiful as good food, and everything tastes good and really nourishes. Let me say it again: *Eat slowly*. As a Chinese cook once told me, "Amelicans eat lickety split—Chinaman enjoy food plenty." Overweighters especially are prone to be food-bolters and unconscious eaters; it is one reason why they have to eat more than they really need to feel satisfied. I do not recommend throwing away knives and forks and eating with chopsticks, but we can learn from the Chinese. They have practiced lean cooking and leisurely lean eating for centuries.

Of course you will *never* say "diet." When you introduce new and more nutritious lean foods, never say, "It's good for you." Just say, "It's good." Change family eating habits gradually and casually. Introduce new dishes as something novel and delicious that you dreamed up as a treat. If you are the one person in the family who is reducing, be nonchalant about your smaller portions or the foods you skip. Eat more slowly than the rest of the family, and nobody will know you are on a diet. If you truly want to trim down to better proportions, you are embarking upon the greatest adventure of your life—approach it in that spirit and your goal is half won. You are not depriving yourself. You are treating yourself to new and interesting experiences in eating.

Make creative cooking your hobby, and let your husband try his hand at it, too—not just at the backyard barbecue pit but in the kitchen. A surprising number of men have a real flair for gourmet cookery. Do encourage your man to develop his culinary creativeness, especially if *he* is reducing.

A good example of how an overweighter can "cook himself thin" is the story of how Tom Donnelly, Washington columnist, lost 175 excess pounds in eleven months. Mr. Donnelly loved good food, and overdid it to a total of 350 pounds. To get the kind of reducing menus he wanted, he turned chef, and thus discovered a fine talent for cooking that is a delight to himself and his friends. The friends, incidentally, proved his biggest handicap—at first they worried him because he didn't reduce, then they worried him because he did. He didn't worry; he kept on cooking. So take heart from his example, if friends and family try to discourage you. Keep on quietly and steadily with your reducing plan.

LEAN COOKERY

For years I have been advocating what I call *lean cookery*. Not just to help my students keep slender (this happens automatically), but to help them to keep healthy, stay youthful, live long, and enjoy all the best food in the world.

What is lean cookery? It is *your* cookery, for the rest of your long, healthy, slender life. It means, first of all, using wholesome, natural, lean foods. It means no overcooking; food should be cooked as long as necessary for maximum goodness *and no longer;* in the case of almost all vegetables, this means only a few minutes. It means being miserly in the use of animal fats, sugars, and thickeners, wasting no time or money on pastries and rich sauces. Instead, we use our money for lean meats, lean fish, poultry, lean milk; for golden vegetable oils; for tasty, nourishing bread; for fresh vegetables and fruits. And these foods we do not spoil with rich additions; but we do make them tastier by spiking them with non-irritating spices, vegetable salt, sweet paprika, and all kinds of fragrant herbs. We use no synthetic sweeteners; instead, we use dark molasses, honey of all kinds, natural brown sugar, and the newly discovered caruba. I cannot conscientiously advocate synthetic sweeteners, though they are widely advertised and recommended; I believe only time will tell whether they are or are not harmful. And, what is more important, I am convinced that only natural foods can help you *retrain your appetite*.

SALAD DAYS ARE HERE AGAIN

Serving salad as the first course is not only the smart Continental and California way of dining; it is the smart way to eat, especially if you are reducing. But not a skimpy little dab of lettuce with perhaps a slice of tomato and a lot of thick dressing sloshed over it. That's a poor imitation of a salad; and if your family balks at it, I do not blame them. Make it a generous bowlful of live, crisp greens and vegetables, lovely to look at and delicious to eat. "Salad days" are youthful days. To help you get started on yours, you will find my favorite salads and lean salad dressings on page 477.

LEAN MEAT IS A MUST

During the course of my television reducing class, I received this letter (in different words) from hundreds of people all over the country:

"Dear Gayelord Hauser: You tell reducers to eat plenty of lean meat, roasted or broiled. How about telling us where to get the money to buy all these prime ribs, tenderloin steaks, and chops?"

I was always glad to get these letters because they gave me a chance to tell my students two pieces of good news: First, that the tough, muscular cuts of meat such as round steak, chuck, rump, and shoulder are more nourishing than the more expensive prime ribs, tenderloin steaks, and chops. Second, that these cheaper cuts of meat can be made tender enough to roast or broil nowadays (and in a matter of minutes) by using the newly discovered meat tenderizers.

Newly discovered? I should say, newly *rediscovered*.

"Señor," said my Mexican cook in Taxco some years ago, when I protested because she brought home a tough old rooster, "this is a special bird, an educated bird, father of many chickens, full of nourishment and wisdom. Its muscles will make muscle and strength for Señor and his distinguished guests; its toughness I take away." And, to my great surprise, she did. The educated old bird was tender and delicious (I did not taste the wisdom). I learned later that she had cut him up, wrapped bruised papaya leaves around each piece, let stand in a crockery jar overnight. I learned also that, for centuries, primitive cooks have been tenderizing their tough wild game by wrapping it in green leaves, especially papaya. No doubt they thought these leaves contained magic, but modern chemistry explains their tenderizing properties more prosaically by telling us that papaya leaves contain a digestive enzyme. Some of my California and Florida students have long been using papaya leaves for making digestive teas and for tenderizing tough meat; the only drawback was that the meat-tenderizing process took so long.

Nowadays this digestive enzyme has been extracted and put into all sorts of liquid sauces for tenderizing tough meats quickly. I find it easiest and most satisfactory to use a dry, sprinkle-on variety; there are many on the market. The one I use is a delicious blend of sea salt, vegetable extract, papaya, and some herbs for flavor. Sprinkle this on your meat thirty minutes before you broil, bake, or roast it. It will be, as my Mexican cook would say, "tender as a Señorita's heart." In addition, the cooking time is reduced and there seems to be less shrinkage.

Meat plays an important part in any scientific reducing program; we eat a good, lean portion at least once a day. And meat need no longer be the most expensive item in the budget. But whether it is or not, let us get all possible nourishment from it. Let us prepare it in the modern, healthful, and flavorsome way. Here are three things to remember:

First, *always buy lean meat.* Have the butcher remove all visible fat. Naturally there will be some invisible fat which emerges as drippings during the cooking process.

Second, *get rid of all these drippings.* You have no use for them, no rich sauces or gravies to prepare.

Third, *cook your meat correctly.* This means broil steaks and chops. Larger cuts of meat should be roasted (not too well done, you know) in a *slow* oven. A research experiment in meat cookery recently was conducted on a grand scale by the U. S. Department of Agriculture. More than twenty thousand cuts of every kind of meat were cooked by every imaginable method, and thousands of professional opinions were recorded. The verdict was that meat is juicier, tastier, and most healthful when roasted at low temperature.

PROTEIN FOR BREAKFAST

A few years ago, when the Argentine government asked me to teach their people better health, I made several discoveries about protein breakfasts. The men told me they could work better and think more clearly when they had meat for breakfast. The women claimed that when they ate meat for breakfast they felt better, did not get nervous during the day, and did not gain excess weight. I realized that intuitively these South American men and women knew that a protein-rich breakfast can make or break the whole day. One of them said to me: "Señor, we eat breakfast like a king, lunch like a princess, and dinner like a pauper."

No, I am not going to ask you to eat steak for breakfast—unless you can afford it. Thousands of experiments have proved that after a skimpy breakfast the blood sugar falls lower and lower, and that this is responsible for much nervousness, fatigue, and even headaches. (See also page 67.) A stick-to-the-ribs breakfast is your best protection against overeating during the day; make this a habit and see for yourself how much better you feel. (I strongly recommend that you read "Breakfast in Relationship to Blood Sugar," by E. O. Keiles and L. F. Hallman, U. S. Department of Agriculture Circular 827.)

FRIDAY IS FISH DAY

There are many good reasons for eating fish; it is a wonder food containing first-class proteins and packed extra-generously with vitamins and minerals, especially iodine. When I lectured recently in Buenos Aires, I gave my audience all these good reasons why, instead of concentrating on their Argentine beef, they should also take advantage of their bountiful fish supply. Nothing happened, until I told them that fish is one of the best foods for *"una bella figura."* Next day, the fish markets were sold out.

SHORT-COOK YOUR VEGETABLES

In lean vegetable cookery, just remember that the quicker vegetables are prepared and cooked, the better your family will like them. Also, the less is the loss of vitamins B, C, P. These vitamins, like salt, dissolve in water; therefore we never pour off any vegetable water. Better still, we short-cook vegetables in such a way that all the goodness and nutrients remain. I have said it a thousand and one times and I'll say it again—when vegetables are cooked half an hour or more in pots full of water, you'd be wiser to throw out the dead vegetables and drink the water they were cooked in, for that's where the precious vitamins and minerals have gone.

Any vegetable can be short-cooked in a matter of minutes. All you need is a heavy cooking utensil, preferably heavy enamelware, and one of those handy vegetable cutters, or "snitzlers" as they are called. Or use an ordinary shredder (the coarse one). Or cut vegetables into thin slivers. Do your shredding or slivering as quickly as possible to prevent vitamin C loss.

Have your cooking pot piping hot; use a small one so it will be filled to the top; the less space for air, the better. In the bottom of the pot have three tablespoons of water; when this boils and the pot is filled with steam, put in your cut-up vegetables and cover the pot tightly. Let the vegetables cook on low flame for two minutes; then shake the pot (without lifting the lid) so there is no possible chance of sticking. After about four minutes, remove the cover and taste one of the vegetable slivers; if it is soft but still a bit chewy, as the vegetables are in Chinese restaurants, it is at its best. Now all you add is a sprinkle of vegetable salt, some herbs, and a bit of vegetable oil; or, if you prefer, you may use half vegetable oil and half butter as my Italian students do. Such short-cooked vegetables have a wonderful, natural flavor and keep their attractive color. When you use vegetable salt last, the juices are not extracted during cooking.

For *extra* lean short-cooking, here is a trick: Instead of water, we steam the sliced vegetables in flavorsome broth—left-over "pot likker," Hauser broth, canned or dehydrated vegetable broth, or chicken or beef broth made with bouillon cubes. Cooked this way, with the addition of vegetable salt and sprinkled with herbs, short-cooked vegetables can be enjoyed without the addition of extra fat. You'll be amazed how soon you and your family will begin to like, and even prefer, the nutty flavor of these vegetables short-cooked *extra* lean.

Here are three easily remembered pointers for successful vegetable cookery: (1) do not peel; just wash thoroughly, or scrub with a vegetable brush; (2) boil or bake whole vegetables in their skins; (3) short-cook sliced or shredded vegetables in the smallest amount of water or broth, and add a bit of vegetable salt *after* they are done. If your family insists on a "buttery" taste, add a pat of sunbutter just before serving.

FRUIT FOR DESSERT

The ideal dessert is fresh fruit, and with all the tempting varieties from all parts of the world piled in our markets there is a new and delicious fruit treat available for every day in the week. Some fruits we stew sometimes with a little honey. Some we serve, on special occasions, as open-faced pies or tarts on a delicious lean whole-grain or wheat-germ crust.

For some of my favorite desserts, see page 512. And if you are looking for pastries, puddings, and gooey desserts, close this book and take a walk. Go to your nearest pastry shop, take a good look at everything in the window, and say: "You will be a few seconds in my mouth, two hours in my stomach, and a lifetime on my hips. You are not for me!"

DRINKING ROBS YOU OF VITAMINS

ALCOHOL STEALS VITAMINS. That is not a news headline. It is an everyday fact. The highball or cocktail that you enjoy before dinner, when the day's work is done, is a B vitamin thief. Don't misunderstand me; I am not a teetotaler or a killjoy. I just want to caution you that alcoholic beverages increase your need for vitamins. Why? Because alcohol is a carbohydrate and, like the candy and pastry carbohydrates, it requires B vitamins for its metabolism. So the body borrows from your daily stores, and then you need more B vitamins to offset the loss.

In a remarkable little book entitled *Nutrition and Alcoholism*, Dr. Roger J. Williams relates the discovery of how alcoholism is tied up with nutrition. Experimental research and clinical trial showed that lack of vitamins was a factor in the overwhelming urge to drink, and that large amounts of B vitamins plus good nutrition eliminated the urge to drink. As long as Dr. Williams' patients abided by his nutrition-plus-vitamins plan, they could drink in moderation or leave it alone, as they preferred. When they neglected their established requirements of vitamins, the old alcoholic urge came back. As with other aspects of the nutritional picture, it was pointed out that there are wide variations in the individual requirements for B vitamins, and this in turn influences the wide variations in individual reactions to drinking.

Alcohol and sugary desserts and candy are remarkably similar: you can "get drunk" on any of them, all are carbohydrates, all are B vitamin thieves, all are loaded with hidden calories that carry excess weight.

Have a relaxing drink, if you wish it. Make it wine rather than hard liquor, if possible. Wine is festive and it contains digestive enzymes, a factor in its favor. But do not make the mistake of having an extra drink because you are reducing and want to reward yourself for eating less. To help you make your own decision on this point, here is a chart that will show you that alcohol, though it does not nourish, definitely can add poundage.

Beverages	Calories	
Beer (12 oz.)	170	
Brandy (1 oz.)	75	
Cocktails (3 oz.)		
Daiquiri	130	(more, if you like them sweet)
Manhattan	170	
Martini	145	
Old Fashioned	185	(more, if you like them sweet)
Eggnog (1 scant cup)	200	
Rum (1½ oz. jigger)	105	
Tom Collins	180	(more, if you like them sweet)
Whiskey (1½ oz. jigger)		
Rye	120	
Bourbon	120	
Irish	120	
Scotch	110	
Wine (3½ oz. glass)		
red	75	
white	90	
Port	160	

SMOKERS NEED MORE VITAMIN C

I myself do not smoke, but this does not mean that I am entirely against it. In fact, sometimes I envy my friends who, after a good meal, relax over their coffee with a cigarette. I imagine that for some people tobacco, used temperately, may fill a certain need.

Many people, however, use cigarettes as a substitute for food; and because overeaters are persons with strong oral cravings, it is possible that, if you are a smoker, you may find yourself wanting to smoke more and more. For this reason I commend to your attention the words of Dr. Clarence William Lieb in a *Reader's Digest* article: "Tobacco contains as nice a collection of poisons as you will find anywhere in one small package. The least you can do, out of respect for the only body you will ever have, is to use these poisons, if use them you must, in moderation."

Dr. W. J. McCormick of Canada insists that heavy smokers increase their intake of vitamin C. So remember, extra vitamin C for Cigarettes (and extra vitamin B for Brandy or other alcoholic Beverages).

BE A SMART HOSTESS

Since eating at home is more than just feeding yourself and your family, let's say a word about entertaining. Here is where you can give full rein to creativeness and really build up a gourmet reputation. But be considerate and don't serve overgenerous portions or insist on second helpings. Just as compulsive social drinking went out with prohibition, you will find the modern trend is also away from compulsive social eating. Remember that some of your guests may be reducing. Or they may be on the wagon—not necessarily because they have an alcohol problem but because they like it that way.

Nowadays more and more smart hostesses are serving fruit and vegetable juices as well as cocktails and highballs at their parties. (See page 503.) They offer a choice casually, and thus relieve guests both of embarrassment of refusal and of the social necessity of taking a drink they really don't want.

Also, more and more smart hostesses are serving Finger Salad instead of (or in addition to) over-rich canapes. I introduced the Finger Salad years ago in Paris and have been serving a big tray of these crisp fresh vegetables at my parties ever since. You should hear my guests—men and women both—rave over them.

How to make Finger Salad? Simply cut up the youngest and tenderest vegetables you can find in your market. Everyone knows and likes crisp carrot sticks, chilled radishes, tender celery; in addition, try strips of green and red peppers, bits of fresh cauliflower, slices of cool unpeeled cucumbers, nutlike kohlrabi, small whole ripe tomatoes (these can be stuffed with cottage cheese) and a delicious, less-familiar vegetable, finucchio or Italian celery, cut in wedges. Be adventurous; use whatever succulent vegetables your market offers. And—you can enjoy these crisp vegetables without a fatty dressing. All I serve with Finger Salads (it's very smart to eat them with your fingers) is a shaker of vegetable salt.

For those who are reducing, these crisp vegetable hors d'oeuvres keep the stomach busy and filled. You can eat them to your heart's content. For extra-special parties serve several of these big plates of crisp vegetables with a bowl full of my special lean dressing in the middle of each tray, for "dunking" (page 482).

Fresh Vegetable Juices—Espressos

In Czechoslovakia, in the years before the Communists, there was a famous sanatorium in Carlsbad. People flocked from all over the world to drink the laxative waters, take long walks in the woods, listen to Strauss waltzes and—instead of eating fresh fruits and vegetables, they *drank* them. Many of these people had intestinal difficulties. The brilliant Doctors Mayr and Zukor realized that they needed fresh things but could not tolerate the roughage; so they extracted the "blood of the plant" and gave their patients fresh juices. The results made history.

It was in Carlsbad that I first learned about drinking fresh fruits and vegetables, and many thousands of my students have benefited. Fortunes have been made in the United States and Europe by companies putting out canned juices; and this is all to the good, especially if the juices are put into specially lined tins. But nothing can compare with the deliciousness of fresh, fresh juices. These vital juices contain vitamins, minerals, chlorophyll, enzymes, and many as-yet-undiscovered food factors in the most appetizing form. I have often seen people who refused to *eat* salads, enjoy drinking them. I hope they will soon be obtainable, not only in the few health food shops, but in every restaurant and corner drug store.

It will pay you to invest in the best juicing machine you can buy. It can become a veritable health mine for you and your family. There are several types on the market. Make certain that all parts which come in contact with the juice are made of stainless steel or plastic. This is important if you want to keep the appetizing color of the juices. Also, be sure that the machine you buy does not vibrate and is easy to clean. The machine I use is so lightweight that I take it with me wherever I go. Now turn to page 503, and learn how to make your own fresh vegetable drinks, or espressos, as they are now called.

FORMULA FOR REMOVING POISONOUS SPRAYS

Nowadays all sorts of poisonous sprays are used by farmers on our fruits and vegetables to keep pests away. And, unfortunately, these sprays still cling to some fruits and vegetables when they reach the kitchen. People with normal, healthy digestive juices need do no more than wash fruits and vegetables thoroughly. But those with a lack of hydrochloric acid or those with ulcers or colitis (whose doctors have ordered them to drink vegetable juice) should by all means remove all traces of these sprays. The simplest and safest method, one used in many sanatoriums, is this:

Buy a large earthenware crock and fill it with a one percent hydrochloric acid solution. This is made by mixing one ounce of chemically pure hydrochloric acid with three quarts of water. The solution can be used for a week. Place all suspicious fruits or vegetables in this solution, leave in for five minutes, and rinse well. This solution should also be used in health bars and restaurants where fresh juices are served, and in all lands where dangerous fertilizers, as well as dangerous sprays, are used.

Now Let's Talk Raw

No, we are not raw-food addicts. We deplore all faddists of the gloomy "Nuts and Berries" school who still munch on and on under the influence of the raw-food movement which swept Europe sixty years ago. We know that some foods are much better for the human stomach when they are cooked.

But we did learn one very important lesson from the raw-food faddists which is of immense value to overweighters: raw foods, liberally included in your diet, are a powerful ally while keeping your weight down. Never in all my forty years of traveling over five continents have I seen a fat raw-food faddist. (Don't jump to conclusions, now. I said raw foods *liberally included in an otherwise balanced diet* or, as the happy Italians so wisely put it, *"un Giorno senza Verdura e un Giorno senza sole."* (A day without greens is a day without sunshine.)

Now, would you like to try raw meat? It is an excellent food, if you can eat it; and when it is fresh and lean it becomes a wonder food. Many Europeans habitually eat raw chopped meat ("Rohsteak") once a week. It can be served in all sorts of variations, but Steak Tartar probably is the most appetizing.

I remember having my first Steak Tartar at Chasen's Hollywood restaurant with Greta Garbo and Erich Maria Remarque. Mr. Remarque wanted his meat mixed with chopped green onions; Miss Garbo wanted hers with dry onions; I preferred mine with chives. Mr. Chasen supervised our order himself and settled our problem, needless to say, in favor of the lady. He used the leanest beef (put twice through the chopper) and mixed with it lots of chopped dry onions, an egg yolk, some vegetable salt, a dash of paprika, and a few drops of lemon juice. With it we ate dark rye bread and unsalted butter and a huge mixed green salad with a light dressing—a nourishing lean meal fit for a king (though I still prefer chives).

Raw Fish Is Terrific—If You Can Eat It

Raw oysters, clams, mussels, and other foods fresh from the sea are wonderfully nourishing and, sprinkled with just a little lemon juice, make delicious lean eating. And how about joining some of the leanest and most vigorous people in the world and experimenting further with raw fish dishes? The Japanese are probably the world's greatest raw fish gourmets; they especially love finely cut cuttlefish mixed with fresh sea greens. But I believe that Americans and Europeans prefer my "seaburger," which is easy to make and can be flavored in many ways. The best-tasting raw fish are mackerel, bonita, sea bass, and, when obtainable, fresh tuna, and the delicious "conk" (Florida's name for conch). It is important that the fish be young, fresh, and tender. In some places you can buy lean fish fillets all ready to be used. Remove all bones. Chop the fish into small pieces; you could put it through your meat grinder, but connoisseurs frown upon that. Chop it to the size of raw chopped onion, marinate with plenty of lemon or lime juice and add as much raw chopped onion as you like (for variety, try chopped radishes, green peppers, or any other flavor you like). Spike with vegetable salt to taste, place in the refrigerator and let it stay three hours. Eat it with a piece of toast or pumpernickel or add a tablespoonful of light dressing to this mixture and serve as a chopped fish salad with lots of fresh greens.

Good News for the Busy Homemaker

There is now on the market a marvelous American invention called the "Scotchpak" food-packaging sealer. This wonder gadget can save many dollars in time, energy, and nutrition. Farsighted purveyors of first-class frozen foods, such as Seabrook Farms, Green Giant, and Armour, are packaging their foods in these clear, appetizing-looking, absolutely airtight envelopes that seal in all the flavor, natural color, and vitamins and other important nutrients. Old-fashioned frozen foods are definitely damaged by long exposure to air by the time they are cooked. This cannot happen with frozen foods in "Scotchpak" envelopes because they are promptly sealed in these envelopes and frozen, ready to be dropped into boiling water; and only then are the airtight envelopes opened and the food poured into serving dishes. Just one whiff, plus the natural color and the farm-fresh flavor, is proof that here, indeed, are freshly frozen foods at their best. Most important of all, you can be sure that you are getting the nutrients so necessary for good health and good looks.

Now there is a wonderful compact home "Scotchpak" food-packaging sealer. About the size of a box of cleansing tissue, it can be kept on your work counter, hung on the wall, or stored in a drawer or cabinet. Plug it into an electric outlet, and it provides the heat that seals the envelopes. And with the sealer comes an assortment of those magic plastic envelopes. With these, a new era of delightful cookery is making its debut in the American kitchen. There is no more excuse for unappetizing, flat-tasting meals that so often result from poor planning, overhasty preparation, or three-day-old leftovers. The busiest homemaker can now prepare several favorite meals, a week or more in advance, and simply seal them in these envelopes. They can be kept for a day or two in the refrigerator and for weeks in the freezer. And all the appetizing color and the vitamins and other important nutrients are safely sealed in. Working wives, especially, can now prepare in advance, evenings or weekends, such gourmet dishes as beef Stroganoff, chicken paprika, and lamb stew with spring vegetables. These sealed-in foods are ready to eat in a matter of minutes. You simply drop the envelope with your gourmet main dish into a pot of boiling water. Add another envelope of fresh-frozen vegetables. When thoroughly heated, open the envelopes, serve, and enjoy.

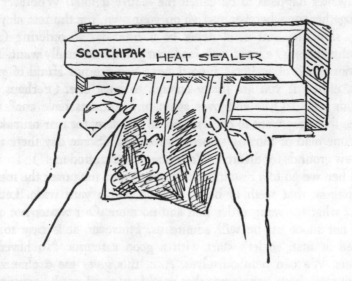

SCOTCHPAK HEAT SEALER

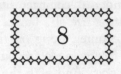

8

Let's Dine Out

We are going to dine out, here, there, and everywhere. I want to show you that the world is yours—that you can eat wherever you want, whenever you want. Before we start, there is something I want to tell you. Listen: *Waiters don't bite.*

Neither do headwaiters. Not even in restaurants where the headwaiter happens to be called the *maître d'hôtel*. Wherever we go together, or wherever you go on your own, for the rest of your long, slim life, you need never be overawed into ordering (and therefore eating) a lot of rich food that you do not really want. You are not afraid of waiters? Fine. I hope you are not afraid of your cook, either, if you are lucky enough to have one. (Perhaps she is your wife.) Over and over again, my students have confessed to me that they want to eat less and do not dare, for fear of making someone mad or hurting someone's feelings. (Some day there may be new grounds for divorce: "Your honor, she stuffed me!")

When we go to a restaurant, let us take our time over the menu, even those that seem to be all French and a yard wide. Let us select what we want, order that and no more. Our waiter not only will not snoot us; he will admire us. However, it is easy to get rattled at first, so let's start with a good cafeteria. No hovering waiters. We can help ourselves. Also, this gives me a chance to repeat something important: that good food need not be expensive. And while we stand in line, I have time to remind you that there are just Five Points to remember, whenever and wherever you dine:

1. Eat something fresh, preferably to start the meal.
2. Eat lots of first-class protein, not less than 20 grams with each meal.
3. Eat some carbohydrates, but let them be natural. If you are overweight, skip bread, rice, and potatoes.
4. Avoid hard fats and use golden vegetable oils, or margarine made with golden oils.
5. Eat fresh or stewed fruit for an ideal dessert.

Our cafeteria happens to be in Chicago, but it could be in any large American city. Let me go ahead. The food all looks good. We cannot dawdle; people are piling up. Quick, what are our Five Points?

First, start with something fresh—a large bowl of crisp salad greens would be ideal. Or perhaps you would prefer sliced tomatoes and cucumbers on a bed of lettuce. Use a bit of golden oil dressing, with vinegar or lemon juice.

Next, protein. Here is lamb stew with lots of vegetables. But there is too much fat floating around in it, and right alongside is good hot roast beef, not too well done. Let's buy that. The man behind the counter gives us an extra big slice, as if he knows we need lots of protein.

And now, automatically, the next counterman is going to give us a big blob of smashed potatoes (there are no baked potatoes). How could he know that we do not like foodless food? He probably does not even know that when the potatoes were peeled most of their vitamins and minerals went down the drain. We say no to him. The rest of the vegetables do not look too good (cooked vegetables exposed on steam tables rapidly lose vitamin C and with it their flavor). Just then another counterman brings in steaming golden corn on the cob; we take this for our carbohydrates.

Now we stand in front of our worst enemy—the dessert counter. Do you want a piece of pie piled-up with white fluff? To me those look like flying discs made of plaster of Paris. Here is anemic-looking cake coated with sticky goo. Not for us. We can have a piece of fruit pie if we leave the greasy bottom crust, but why bother? Here is a large bowl with all kinds of fresh fruits cut up. Let us have that!

Let's check our Five Points. We have salad greens to start, roast beef for protein, corn on the cob for carbohydrate. The salad and fresh fruit cup provide vitamins and minerals and bulk. Here are whole-wheat muffins; let us take one and enjoy it with a bit of fresh butter or margarine. Our dinner is complete, and here is a quiet corner where we may relax and enjoy it. So that there is no possibility of any kind of shortage, vitamin and mineral tablets are in order when we get home, and with them, perhaps, a glass of fortified milk or a hot drink for an excellent nite cap.

Because we selected this dinner in terms of our Five Points, don't think we are going to harp on them. Keep them in mind only during the first few weeks; after that you will order in the modern manner, *automatically*. And here's another tip for your first few weeks of intelligent eating. Instead of munching bread and butter and sipping icewater while you wait for your main course, ask the waiter please to bring your salad *first*. Millions of pounds of fat could be prevented by just this simple habit of satisfying the first hunger with a big, fresh salad.

Le Petit Gourmet

One of my favorite restaurants is Le Petit Gourmet. In my early days in Chicago I went often to this restaurant to sit in the charming patio and enjoy the salad bowls, broiled meats, and short-cooked vegetables. At this restaurant they specialized in serving lean, healthful foods long before it was popular to do so.

I well remember the last time I was here. It was a party given in honor of Monsignor Scammacca of Sicily and myself by Virginia Fox Kennady and ten of her Beautymasters—a charming group of women who knew the secret of eating intelligently. This was a late supper, after my lecture, and because it was a party we were greeted with cool champagne cocktails. The menu was:

Chicken Salad
Ripe Strawberries
Coffee

That was a small but delicious meal—a huge bowl filled with chopped young cabbage mixed with big pieces of breast of chicken and fresh pineapple chunks. The whole thing was marinated with a delicious dressing made of fresh pineapple juice and fresh yogurt. With it we ate crisp rye bread and very dark pumpernickel. For dessert, the luscious ripe strawberries were served *au naturel* —unplucked and arranged on a dessert plate in a circle with a teaspoonful of fragrant California honey in the center. A steaming cup of cafe espresso ended this memorable meal.

THE PUMP ROOM

While we are in Chicago, we'll go to the Pump Room of the Ambassador East Hotel, internationally known for its good food and interesting people. This was Ernie Byfield's pet project; for years celebrities have stopped there en route to New York. Our menu?

> Pump Room Special Salad
> Butterfly Steak
> Fresh Pineapple
> Demitasse

It was Irene Castle—the still slim, vital lady—and Pat Dougherty, the society editor who had lost forty pounds by eating intelligently, who introduced me to the Pump Room's famous butterfly steak. This is a small sirloin split in two with the bone in the middle; it is shaped exactly like a butterfly. It takes only a few moments to broil such a steak; when it arrived, piping hot, all three of us, in unison, automatically cut off the outside fat.

With this we had the Pump Room special salad made of that very tender Kentucky limestone lettuce, mixed with bits of hearts of artichoke; and when Philippe, the *maître d'hôtel*, asked what kind of dressing we preferred, we three, again almost in unison, asked for a light dressing—which meant olive oil well mixed with the greens, some wine vinegar, a pinch of vegetable salt, and spiked with salad herbs. This salad bowl was unbelievably delicious; we devoured it all with our butterfly steaks. The perfect dessert, after this, was a slice of juicy, ripe pineapple, and with it we enjoyed a small cup of black coffee. (Who could possibly want sugar and cream?)

TWENTY-ONE

You do not see many overweighters at the Pump Room. The people who go there are really smart. This is true of most famous restaurants where people go not only for good food but also for interesting people—Jack and Charlie's "21" Club, for example, which is one of my favorite restaurants in New York.

By all means, let us go to "21." I was first taken there long, long ago by Adele Astaire, and throughout the years Jack and Charlie have maintained their high standard of excellent food. Let's go after the theatre; in New York we are so busy that many times we haven't time for dinner at the usual hour. We will see many celebrities. Last time I was there, Helen Hayes, and my friend Anita Loos, were at the tables on either side of mine, with their big after-theatre parties. I was with Jessica Dragonette, affectionately called the "vest-pocket Venus" by her friends. Busy as she is with concerts and lectures, she always looks fit and trim. This night I let Jessica do the ordering and she chose the famous "21" hamburger sandwich. We started with honeydew melon, sprinkled with lime juice. When the hamburgers came, they were sizzling hot, deliciously brown, served on a piece of rye bread toast. With the hamburger we munched celery and olives, and since it was late we ended our meal with a cup of Swiss coffee—half hot coffee and half hot, hot milk.

MERCURIO'S

I have lived so much in Italy and know the Italian cuisine so well that it hurts my feelings to hear, as I so often do, "All Italian food is fattening." There are many so-called Italian restaurants in America; they serve too much pasta, and some of them specialize in a rather awful dish called Italian spaghetti and meat balls, which is unheard of in Italy. But, believe me, smart Italians, like smart Americans, know the secret of good eating.

Let me take you to a truly fine Italian restaurant—Mercurio's in New York. There they have a chef, a real Genovese, whose meals are out of this world. Here is our menu:

Large Salad Bowl
Saltimbocca
Cooked Greens
Fruit Dessert
Cafe Espresso

Madame Fontana, the famous designer—the slim and chic Roman lady who designs clothes for the smart, international set—was my guest the last time I ordered this dinner at Mercurio's. In her honor, the *maître d'hôtel* himself brought out the biggest salad bowl I have ever seen and placed in it dark green lettuce leaves, escarole, dandelions, and ripe tomatoes. With loving care he marinated the whole with golden olive oil; then he poured on some wine vinegar, and, last, a pinch of fragrant herbs. Madame Fontana and I had double portions while we waited for our main course; we agreed it was one of the best salads we had eaten since last we dined together in Italy.

Saltimbocca is made with thin slices of veal, each covered with a slice of lean ham, about the same size. Add a pinch of herbs, preferably fresh sage. Roll up and secure with toothpicks. Then sauté in butter or olive oil until golden brown. Add a little bit of wine, cover, and cook a few minutes until tender. How appetizing it smells and looks! With this delicious fare we have our cooked mustard greens (Italians know so well how to prepare them). After such a meal it would not occur to me to offer a guest a rich dessert. We end with fresh fruit cup, and, of course, cafe espresso.

LINDY'S

Would you like to go to Lindy's while we are in New York? You will eat well there.

We start with Lindy's special hors d'oeuvres—old-fashioned dill pickles, the best you ever ate; beet relish; and raw sauerkraut, not out of a can, but homemade and wonderful. We can have all we want; they are appetizing, satisfying, and lean.

Now, what else? Suppose you do the ordering this time. Goose? Duck? Come, now. This menu is full of wonderful dishes—lean corned beef or a delicious breast of chicken, cooked with many fine vegetables—a sort of *pot-au-feu*, which I recommend highly. What?

You're still thinking of roast goose? Don't be a— Here, I'll do the ordering.

"Waiter—bring us boiled beef with horseradish for two."

It's the best and heartiest dish on the menu. They serve a big portion and we can eat it all without conscience trouble, if we cut away the outside fat. For dessert, fresh, ripe pineapple. . . . No, let's have a big half-grapefruit—broiled, this time.

You think Lindy's is tops? I knew you would.

BUENOS AIRES

You will be amazed at the superabundance of meat, milk, eggs, and cheese in Buenos Aires; and when I tell you that in the markets calf liver costs fifteen cents a pound, you will see why, in this charming city, you can dine like a king without paying a king's ransom.

We will go to the Alvear Palace Hotel. I lived there when I was lecturing in Buenos Aires, and I ate most of my meals in the Grill Room, with government officials and with friends. One meets many North Americans there, and many celebrities. I remember that, among others, the flier Jacqueline Cochran and her husband, Floyd Odlum, found it their favorite place to dine and to entertain their friends.

Meats are prepared wonderfully well here and—can you believe it?—it is not unusual for an Argentine to eat a two-pound steak for lunch. However, we'll settle for half of that. With our big steak let us order a big salad made of leaf lettuce, unpeeled cucumber, chopped-up radishes, and green peppers. We also will have artichoke hearts, which are so plentiful in the Argentine. These are topped with a bit of butter and taste unbelievably delicious. Once again there is no room for a big dessert. We end our meal with a big slice of juicy pineapple, sprinkled with a bit of kirsch, a demitasse, and a salute to the cuisine of the Argentine!

LONDON

Now we are in London, and London has good food again. We will go to the Restaurant Caprice, which I learned about from Anna Meyrson, the famous Austrian-born British painter. She has much talent and a heart that is typically Viennese; she looks like a combination of Luise Rainer and Audrey Hepburn. Anna and I have two loves in common. One is the beautiful town of Taormina, Sicily, where she has a studio, and the other is good food. We happened to be in London at the same time, and Anna invited me to dine with her.

We arrived at the Caprice, and sat side by side on a banquette, studying the menu; my eyes fairly popped at its size and variety. Slim Anna does not diet. She knows how to eat, and she proceeded to order a meal I will long remember:

> Belgian Endive
> Steak Diane
> Green Asparagus Amandine
> Wild Strawberries with Yogurt
> Demitasse

We were treated like royalty. The headwaiter himself cooked the special steak right at our table. He put just a little oil in a heavy skillet and in less than five minutes the Steak Diane was tender and delicious. With this we had the green asparagus, sprinkled with a teaspoon of toasted almonds. The wild strawberries were the last of the season and tasted especially delicious. We ate them with yogurt and honey—who could possibly prefer heavy cream?— and ended the meal with a steaming demitasse.

PARIS

Yes, I know. French cuisine is heaven to eat but can be hell on the waistline! But here is good news: Slowly and cautiously the wonderful chefs of France are changing their ways. They are not getting less wonderful—perish the thought. But they are being influenced by the *"Societé d'études pour l'application des Méthodes Gayelord Hauser"* which has offices at 4, Faubourg St. Honoré in the heart of Paris.

This new center was formed by a group of influential Parisians, headed by Philippe de Rothschild, a member of the famous Rothschild dynasty. Through their efforts, intelligent eating in all its branches is being taught to thousands. French chefs are listening and learning that they can cook leaner foods without sacrificing a soupçon of flavor or deliciousness. I have high hopes for this new awakening. Those miraculous chefs of France are among her best goodwill ambassadors; I believe that Paris, in addition to being the world's high fashion center, may yet rule the world of intelligent eating.

While we are in Paris, let us go to France's beloved Maxim's. There was great excitement here one day. The entrance was garlanded with great festoons of fresh vegetables in a riot of colors. People passing exclaimed, "*Ça, c'est fou!*" But it was no crazier than I am. In fact, it was a party given in my honor.

This was a novelty for the conservative French people; more than five hundred turned out to see "*Qu'est-ce que c'est que ça.*" On one side of the famous restaurant was a Hauser bar, where fresh vegetable espressos were served in champagne glasses. On the other side was a champagne bar, where the driest (which is the leanest) champagne was served. Most of the Frenchmen had first a glass of freshly made vegetable espresso and then a glass of champagne; and *Figaro*, the Paris newspaper, the next day called me a wise man. Why? Because I featured not only my vegetable juice (which they liked) but also their French champagne, which after all is, as *Figaro* said, one of the most delicious fruit juices in the world!

After this cocktail party, I dined at Maxim's with Madame de St. Hardouin, the French Ambassadress who entertained me so royally at the French Embassy in Istanbul. Our menu was a celery-shrimp cocktail, followed by delicious *poulet* (tender chicken) surrounded by many small white roasted onions and served with tender *haricots verts* (green beans). For dessert, Madame de St. Hardouin, who knows exactly what I like, ordered a *coupe de fruits* made with small, wild strawberries, fresh peaches, and bits of toasted almonds, to which was added just a touch of kirsch for its delicate flavor.

VENICE

It was festival night—the last time I saw Venice. The hotels were packed with people from all over the world. I had arrived by plane from my holiday in Taormina to be a judge at one of those fantastic celebrity parties given by Earl Blackwell, Mr. Celebrity himself. There were many attractive and interesting people to meet—Maria Felix, the Mexican star, Isa Miranda, Sylvia Gable, Lorelle Hearst, Princess Pignatelle, Count and Countess Rudi Crespi, Greta Keller from Vienna, dukes and princesses—but the lady who interested me most was Gloria Swanson, who also was one of the judges. She was tiny and slim in her maharanee costume, full of life and radiant with the spirit of tomorrow.

Gloria and I dined at the Taverna de la Fenice in one of the small, intimate squares—one of the world's fine restaurants, where good food has been served for more than a hundred years. We sat in a comfortable corner where we could relax and talk. Here is what we ordered from the big menu:

> Italian Salad Bowl
> Grilled Scampi (shrimp)
> Peach Flame
> Cafe Espresso

While we waited for dinner, Gloria told me the why and wherefore of her great interest in food. I was amazed at her knowledge; she is a real crusader and knows from personal experience what good food can do for you. She eats little and is a connoisseur; so much so that, wherever she is, she has organically grown vegetables and fruits flown to her from California. One of her favorite meals is a salad bowl which is a complete meal; occasionally she makes this for her friends.

As we sat in this cozy square in Venice I could not help marveling at her. Twenty years had passed since I last saw her, but she looked the same. No—I take that back. She looked even better than she had twenty years before when she was the reigning queen of Hollywood. Nowadays her face looks softer, gentler, more radiant and understanding. Her small body is the same; no cushions and rolls to mar her tiny figure. Viva Gloria!

Dining with Friends

During the first weeks of your new eating program, you probably will not accept invitations from friends to dine in their homes— unless they are following the same program. But sooner or later you will face a menu that you had no hand in preparing. Suppose the menu consists of cream of mushroom soup, roast beef, smashed potatoes, greasy gravy, overcooked green beans, fruit gelatin salad, and chocolate cream pie. Surely any friends who invite you to dinner should know about your eating habits, so they should not be offended if you skip the soup, potatoes, gravy, and pie. Roast beef and green beans will be enough at this time, with the gelatin salad for dessert. Not exactly an ideal menu, but it will sustain you until you get home, when you can have some fresh fruit, a vegetable espresso, or a dish of yogurt.

If someday you find before you nothing but a greasy patty shell loaded with gooey chicken à la king and a tired salad already smothered with pink dressing, cross your fingers, eat two or three bites, and keep yourself busy as the Duchess of Windsor does under such circumstances—playing with her fork, taking sips of water, and chatting with the other guests—and never accept another invitation to eat at that house! Of course, if you particularly like your hostess, you might do some missionary work: Return the invitation, and give a practical demonstration of good, lean food, attractively served, in *your* home.

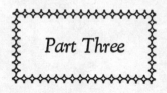

Part Three

YOUR GOOD HEALTH

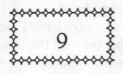

9

Know How Your Body Works

You are a free, adult human being, entitled to life, liberty, and the pursuit of happiness. You have a reasonably healthy, reasonably active, reasonably good-looking body. But do you really know how it works?

Now—pack up all the curiosity you possess. Open wide your mind's eye and the door of your imagination. Come along on a sightseeing trip with me. Let's see what your body is. This knowledge will help you to understand *why* the principles of nutrition are so important to you.

Are you ready? Just a moment. You will need a pair of X-ray glasses. Now—all set?

YOUR BODY ARCHITECTURE

Everybody can visualize the skeleton. (Perhaps you have one in your closet.) What I want you to do now is to "see" *your own* skeleton—the warm, vibrant, living armature on which the Master Sculptor has constructed, with flesh and blood for clay, the masterpiece, YOU. It is far more interesting than the rattling armful of dry, chalky bones so familiar to anatomy classes, art students, and to all of us at Halloween. Anything but ghostly, it is *very* much alive.

Your skeleton is composed of 206 bones—count 'em. They are

pinkish-white on the outside; deep red inside. Their surface is very dense in structure and very hard. Examine them closely, however, and you will see that they are full of minute openings through which intertwine the living network of arteries, veins, nerves, and connective tissues which activate and sustain them. Inside the bones is spongy latticework containing bone marrow—fat and tissue engaged in the production of blood.

Your bones contain living cells, which determine their tenacity and elasticity, and mineral component (calcium phosphate and calcium carbonate) which gives bones their hardness and rigidity. You know how light your bones are; but have you any idea of their strength? It has been calculated that bone, weight for weight, is about as efficient as steel.

Straighten Your Spine

Visualize your spine. When you do, you automatically "brace up," do you not? It is not by accident that we speak of moral strength as "backbone," of weakness as "spinelessness"; that we call an honest person "upright" or "straight." It is your spine that makes you superior to the lower animals, or invertebrates. It is your erect backbone, plus your well-developed hand (particularly the thumb) that makes you superior to the higher animals. Be proud of your spine and bid it carry your head high; it has been called the physical embodiment of character.

Visualize a flexible column a bit over two feet long, consisting of thirty-three separate vertebrae—cylindrical bones all containing a central canal and strung on the spinal cord, almost like beads of a necklace. Almost, but not quite—since the support which holds the vertebrae together is not the spinal cord running through them but the ligaments which run along their outside, and the very close fit which they have upon each other, due to the presence, between each vertebra and the next, of a spongy, elastic circle of cartilage called a *spinal disc*. The fact that the vertebrae are so separated gives the spine its remarkable flexibility and helps it absorb shocks, such as the impact of the body weight hitting the ground with each step in walking.

Let us begin our tale at your tail. The lowest four vertebrae are fused into one bone, the coccyx, or vestigial tail, whose office is to close the floor of the pelvis. By the time you are twenty-five years old, the next five vertebrae also have been fused to become the sacrum or "sacred bone"—so called because at one time this was thought to be the seat of the soul. Next come the five lumbar vertebrae which support the abdominal organs; next, the twelve dorsal vertebrae, to which the ribs are attached; and at the top are the seven cervical vertebrae, which I have saved for the last because they particularly concern us.

Let's Turn Your Head

Turn your head to the left. And to the right. Nod it up and down. Now rotate your head slowly. How is it that you are able to do this? Because of those seven cervical vertebrae, particularly the last two —the topmost, or atlas vertebra, named after the mythological giant who supported the globe (in this case, your skull) and, just under it, the axis vertebra, so called because your head turns on it as the earth turns on its axis.

Here is the crossroads between your body and your mind. Here, in these bones, muscles, and nerve cells, is where, in time of danger, you instinctively thrust forward to initiate action or draw back to defend yourself. Here, in the simple gesture of nodding your head or shaking it, is where you register your opinions, reactions, and decisions. Is it any wonder that human beings, who so often are tense, confused, and flooded with conflicting desires (in other words, whose yes-no signals get jammed at the crossroads) so often suffer from stiff neck?

Now we have reached your skull. Its top part (cranium) is the container for that vast and powerful organ, your brain. It is egg-shaped, but it is no eggshell. It is one of the toughest bone structures you have; and, though it gives the impression of surface smoothness, it is a complex jigsaw puzzle of eight different bones, fitted together with incredible precision. The lower part of the skull is the part organized for the purpose of eating—mostly cheekbones and jaws. It is interesting that the teeth are not considered a part of the skeleton, but, like the fingernails, are derived from body cells related to those which produce skin.

Your Torso, Arms, and Legs

Attached to the spine is the bone framework of the chest—twelve pairs of ribs and the breastbone, which form a protective cage for the heart and lungs and give the latter "houseroom" to expand and contract during breathing.

The bone structure of arms and legs is basically the same—a single long bone (upper arm, thigh) and a pair of bones (forearm, leg) to which are attached the hand and foot. Both extremities are fastened to the spinal column by special bones of their own—the shoulder blades (scapulae) for the arms and the pelvis for the legs. You can easily visualize your joints and the "ball-and-socket" principle on which they are constructed, giving you freedom of movement and activity.

But stop a moment to pay homage to your two forearm bones, the radius and ulna, whose rotation around each other allows for the extra action-capacity of your hand. There is evidence that, in the course of evolution, the exploring function of the ape's hand was one of the major factors in the development of the higher centers of the brain, contained in the cerebral cortex. This started something, evolutionary scientists tell us. It led to the development of the human animal, man, and eventually of civilization and culture—all of which are the result of co-ordination of the hand with the brain, of using the hand for intelligent purposes.

YOUR MUSCULAR BODY

With the mental picture of your skeleton in mind, follow with me the handiwork of the Master Sculptor who has fashioned on this framework (helpless in itself) the glistening forms of reddish muscular clay that give it shapeliness and make it capable of movement. Two materials have been used—muscle fibers and connective tissue.

Muscles, generally speaking, are of two kinds—voluntary and involuntary. The voluntary muscles perform as your conscious mind directs them, ache when you are bruised, rest when you rest. These have been attached to your bony armature in broad or narrow bands or crisscross like basketwork. They are the instruments of your power, strength, skill, mobility, and self-defense.

Stop reading for a moment and clench your hands, feet, and jaws; wrinkle your forehead and tense your belly and buttocks. Then let yourself relax. You have just brought into play virtually your entire equipment of voluntary muscles, and these muscles, incidentally, constitute 42 percent of your body weight.

The Independent Muscles

How would you like to give your involuntary muscles a similar workout? Sorry. It cannot be done. (Unless you happen to be a Yogi.) Hidden deep in the recesses of your body structure, these muscles are entirely controlled by your involuntary nervous system. You can neither set them in motion nor stop them, though they are responsible for all your internal bodily activity except chemical action. You cannot relax or regulate them, for they relax and regulate themselves, independent of your will. Throughout your life their steady contraction-and-release is slow, rhythmic, and perpetual, pushing food through your digestive tract, milking body fluids and glandular secretions along to their appointed destinations, moving your blood stream, and collecting and disposing of waste material. You yourself are unaware of their action unless something gets blocked—a kidney stone in the ureter, for example—in which case you feel rhythmic pain as the muscle strains to dislodge the obstruction. No—I take that back. There is one normal and natural way in which you may become aware of the action of your involuntary muscles. This is in the "hunger contractions" of the empty stomach.

A Natural Corset

Just as your skeleton would be useless without its muscular "clay," so would your muscles be useless without their "cement" of connective tissue. What you think of as a muscle actually is a bundle of muscle fibers bound together in sheaths of connective tissue. Muscles, in turn, are fastened to your bones by more connective tissue in the form of tendons and bursae (little bags filled with semifluid material which serve as pulleys at some of your joints). Bones are joined to other bones by connective tissue in the form of ligaments. Connective tissue fibers, knitted into open webbing, form the groundwork for the construction of your skin and membranes. Spread out into great flat sheets, connective tissue wraps your viscera, heart, and lungs in a strong winding-cloth; it forms a large part of the wall of the digestive tract and lines the entire body cavity with a firm, elastic underpinning. When I speak of the "natural corset" which my Stomach Lift exercise (page 175) helps you to develop, I am talking about connective tissue.

Your Amazing Digestive Laboratory

For years I have been saying, "You *are* what you eat." Now I invite you to see for yourself exactly what this means. Imagine that you are standing outside your body, wearing your X-ray glasses, and watching that amazing, completely automatic laboratory, your digestive system, in operation. You are watching what you eat become YOU.

You'll have to make a day of it. What you eat is still being digested by your small intestine eight or nine hours after being swallowed and may remain in the large intestine at least ten (or as long as forty) hours after that. Ready? All right. First, a few general remarks.

Food and Energy

Your body needs energy for operation, and building blocks for repair of structures involved in its operation. To supply this energy and these building blocks, you must eat; and, as the old jingle has it, "there's nothing to eat but food." But food, as is, won't nourish you. It must first be changed into the smaller building blocks (glucose, amino acids, fatty acids, and glycerin) which can pass through the narrow portals of the intestinal wall. These changes take place in the digestive tract, which has the following functions: to take in food; to break down the more complex foodstuffs into small particles by (1) mechanical and (2) chemical processes; to assimilate these particles, store them, and finally eliminate from the body undigested waste material. The digestive system consists of (1) the alimentary canal, through which food passes while it is being processed and (2) the accessory glands (liver and pancreas) which aid this digestion.

Tubes within Tubes

Your alimentary canal, a hollow tube which begins with the mouth and ends with the rectum, is anywhere from twenty-five to thirty feet long. In other words, it is more than five times as long as you are. While you are "digesting" this remarkable fact, here comes another: The inner lining of your small intestine, because of the way it is made, presents an absorptive surface of well over one hundred square feet. (You probably know nightclubs whose dance floor is not much bigger.)

Actually, your alimentary canal is composed of four tubes, one inside the other. The innermost tube, called the mucosa, supplies many of the glands which produce the digestive juices (there are 35,000,000 of these glands in the stomach alone) and also contains the blood vessels into which the food is finally absorbed. The next tube, proceeding outward, is the submucosa, composed of connective tissue and mainly protective and supporting. Outside of this is the muscular coat, with smooth muscle fibers running both circularly and longitudinally. This allows the two basic types of motion to grind up and mix food with the digestive juices, and the long sweeping wormlike peristaltic waves which move food down along the tract. The outermost layer, called the serosa, is smooth, glistening connective tissue, continuous with the lining of the body cavity.

Chew It Well

Now, watch. Food goes into your mouth, which bites it off and grinds it into pieces small enough to swallow. Digestion starts here, in the action of saliva which contains an enzyme called ptyalin. (There are twenty or more digestive enzymes, agents which promote chemical reactions without themselves being changed.) Ptyalin converts starch partway into sugar; that is why, when you chew up a piece of bread it begins to taste sweet; it is also one reason why you are urged to chew food well.

The tongue pushes the food into the pharynx (back of the throat). While you are eating, the soft palate rises to close the nasal passages, and the lidlike epiglottis drops to close off the entrance to the lungs, so you won't choke. Now the food is propelled by muscular contractions down the ten-inch-long esophagus and into the stomach. If you have overeaten and feel "stuffed," I'll tell you why: The stomach has had all it can hold, the valve at its entrance has closed, and food is massed in the esophagus.

A Full Stomach

Now the food has reached the stomach, which lies under your left rib margin, not in the center of the abdomen, as often is supposed. Empty, the stomach is more or less tube-shaped and rather small; distended by food it is pear-shaped and has a capacity of one to one-and-a-half quarts. Its functions are storage, mechanical mixing, and chemical digestion. It operates like a churn, producing three wavelike motions a minute. Tea, coffee, and broth pass through the stomach almost as soon as they are swallowed. Milk takes somewhat longer; it gets mixed with rennet which curdles it for digestibility. Thin cereal may pass through in two to three hours; a heavy dinner may linger six hours. The digestion of protein goes on apace in the stomach; that explains why bulky vegetables and fats "stay with you longer" than most proteins; they do, literally, stay longer in the stomach. Stomach activity reaches its peak about two hours after you have eaten; in about four hours' time you begin to feel the "hunger contractions" which tell you it is getting empty.

Twenty-Foot Trip

From the stomach, food passes into the small intestine, which is certainly one of the most wonderful parts of the human body. It is more than twenty feet long. Its actions are both mechanical and chemical. If you have had a hearty meal, the small intestine is in for five or six hours' ceaseless activity—squeezing shut to break food into smaller and smaller bits, churning it, moving it by peristalsis along the tract. The innermost lining of this intestine has rough, ridgelike folds covered with millions of tiny hairlike protuberances called *villi*; this provides the huge surface area I mentioned, necessary for the body to absorb all the food it needs, either directly into the blood stream or (especially in the case of fats) into the small canals called lymphatics which then empty into the blood stream.

Now take a side glance at your liver and pancreas, which went into action the instant food began passing through the pylorus, or gate, between the stomach and the duodenum (the first nine inches of the small intestine). The secretions of the stomach are acid; of the intestine, alkaline. To achieve this acid-to-alkaline change, the liver pours in bile. The pancreas also helps, and the intestine itself secretes alkaline fluid.

The food, as it has been traveling along hour after hour, has been churned and mixed into a sudsy froth; by the end of its twenty-foot journey, almost all that is usable has been absorbed into your body. It has been transformed into the four essentials of life: glucose, amino acids, fatty acids, and glycerin. The fatty acids and glycerin have been picked up by the hairlike villi and passed into the lymphatic system; glucose and amino acids have been passed through the intestinal wall, picked up by the blood, and carried to the liver. Each of your body cells knows what it needs—to build skin and hair cells, repair muscles, kidneys, etc.— and picks it up in exactly the right combinations from the blood stream. The miracle has happened: Your food has become *YOU*.

What is left? Waste products—dead bacteria, shed cells, mucus, and indigestible cellulose such as vegetable fibers, peel, seeds. Still in very fluid form, this passes into the large intestine (between five and six feet long) where it is compressed into feces, thus saving the body water that would otherwise escape (as in diarrhea) and lead to body dehydration. The large intestine takes its time over this—ten to forty hours.

Don't Challenge the Efficiency

Now note this well: As I said, by the time the contents of the small intestine reach the large intestine almost all the potentially usable food content has been absorbed into the body. I repeat this because it is important to overweighters; it upsets forever the outdated theory that the fat person is fat because he absorbs more of the food he eats than does the thin person. No matter whether you eat like a bird or only think you do, no matter what you weigh, your digestive system works with the same marvelous efficiency which you have seen in progress. It absorbs just about everything that can be utilized. And any food it *doesn't* need, it stores—as you know—as body fat.

YOUR CIRCULATORY SYSTEM

Perhaps the best way to appreciate the wonders of your circulatory system is to think of your body lying flat and of yourself looking down on it as you might look at a familiar country on an outspread color map, studying its rivers and streams.

Your Rivers of Life

You will see three rivers—one bright red, one dark red (almost black), one white—sometimes running parallel, sometimes intertwined, all traversing the entire country of your body, each intent on its own commerce, yet all three emptying at certain places into one another.

See your bright-red arterial stream spurt along, full of force and vitality, rising in the large aorta of the heart, coursing through smaller and smaller arteries, dwindling at last, just under all your body surfaces, into tiny networks of tributaries called the capillaries. It carries foodstuffs, oxygen to burn them, hormones, and repair material; also, it maintains your body's even temperature and warm, healthy glow. This is your River of Life. Its capillaries flow into the venous stream, which, through veins that coalesce to become ever larger and larger, ebbs back toward the heart. Heavy with waste products, its hemoglobin black with the carbon dioxide (smoke) from burned foodstuffs, the venous stream accurately has been called your River Styx. And the third—the lymphatic stream? White though it is, it transports an even denser cargo of debris than the venous river. Think of it as your body's drainage canal.

Your Heart Is a Pump

Now for a breath-taking experience. Put on your X-ray glasses and look into your heart—a hollow muscular organ, just a bit larger than your clenched fist, lying behind the lower part of your breastbone, a little toward the left. You will see four chambers—two auricles above, two ventricles below. The auricle and ventricle on the left side are filled with bright red arterial blood; the right auricle and ventricle are dark with venous blood. Both your auricles and the right ventricle are thin-walled chambers, but the muscular walls of the left ventricle are about three times thicker than those of the right and develop pressure six times greater—and soon you will understand why.

Your auricles receive blood, force it through very efficient valves into the ventricles, which contract their walls to send it out again —bright blood from the left, which goes to the body for maintenance; dark blood from the right, which goes to the lungs for purification. Both ventricles contract together, and when they do it sends a throbbing wave through your every artery and capillary. This occurs sixty to seventy times every minute of your life if you are in good health, and you know it as your pulse beat.

Your Life Blood

Now, see what happens. Pure, sparkling, oxygen-laden blood, entering the left auricle from the lungs, flows into the left ventricle and is pumped—whoosh!—through the arteries to the capillaries of your head, toes, fingertips, and everywhere in between. (Quite a distance. No wonder the left ventricle needs those extra-powerful muscular walls.) Reaching the venous stream, the arterial river empties into the venous capillaries and turns back heartward. At the upper part of your chest, the white lymphatic stream, fed from tissues all over your body, dumps its entire contents. It has been laving your tissue spaces in a sort of bath of nutrient, and into your venous river, already heavy with waste material, it empties its dishwater. Dreary and black now, the venous river reaches the right auricle of the heart, passes into the right ventricle, which pumps it back into the lungs, from which—presto!—bright and sparkling again from oxygen, it goes back to the left auricle and instantly begins all over.

What has happened? Your blood streams have traversed your entire body. How long did this take? Less than two minutes by your watch. What you have just witnessed happens thirty times every hour, every hour of your life.

There are about ten pints of blood and plasma in your body, and this represents about ten percent of your body weight. Blood consists of liquid plasma and cells, or corpuscles—the red ones which transport oxygen and the white corpuscles which combat infection. Lymph is blood plasma minus red corpuscles; that is why it is white. Your heart pumps five quarts of blood a minute through the circulatory system at rest, and as many as twenty-five quarts a minute during exercise or exertion.

More Tubes within Tubes

The tubes which carry your blood and lymph are similar in structure to your other body tubes—the alimentary canal, for instance, with which you already have become familiar. That is, they consist of tubes-within-tubes—in this case, three: an inner tube of tissuelike cellular membrane, a middle tube of involuntary muscle fiber, and a strong protecting outer coat of connective tissue. Like your other body tubes, they are controlled by the switchboard of your central nervous system, and when this operates smoothly, all goes well with your blood circulation. Let the different telephone exchanges disagree, however, and send contradictory orders from brain to heart about the amount of blood needed in different organs, muscles, and glands, and your whole body feels the effect of the quarrel.

YOUR RESPIRATORY SYSTEM

"And the Lord God formed man of dust from the ground, and breathed into his nostrils the breath of life; and man became a living soul."

Now the work of the Master Sculptor is completed. He has shared with you His own Being, which means the power of constantly transforming death into life; replacing used, dead blood cells with newborn, live ones; exchanging death-dealing carbon dioxide for life-bringing oxygen. He has made you self-sustaining, self-healing, self-regenerating, self-resurrecting. Stop and think about your breath for a moment, inhaling and exhaling regularly. Has it ever occurred to you that with every breath you draw, throughout your entire life, your body re-enacts the mystery of Easter?

I think I hear you sigh with wonder, or give a small gasp of awe, at this concept of your breath of life as initiating a continuous process of death and resurrection. Am I right? Then sustain awe and wonder with me as we look to see what happens whenever you sigh, gasp, or simply inhale and exhale regularly.

The Air You Breathe

Air (oxygen) is taken into your nasal cavities, where it is warmed by contact with the warm vacular structures of the nasopharynx and cleaned by the hairs at the entrance to the nose and by the very tiny hairs deeper inside it. Mucus cells in the nose help humidify the air to make it more acceptable and less irritating to the more delicate structures inside the chest. Passing through the nasal passages the air enters the pharynx, a fibro-muscular structure about five inches long, through which, as we have seen, your food also passes. Now air and food passages separate, food continuing down the esophagus at the back of the throat and air entering the larynx or voice box at the front of the neck (from the outside, this is seen as your Adam's apple).

Next, air proceeds into the trachea or windpipe, an elastic tube about five inches long, about as big around as your index finger. Behind the important Angle of Louis, the bump on your breastbone, the windpipe branches into the two main bronchi and thence into the much smaller bronchioles which divide into small ducts that lead into the lungs proper—large, spongy half-cones occupying the chest and consisting entirely of alveoli or air sacs, so called because they resemble a bunch of grapes and *alveolus* means "bunch of grapes" in Latin. The walls of the alveoli are a busy network of capillaries through which your blood cells continually hurry in single file, giving off carbon dioxide and then taking up the oxygen you have just inhaled.

As you breathe in, your diaphragm, a large flat muscle separating your chest from your abdomen, contracts, moving itself somewhat downward and thereby increasing the capacity of the chest. Also, your ribs rise from a sloping to a more horizontal position, increasing the front-to-back diameter of your chest. It is this creation of a partial vacuum in the chest, followed by the inrush of air, which fills the alveoli of your lungs. For exhalation, your diaphragm relaxes and is pushed upward by your abdominal viscera; the ribs return to their former position. And thus your breath (now carbon dioxide) is squeezed out of the alveoli and into the conducting tubes and out into the world again.

(You know, I am sure, of the wonderful way in which animals—

including man—share the air with plants, interdependently: In animals, oxygen is breathed in to burn up carbon and be breathed out again in the form of carbon dioxide. Plants do just the opposite: by *photosynthesis* they take the carbon dioxide from the air, use it to form carbohydrate, and give off oxygen.)

Your Cells Must Breathe Too

All right. You have drawn breath and released it. Now watch the way your circulatory and respiratory systems combine in your best interests. Every living cell in your body—organs, glands, tissues, bones—must do what you are doing: It must breathe and keep on breathing. That is, it must maintain constant interchange of health-giving oxygen and death-dealing carbon dioxide. In those moist, membranous air-filled sponges—your lungs—is accomplished this transfer of the two gases in and out of the solution in the blood stream. Your lungs have breathed the breath of life on every drop of bright red blood in your arterial stream. Moreover, the suction of your breathing is felt by all the branches of your venous system, whose muscular walls need the extra power of this suction to return their dark blood from the peripheral tissues to your heart. And think especially of this: So perfectly do the speeding and slowing of your respiration, the shallowness and depth of it, respond to your various *emotional* states that they transmit your every mood and temper to the remotest recesses of every one of your bodily structures.

World's Most Potent Cocktail

In this whole big, wide, confused world, there is nothing that can give you a greater instant lift than an oxygen cocktail. We could live without martinis a lifetime, without food for weeks, without water for days, but only a few moments without air. Yes, plain fresh air is one of the most important elements in your life. Air contains the vital properties that cleanse the body. Yes, the thoroughness with which those thirty trillions of cells of your body are pepped up and energized depend on the way in which you breathe. Just as air is the most important element of nature, so breathing is the most important function of your whole body.

The Hindus, more than any other people, took their breathing seriously (perhaps because they had so little food). Their yogis were the first to develop breathing into a vital part of their daily living. The respected Vivekananda taught his millions of followers that all the good things in life—inner peace, poise, good health, and longevity—depend on right breathing. Yogis are also taught that fresh air contains "*Prana,*" which contains the vital spirit. Whether this is so, we Westerners are hardly in a position to tell. What we do know, and scientists have been able to prove this, is that deep rhythmic breathing, charging the body with as much fresh air as possible, is the quickest way to pep up, vivify, and energize a tired body. There are many systems; in England, France, and Germany many schools of "breath culture" have sprung up. Some doctors also teach diaphragmatic breathing, which I believe is the best and most successful method for us Westerners. My pupils call it "belly breathing," because that's where deep breathing starts.

Whenever your spirits sag, when your thinking becomes foggy, or whenever you feel tired, tank up with more oxygen. Step outside, or at least open a window, and inhale as much fresh air as possible through the nose. (As you do this your stomach pulls inward and your chest expands.) After you have inhaled all you can of fresh air—through the nose, remember—exhale the air slowly through the mouth, making a slight whistling sound. The longer you can make the exhalation last, the better. I believe the million dollar secret of the yogis, who have perfect breath control, is their long exhalation. Do this inhalation through the nose and longer exhalation through the mouth about five times. Do it quietly, in a relaxed manner. You will be amazed how mental cobwebs and fatigue disappear almost instantly. Professor Tiralla, in Vienna, discovered that even the tension that causes high blood pressure is reduced by slow, rhythmic, deep breathing. Where nostrils are congested, and for getting an extra amount of vital oxygen into the system, some doctors recommend that you take both hands and pull the nostrils wide open as you inhale slowly.

You have seen, in this personally conducted tour of your real body, that your bony frame and muscular structures are YOU, your food becomes YOU, your blood is the liquid YOU. Marvel with me at your respiratory system, remembering that in addition to all we have just seen about it, it is also responsible for your function of speech. Most certainly, both bodily and mentally, and also in a very special spiritual sense, your respiratory system is YOU.

YOUR NERVOUS SYSTEM

To visualize your nervous system, we will use the classic analogy of the telephone exchange. This vast and busy mechanism not only consists of visible brain cells, tissues, and nerve fibers but also is the invisible stuff your awareness, knowledge, memory, emotions, and experience are made of. So I want to present it to you, first, not as a bodily structure but as an over-all concept.

Your nervous system has two parts—the voluntary (or cerebrospinal) system and the involuntary (or autonomic) system. The voluntary system controls your conscious activities; it serves your voluntary muscles (biceps, triceps, muscles of the eye and jaw, etc.); it needs about eight hours in twenty-four for rest and recuperation in sleep. The involuntary system controls your unconscious activities; it serves your involuntary muscles (those which accomplish digestion, gland secretion, blood circulation, etc.); from the moment you are conceived until the end of your long life, it never sleeps.

Voluntary nerves activate your five senses and your external physical response to the outside world; they get their signals from your conscious mind. Involuntary nerves activate your internal bodily processes and your emotional responses; they get their signals from your unconscious mind. I like to think of it this way: Your voluntary nervous system says, "I see, I hear, I smell, I taste, I touch; I think, speak, decide, act." Your involuntary nervous system says, "I am."

A Living Telephone Exchange

Now let us look at this central nervous system—your personal, built-in telephone exchange. "Central" is your brain, which fills your skull and, at the base of the skull, narrows to become your spinal cord, which is about one-half inch in diameter and is threaded through the vertebrae of your backbone down as far as the small of your back (about eighteen inches). From this switchboard Central sends out wires (peripheral nerves) to every part of your body—voluntary or fast nerve fibers, over which messages travel more than 500 feet per second, and involuntary or slow nerve fibers, which carry messages at 15 feet per second. This network of trunk lines establishes and maintains contact between you and your environment. In addition, it has local telephone exchanges which keep the different parts of your body in communication with one another. Also, it has private telephones connecting one portion of the brain with another. Most remarkable of all, perhaps, it has a two-way "intercom" phone over which your conscious and unconscious minds talk back and forth—and how they argue, at times!

A Little on Your Nerves

The brain and spinal cord weigh about three pounds. They are fashioned of spongy gray matter and bundles of incredibly fine white fibers—the nerves. For a fascinating few hours, borrow an anatomy book and study the structure of your nerve cells and fibers; see how they are grouped according to the work they do and the portion of the body they activate; how their cells and fibers are so arranged that one set responds to vibrations of light, another to sound, taste, etc.; and how they aid and supplement one another. Study the different parts of the brain and how they control your various functions—voluntary functions such as walking, chewing, smiling; and involuntary functions such as sorting impressions and comparing them with previous such impressions (memory) and interpretation of things seen, heard, tasted, felt.

Truly your body is one of the great wonders of the world of nature. Do you now see why it must have good nutrition to function efficiently?

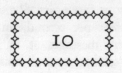

10

Build Up Your Body's Resistance

If you have a health problem, be sure to discuss it fully and openly with your family physician. He alone is in a position to advise you specifically. In the next few pages, let us consider how certain food elements help take care of some specific needs. Whatever vitamins and supplements your doctor prescribes, be sure to take them faithfully. And buy the best and freshest high-vitality foods your budget permits.

INFECTIONS

By building up your body resistance, you can reduce your susceptibility to many infections that are commonly accepted as inevitable in later life.

As you know, your blood stream is the river of life which can bring health and nourishment to every part of your body. This stream is a two-way river and (believe it or not) it is about 62,000 miles long. Flowing in one direction is your arterial blood stream, which carries nourishment, together with the oxygen needed for its utilization, to every cell of your body. Flowing in the other direction is your venous blood stream, which removes carbon dioxide and other waste matter from your body cells.

For the proper nourishment of every organ in your body and for building resistance to infection, the arterial blood stream must contain an adequate daily supply of nutrients.

Protein is of first importance. The body needs proteins containing all the essential amino acids, if it is to produce its own army of antibodies and cells known as *phagocytes* which destroy bacteria and viruses invading your life stream. *Experiments have shown that when a high protein diet replaces one low in protein, as much as a hundred times more antibodies are produced within a week.*

Not less than 60 to 80 grams of complete protein should be consumed daily. One of the cheapest, most palatable, most concentrated, and most completely digested of all protein foods is powdered skim milk. The addition of half a cup of dry skim milk to such dishes as cream soups, milk drinks, junkets, and custards will give you an unbelievable amount of protein value to fight foreign invaders.

Remember that your body's life stream cannot be vitally healthy without the necessary amino acids contained in proteins. (See page 27 for high protein foods.)

Of all the vitamins, A and C are the two most important for building up resistance and combating infections. It is a well-known fact that epidemics are rampant during famines and wars when the diets are deficient in proteins and vitamins A and C. Doctors King and Menton have reported that resistance to diphtheria is increased by taking large amounts of vitamin C, and Kaiser reports that streptococci are less likely to be found in the tonsils of patients who have been given large amounts of this vitamin. Vitamin A is of value in combating infections of the lungs and bronchi; it maintains the health of the lining of the respiratory tract. As Dr. Walter Eddy has pointed out, "Vitamin A is necessary for resistance to germ invasions."

Vitamin A is found in all yellow and green vegetables and fruits, and in liver, cream, and butter. It may not be possible to eat these foods in quantity during illness, in which case vitamin A requirements can be supplied by taking fish-liver oil capsules (of 25,000 or 50,000 units) immediately after meals.

For a list of other sources of vitamin A, see page 41. Make sure that your daily diet contains adequate supplies of this life-giving nutrient; it is "A" must for a healthy life stream.

Vitamin C, equally important to healthy resistance, is found in all fresh fruits and vegetables. Two or three glasses of fresh citrus juice daily will give you an adequate supply of the potent vitamin C so necessary to a smooth-flowing life stream. On page 51 you will find a list of other sources of vitamin C.

For those who cannot take that quantity of fresh juice daily, I recommend the substitution, when necessary, of a 100-milligram tablet of ascorbic acid, or still better, rose-hip tablets, nature's richest source of vitamin C.

One hundred milligrams of ascorbic acid (vitamin C) can be taken every hour to good advantage at the beginning of any infection, including the common cold.

In combating any infection, the entire diet must be made adequate not only in protein and the vitamins A and C, but in all other nutrients as well.

FOCAL INFECTIONS

No Look Younger, Live Longer program, be it ever so perfect and ever so perfectly followed, can yield its best results if it has to compete for health with focal infections. These bacterial infections occur in various areas, such as teeth or tonsils; they can trigger other infections, even in remote parts of the body. Certainly, following our program will help you in your fight against them, and there will be need for a superabundance of certain factors; but why prolong the fight when your physician can help you track down the seat of your difficulty, and in many cases offer measures that lead more quickly to its elimination?

The subject of focal infections has been much mooted. They have been accused of many disorders that did not always disappear when the suspected foci were removed. But, notwithstanding, when they are to blame, their elimination is followed by such dramatic results that the effort always is justified. If the infection starts in the teeth, it can be discovered through X-ray photographs. If it starts in the tonsils, this can be discovered by direct examination by your physician. But, alas, the location is often remote or hard to discover. Teeth in which the nerves have died can easily become infected—they have nothing with which to fight back. If you are fatigued and "all dragged out" from toxins pouring into your blood from infections at the roots of devitalized teeth—get rid of them. Even if at one time you were so bent on keeping them, at any cost, that you let your dentist fill, cap, or inlay them with gold, such gold is not riches; get rid of them so the pus can drain away, and you can be on the road again to richer health.

Focal infections long were blamed for arthritis. In some cases, the elimination of the focus is accompanied by a dramatic subsiding of the arthritic symptoms. In many other cases, the focus may be eliminated but the arthritis remains. What does that mean? Is the theory of focal infection, as the cause, wrong? Perhaps yes— in an individual case—perhaps no, even for the particular case in question. There may be other foci present in the body. A focal infection of long standing not infrequently migrates to remote parts of the body to set up new foci.

Should you be so unfortunate as to have teeth and tonsils infected at the same time, talk it over with your physician; try eliminating the infection of the teeth first. A clearing up of the infection in the tonsils soon may follow, by itself.

Focal infections are sometimes responsible for neuritis, which can be most painful. The foci also may be located in the blood vessels themselves. This condition occurs most often in the veins of the extremities, producing phlebitis. Sinusitis, or "sinus trouble," represents a discomforting and sometimes very painful infection, stubborn in responding to treatment.

Quite apart from any direct kind of treatment, the most valuable measures in combating focal infections are those that build up the general health—diet, rest, sunshine, and fresh air. The High Vitality Diet given you on page 80 should be followed. Moreover, you should give special attention to vitamin C. Eat as much as you can of foods that are rich in it. Eat your green vegetables raw in salads, or short-cooked, to preserve as much vitamin C as possible. Your physician may recommend fortifying your diet with vitamin C tablets. It is an established fact that in the presence of bacterial infections the vitamin C content of the body fluids is greatly decreased. Moreover, both vitamins B_1 and C are excreted in perspiration, and you must make up for this loss, particularly in hot weather.

Of the many conditions which may be caused by venous congestion, arthritis and apoplexy, generally regarded as conditions about which little can be done, deserve to be given greater consideration. A fatalistic attitude is no longer justified, since it has been shown that in some cases arthritis can be overcome by restoring a balanced circulation in the arthritic joints, and that apoplexy can be prevented by removing the cause of congestion in the brain area.

Summarizing the treatment of infections caused by disturbances of the blood circulation, we find that the first step is to locate and remove focal infections. With these sources of infection removed, the blood stream, freed of pollution, can re-establish a balanced circulation in all organs of the body, especially when all of the vital food nutrients are used not just for a week or two, but for all the rest of your long life.

DIABETES

All diabetics should be under the care of a physician. Each person's tolerance for carbohydrates is governed by the state of his insulin sufficiency, and the patient must be guided accordingly. As practically all foods, apart from meat and fats, contain varying amounts of carbohydrates, proper diets can be furnished only by direct medical supervision.

There are, however, several general comments that I would like to make about the diet in diabetes. Frequently it is reduced to such a preponderance of protein and fat that little room remains for foods that are rich in many of the vitamins and minerals. I would advise the patient to discuss with his physician the use of as many vegetables as possible. The low-carbohydrate vegetables generally can be used, and most of them provide important sources of vitamins; try, with your physician, to select the vegetables that give you as many and as much of the various vitamins and minerals as possible. Then, if the diet is not adequate in vitamins and minerals, ask your physician to recommend a proper vitamin and mineral supplement for you to use. In our discussion of hardening of the arteries, I make clear the role played by dietary fat in atherosclerosis. We find also that choline and inositol have been shown as effective in preventing hardening of the arteries. Discuss this matter with your physician. His purpose is to help you, and he will welcome your intelligent interest in your own care and what he is doing for you.

Our great task in the Look Younger, Live Longer program is

to *prevent* diabetes. Overeating of refined sugars, for years and years, well may overwork and depress the insulin-producing cells until they finally break down. I have said many times that the "human machine" is wonderfully made, but it cannot work efficiently under constant abuse. In 1900 the national consumption of white sugar was about ten pounds per person in a year. Today, what with our mountains of cheap candies and candy bars, and our oceans of soft drinks, the national average of white sugar consumed yearly is more than 150 pounds per person.

The prevention of diabetes will be a part of the program fostered by our "human machine shops," changing the eating habits of those with diabetic tendencies and including an abundance of the B vitamins. These are extremely important. In Europe vitamin B is sometimes called the poor man's insulin.

CANCER

Nothing is more gratifying or more worthy of support than the tremendous drive, now well under way in America, against cancer. This is a dreaded disease. It recognizes no age, no station in life, but takes its victims where it finds them.

Of utmost importance is the diagnosis of cancer *in its early stages*. Much can be done then that is not possible once the growth has gotten out of control. The cancer cell is a runaway cell, one that has lost all restraint. It goes on, at an accelerated rate, producing new cells, proliferating new tissue, until it crowds out the surrounding tissues, impairing and ultimately obliterating them. Treatment in the earliest possible stage, therefore, is of prime importance.

In the past few years we have learned a great deal about the characteristics of cancer, much about means of its identity and diagnosis, and something about its treatment in the early stages. Its cause, however, remains elusive. There are theories galore. They run the gamut, from diet to the endocrine glands, highly involved aspects of physiologic chemistry, and even the very genes that pass on to us our total heredity. Guesses and hopes are abundant, but facts are scarce.

The study of cancer is a subject for the layman in that he should know that this is not a disease to be temporized with. Early diagnosis and treatment is so important that it should not be neglected for one single moment after suspicion of it arises.

But cancer is not a subject for the layman to try to solve. Implications should not be made that may raise hope in cases that may be in their terminal stages. Here we are dedicated to the proposition of living longer and looking younger through diet. A sound, well-balanced, vitality diet is *essential to optimum health.* That and an optimistic outlook, with a will to be young in spirit, can do much to help us achieve our goal. The will and the spirit, never forget, are important allies in the quest of good health. I ask your forgiveness for having introduced a depressive note, but the matter is of such importance that I felt that it should not be completely ignored here.

THE KIDNEYS

Like the heart, the kidneys are sturdy and can take abuse. Their performance in emergency is magnificent. If given, through adequate diet, the nutrients they require, the kidneys can be depended upon to do their share and more, to function faithfully throughout a long life.

There is definite relationship between good kidney functioning and good heart functioning. The normal blood pressure of the kidneys is necessarily higher than that of other parts of the body in order to force blood plasma into the kidney tubules, in the urinary processes. An abnormally high bodily blood pressure, superimposed, over a period of years, on the already high but normal pressure in the kidneys, can readily bring about deterioration of these delicate tissues. There are also many other causes of kidney troubles, and much damage is caused by the presence of kidney stones, or gravel. In experimental animals, kidney stones can be induced through severe deficiency of vitamin A, and when vitamin A again is supplied in rich quantities, the stones slowly dissolve and pass away. A lack of vitamin A may be involved in the formation of the stones, but the affliction is one that should be treated by your physician.

The accumulation of minerals in the formation of kidney stones is often accelerated in vegetarian diets when too large amounts of fruits and vegetables and too little meat, eggs, and milk are eaten, thus making the urine too alkaline.

Infections of the kidney can bring about destruction of the tissues, so that the walls of the kidney tubules become somewhat like a sieve, or strainer. In that event, blood proteins, which normally cannot pass into the urine, go through the damaged tubules and are lost. In normal health, these proteins attract into the blood stream the waste materials from all body tissues.

When blood proteins are lost in the urine, or the diet is so deficient in protein that normal amounts of blood protein cannot be produced, liquids tend to accumulate in the body, especially in the feet, ankles, and legs. When kidneys are damaged to such an extent that too much blood protein is lost and wastes cannot be collected, the result can be fatal uremic poisoning through failure to excrete uric acid.

URINARY TROUBLES

Having to urinate during the night may be indicative of no more than a naturally small bladder, but if the urges are overly frequent, particularly in older men, a checkup by a physician may be in order, and all the more so if the need is of relatively recent origin. Infection of the urogenital tract, incipient diabetes, and enlarged prostate, among other disorders, may be the cause. Prompt attention is most important, for urinary trouble caught in its early stages is easier to treat, and a very great deal of trouble can be avoided.

In the dietary management, vitamins A and C should be kept high; proteins should be adequate; and the diet should consist largely of whole-grain breads and cereals, meats, and eggs to keep the urine acid. During treatment for such irritation or infection, the use of citrus fruits and juices, and all fruits and vegetables, should be largely avoided as they make the urine alkaline, a condition which allows the multiplication of bacteria. When all infections have been removed, the High Vitality Diet on page 81 should be followed to prevent such troubles for the rest of your long life.

GALLSTONES

The well-known liver and gall bladder specialist, Dr. Roger Glenard of Vichy, France, has been asked thousands of times what causes some people to have constant gall bladder difficulties. His answer has become a famous saying, "Three F's contribute to gall bladder troubles: Female, Fat, and Forty." It seems that women are especially prone to such troubles, often those of calm temperament, rather than the tense, nervous type.

Interestingly, psychiatrists also have pointed out that persons with "inner tensions" but with outer calmness are susceptible to gall bladder troubles.

In any case, gallstones are made up of cholesterol, which is normally excreted through the bile. (In fact, gall bladder difficulties made the general public conscious of cholesterol.) Under healthy conditions, the muscular wall of the gall bladder contracts sufficiently to completely empty all bile from the bladder. When the bile is not emptied, the cholesterol, being a heavy substance, settles in the stagnant bile to form gallstones. As these stones become larger, they cannot pass through the bile duct even though the diet may have been improved and the emptying of the bladder become normal.

Those suffering with cirrhosis (fatty degeneration) of the liver are found to be especially prone to gallstones. There is an obvious connection here, in that cirrhosis of the liver also is recognized to be the result of B vitamin deficiencies, and of choline in particular. If you have gallstones, by all means seek the advice of your physician to be rid of them.

To help avoid gallstone troubles for the rest of your long life, make sure that your daily menu includes more than ample amounts of all the vital B vitamins.

Don't Be Anemic

Keep your blood stream, the river of life, flowing strongly and smoothly. Begin today to revitalize it. It needs iron and copper; the best sources of iron and copper are wheat germ, liver, and molasses. Plan to eat liver once or twice a week. Include wheat germ and unsulphured molasses in your daily meals.

Marginal anemia, a much-too-common complaint among people of all ages, is caused largely by an inadequate diet. Lacking iron, copper, proteins, and the ever-important B vitamins, the body cannot produce enough healthy red blood cells to maintain a healthy blood stream.

Proteins are very important. (See page 25.) As the red corpuscles contain more protein than iron, all the essential amino acids must be supplied for the proper building of blood. Women in general eat less protein food than men do; moreover, they lose blood at regular monthly intervals, and therefore are more prone to anemia than men are. This anemic condition is readily corrected when the diet contains ample amounts of complete protein, supplied by milk, eggs, meat, wheat germ, and brewers' yeast.

All the B vitamins (thiamine, niacin, pyridoxine, para-aminobenzoic acid, folic acid, etc.) are very essential to the formation of healthy red blood cells. In particular, a lack of folic acid and of vitamin B_{12} appears to be the causative factor in pernicious anemia, which is a most serious complaint.

Pernicious anemia (not to be confused with the commonplace marginal types) is closely connected with decreased functioning of the liver. The American scientist George R. Minot, who discovered this connection, found that the blood vessels become saturated with immature blood cells from the bone marrow, but that the total hemoglobin is greatly reduced.

Formerly considered incurable, pernicious anemia became amenable to treatment following the epoch-making work of Dr. Minot and his colleagues. Liver therapy, and later highly potent extracts of liver, saved untold lives. Pernicious anemia was brought so beautifully under control that there were times when it was difficult to find sufferers. Now with the isolation of the active principle, vitamin B_{12}, and its synthesis, the treatment of pernicious anemia promises to become mere routine; and a mere fraction of a milligram of vitamin B_{12} suffices to control the symptoms of the disease.

Returning to the more common, and by no means necessarily dangerous, nutritional anemia, its presence can be readily determined by a blood test which should be a routine part of your regular medical examination.

To help you plan an adequate diet, rich in all the nutrients needed to prevent or overcome nutritional anemia, remember that liver and wheat germ are natural sources of proteins, iron, copper, and B vitamins which the blood needs. Unsulphured molasses is a rich and convenient source of iron. Liver, wheat germ, and brewers' yeast are rich sources of the B vitamins.

VARICOSE VEINS

Although the beating or pumping action of the heart forces the blood throughout the body, its effect diminishes as the blood passes into the thousands of miles of capillaries. The return of the blood to the heart is brought about by contractions of muscles; the back flow of the blood toward the arteries is prevented by valves in the veins. If, however, the muscles fail to contract normally, the blood cannot be pushed on in its return to the heart. Then blood stays in the veins; it clots and remains there. Other blood may be pushed into the clogged veins and if not forced out will likewise remain to form clots. Such clogged veins, filled with stagnant blood, are spoken of as varicose veins. In time, new blood vessels are formed around the plugged veins, but the varicosities themselves remain to become unsightly, perhaps painful, and in extreme cases ulcerous.

There are two methods for removing unsightly varicosities. One is by surgery, which eliminates the difficulty permanently; it is a comparatively simple operation, but requires hospitalization. The other is the injection method which has become very popular in Europe and in America. Discuss these methods with your doctor if you are troubled with varicosities; do not spend the rest of your life trying to hide them.

More pertinent to our purpose is the prevention of varicose veins. Certainly, a vitality diet, rich in body-firming proteins and vitamin C, is going to be help of the first order. And so is relaxation. As we get older, the distance from the lower extremities to the heart remains geometrically the same, but in terms of heart burden it lengthens very considerably. Do your heart, and your veins, a favor. Rest in the horizontal position, or better still with your feet above your head, on the Yoga Slant board (see page 173). Let the blood in your veins run downhill for a change, with the aid of gravity instead of always against it. Added to the pressure available for returning the blood to your heart, this helps flush the veins, keep them clear, and prevent conditions of varicosity.

The bicycle exercise—thirty seconds of lying on your back with your legs in the air and pretending to pedal a bicycle—is recommended by physical-fitness trainers and is very helpful in preventing varicose veins.

MENTAL DISTURBANCES

I am never happier than when I find that the science of nutrition is becoming more and more helpful in preventing mental deterioration and disease. Mental disease does not just happen; it is the end-product of a long series of causative factors. Happily, some of these causes are simply nutritional; *these can be eradicated.*

It has long been known that a severe lack of the B vitamin niacin can result in a type of dementia. Furthermore, when human volunteers have been kept on diets lacking almost any one of the B vitamins, it led to the development of mental confusion, depression, and anxiety states.

When Dr. Sydenstricker, in his studies, kept human volunteers on a diet adequate in all respects except for the B vitamin biotin, the resultant mental depression became so severe that his subjects developed suicidal tendencies and the experiments had to be stopped. Such findings indicate that the lack of the B vitamins may well be a causative factor in inducing certain forms of mental disturbance.

Groups of scientists, particularly in Sweden, have studied the brains of persons who died of mental diseases and have compared them with the brains of normal individuals who met accidental death. They found that four substances essential to the healthy nucleus of brain cells were lacking in the mentally disturbed: adenine, thymine, cytosine, and quanine. These four nutrients are found in multicellular meats such as liver, calf or lamb brains, sweetbreads, kidneys, and in brewers' yeast. Such excellent meats should be eaten frequently, and brewers' yeast should be added to the daily diet.

Statistics show that one out of every twenty persons spends some time of his life in an institution for mental diseases. *Let us change these shocking statistics.* How? By proclaiming a dietary revolution. Hand in hand with the ever-developing science of psychiatry, the science of nutrition can work toward the prevention of mental illness. It can give man the freedom he longs for, freedom from the greatest of all his fears—the fear of losing his mind.

NERVOUSNESS

Eat and stop fidgeting. Nervousness can be a result of unwise diet. That high-strung, jittery feeling, that jingle-jangle of nerves, readily could stem from a lack of B vitamins, particularly thiamine; if your diet is high in carbohydrates, then the effect of thiamine deficiency is all the greater.

If your diet is very deficient in calcium, to the extent that the level of calcium in your blood becomes low, your nerves will become irritated. Fortified milk is the best source of calcium. It is easily prepared. Just beat one cup of powdered skim milk into a quart of fluid milk. A hand egg-beater will do the job, but of course an electric blender is easier. You may consume generous quantities of calcium; but unless you do so in perfect ratio to phosphorus (and you would have to be a mathematician and check every bit of the food that you eat), it will not be absorbed from the intestines unless vitamin D also is present. If you are indoors most of the time and do not eat eggs every day, you may be getting ample calcium and still not be absorbing it effectively. In such cases it is wise to fortify your diet with a vitamin D concentrate. Many nutritionists now also recommend small bone-flour tablets containing the right amounts of calcium and phosphorus, plus the sunshine vitamin D.

Scientific experiments with human volunteers have shown that diets lacking in any one of several B vitamins can lead to nervous tension. A serious lack of thiamine (vitamin B_1), niacin, or pyridoxine (vitamin B_6), separately or all together, may lead to nervous tension.

A balanced, vital diet is essential to general good health and a sense of well being. It follows, therefore, that it is essential to a calm and stable nervous system.

In older people, a sense of tension and fatigue frequently can be caused by failure to take a snack between meals, particularly if the oldster is normally a light eater. The sugar in the blood may have been used up to a sufficient extent to produce "physiological hunger" that often is manifested by a feeling of fatigue and uneasiness. It can be corrected very simply indeed—by a glass of milk or fruit juice, vegetable espresso, cheese and crackers, or almost any light snack. (If you are truly wise, you will see to it that your snack contributes its full quota of vital elements. See page 78.)

In the light of scientific evidence, and personal observation, it is my belief that adherence to a well-planned nutritional diet, plus the ability to relax all parts of the body, would eliminate an infinite variety of "nerves" for which the pace of our modern world conveniently takes the blame. *Remember that it is impossible to be tense and nervous when the body is relaxed.*

To Look Younger and Live Longer, you must be free from "nerves." Learn as much as you can about their cause, about the general laws of mind and body, and about your own mental quirks. If necessary, go to a trained psychotherapist and let him help you uncover those trouble-making parts of your personality which you cannot find and correct yourself.

FORGETFULNESS

Stella Nash, who likes the form of headgear known as a beanie, went into the kitchen, beanie in hand, to get a glass of milk from the refrigerator. She drank the milk, then carried the emptied milk bottle to the hall closet. "Where on earth is my beanie?" she asked, several hours later, turning the hall closet upside down. The beanie was in the refrigerator.

Stella is "getting on," you say? Beginning to be absent-minded? Stella is sixteen. It was her mother who told me the story. Mrs. Nash, a delightful woman in her mid-forties, had gone to the hall closet for a suit that needed cleaning. Seeing the milk bottle her daughter had absent-mindedly left there, she picked it up—and absent-mindedly handed it, instead of the suit, to the waiting drycleaner's man!

Absent-mindedness is a sign of something, psychologists tell us, but it is not necessarily a sign of old age. It can be a sign of dietary deficiency.

One of the Philadelphia hospitals conducted tests for memory, clarity, speed of thinking, and general intelligence among a group of elderly patients living on a standard hospital diet. The tests were made before and after a number of the B vitamins were separately given them, and repeated again when the entire B family was amply supplied by natural foods. There was no change in native intelligence, but the patients showed improvement in memory and ability to think clearly after the separate B vitamins were given. Marked improvement followed, however, when *all* of the B vitamins were amply supplied. If you have difficulty in remembering or find your thinking growing foggy and confused, try adding such food nutrients as brewers' yeast and wheat germ to your diet; it may help.

Recent experimental work has shown that one of the amino acids, known as glutamic acid, is a principal component of an enzyme in the brain. When glutamic acid is amply supplied in the diet, the intelligence has been found to be actually increased, the ability to learn is accelerated, thinking is clearer, and memory becomes more keen and accurate. While glutamic acid is found in all complete proteins, it is interesting to note that milk is rich in glutamic acid. Fresh and powdered milk are excellent sources of this invaluable nutrient.

Glutamic acid now comes also in concentrated form. When Grandma Reynolds, then well into her nineties, was called on to act in a television show, I received a telephone call from her daughter in Los Angeles. It seems Grandma was worried about forgetting her lines. A "cocktail" of milk, yeast, and honey, plus a tablet of glutamic acid, every hour, produced a "miracle" of memory for Grandma Reynolds. She went on-stage to do a "live" broadcast for "Playhouse 90" with complete confidence and success.

If you are forgetful, absent-minded, or slow on the uptake, do not say, "It's my age," and let it go at that. Follow the High Vitality Diet (page 80); it is rich in proteins and B vitamins. It will send you frequently to the refrigerator to get a glass of fortified milk, and help you remember where you put your hat.

ALLERGIES, HAY FEVER, AND ASTHMA

As we have seen, the blood stream is the great transportation system for the cells of the body. Upon it they must depend for all of their nutritive supplies, and also for the carrying away of all the waste products of their metabolic activities. Back of the blood stream, in the stomach and intestines, specialized enzymes and chemicals first process the food—digest it—so that the tissue cells can use it. The body cells have no means of coping with undigested food. When they are confronted with it, they have to reject it; and it remains in the blood stream as a foreign substance. If the kidneys can excrete it, or it can be excreted into the lower intestine, well and good; nothing happens. If not, it must remain in the blood stream.

The blood resents foreigners! It goes to work to produce an army of antibodies to entrap and render harmless the foreign substance. If the same species of foreigner almost daily invades the blood, antibodies are continuously produced and remain in the circulatory blood; the body is then said to be in an immune state, as far as that particular species of foreigner is concerned. If the invasion is spasmodic, say at intervals of ten days and upwards, during the intervening period the antibodies attach themselves to certain cells of the body, remain there, and do not circulate in the blood stream; the body is then said to be in an allergic state.

During the allergic state, should the same species of foreigner invade the blood stream, there are no circulating antibodies to intercept it; and when it reaches the antibodies attached to the cells, an irritation is produced—so-called anaphylactic shock—which is manifested by one or more of the symptoms of allergy, according to what cells of the body the antibodies have become attached to. Nonproteins also can cause allergylike reactions; allergy to drugs is a typical example. But even in such cases, certain body proteins become involved in the reaction. That is the mechanism of allergy, as it is known today. Its cause is the invasion of the body by foreign substances—generally, but not always, proteins.

How do the undigested foreign proteins get into the blood? The details are not entirely known. The evidence indicates that absorption of them occurs even in the mouth, more particularly the nasopharynx. Also, they may be absorbed almost anywhere along the intestinal tract, even as far down as the rectum.

Under what conditions are they absorbed? Air-borne allergens—pollens, dusts, and the like—are drawn into the lungs with the air we breathe, and thus are absorbed into the blood stream. Another condition is absorption from the intestinal tract, which, it is suspected, is more likely to take place following the eating of offending foods in more than ordinarily large quantities, possibly causing the digestive apparatus to become overburdened.

I have made searches of the literature to see if anyone has attempted to correlate the occurrence of allergy with subnormal vitamin A intake, as vitamin A is concerned with the soundness of the mucous lining of the intestines, but no data were discovered. If the diet is continuously supplied with liberal quantities of vitamin A, the general tone of the mucous membranes would be enhanced. The mucous surfaces of the healthy digestive tract are usually not penetrated by undigested food, but this may occur under certain circumstances.

What can be done about allergy? First, it is desirable to know what substance or substances produce allergic responses. A physician specializing in allergies frequently can make the discovery. Once the offending material is known, it is best to completely avoid the offending substance. Or, you can make your own effort at immunization. If it works, you are so much ahead; if not, little if any harm is done.

First, you must know what food causes the allergy. Then try eating daily almost infinitesimal quantities of that food. Slowly and cautiously, over long intervals of at least several weeks, very gradually increase the amount. You may reach a normal amount with no more trouble. This method is a long way from being infallible, but I have seen it work. If you are allergic to any meats cooked in the rare form, the chances are you will be able to tolerate them if they are well done. If you are allergic to ordinary milk, try powdered skim milk. In all cases, if you are concerned with your diet because of allergies, remember that a diet continuously rich in all the vitamins is probably the best possible precaution in maintaining general good health. One of the most helpful books about allergies is *The Pulse Test*, by Dr. Arthur F. Coca, M.D. He says that any food that raises the pulse unduly may be one that causes the allergy.

PSYCHOSOMATIC DIFFICULTIES

Psycho refers to the mind and *somo* to the body; *psychosomatic* therefore refers to the relationship and reaction of mind and body, one to the other. In recent years, much has been written about psychosomatic difficulties. We have all become increasingly aware that worries, emotional upsets, and anxieties can have such a tremendous effect on general health that they can be causative factors in producing severe illnesses.

Such abnormalities as asthma, hay fever, and other allergies, migraine headaches, digestive disturbances, diarrhea, and high blood pressure may be caused by several things. All, however, *can* be induced by psychosomatic disturbances.

The point which I feel has been almost wholly overlooked in the annals of psychosomatic medicine is the role of B *vitamin deficiencies* in producing the original emotional problems at the root of such disturbances. It is just now being recognized that anxiety states develop when the diet contains too little of the several B vitamins, particularly B_1 (thiamine), niacin, and B_6. These anxiety states are characterized by excessive worrying and brooding, mental depression, emotional instability, and nervous tensions.

The person suffering psychosomatic illness all too often has allowed himself to develop multiple deficiencies of the B vitamins to such extent that he is readily upset emotionally. If an allergy also has developed, and a restricted diet supplying even less of the B vitamins is followed, the whole psychosomatic condition becomes worse. A vicious circle then has been set up, for which the obvious correction is to plan a complete diet adequate in all respects and extremely high in all the B vitamins. Such a diet should include, daily, several heaping teaspoons of brewers' yeast, half a cup of wheat germ, and from a pint to a quart of fortified milk.

BRITTLE BONES

Bones need not become brittle and fragile with age. In general, such bones are the cumulative effect of years of eating foods deficient in the nutrients essential to good bone strength. Experiments with animals have shown that when their diet always is rich in bone-building elements, their bones retain strength even in most advanced age. Of course a serious glandular disturbance could upset the calcium metabolism, in later life, but this is not a major cause of brittleness.

The substructure of the bones requires vitamin C to produce collagen, which is responsible for its soundness. Calcium and phosphorus are deposited on the substructure to produce dense, hard bones; therefore, the diet must also supply calcium and phosphorus.

Furthermore, without vitamin D, calcium is not absorbed from the intestines; and so we must have this vitamin, too. However, most foods, other than egg yolks and fish roes, provide little if any vitamin D.

Exposure of the body to the rays of the summer's sun will produce vitamin D in your skin, but unless you receive a great deal of sunshine, you may be highly susceptible to vitamin D deficiency. If you drink two glasses of milk a day, and use only irradiated milk, you can get 200 units of vitamin D; but in my opinion that is not nearly enough, and supplementing the diet with a vitamin D concentrate would be most advisable.

Older people frequently are deficient in calcium. This comes about in several ways. Dairy products, milks, and cheeses frequently are shunned or taken in too small quantities. Many vegetables contain large quantities of calcium, but much of it may not be available to the body, for a variety of reasons. The calcium in spinach, for example, is unavailable because it is present in an insoluble form and cannot be absorbed. Also, vegetables with considerable fibrous matter may not be well chewed, hence poorly digested; with poor digestion the calcium may never be liberated in the intestines. Yogurt is an excellent source of calcium. It is easily digested and its calcium is highly available.

Keep your diet rich in the bone-building elements: calcium, vitamins C and D. If citrus juices, excellent sources of vitamin C, are not liked, many of the vegetable juices can be used to replace them. (A juice espressor is a valuable possession for the home. See page 505.) You will probably not be deficient in phosphorus, so don't worry about that. If you watch your calcium and vitamins, you will have taken the best possible precautions against brittle bones, and can hope for strong ones for the rest of your long life.

ARTHRITIS

Arthritis produces serious disability. It may be infectious in origin. The seat of the infection, whether in teeth, tonsils, or elsewhere in the body, must be cleared up before health can be regained. Sound nutrition always plays a vital part in recovery.

A note of hope for those suffering from arthritis has been sounded by Dr. Walter Bauer of the Harvard Medical School, and by Dr. Philip S. Hench of the Mayo Foundation. Injections of a hormone from the adrenal gland were found to bring dramatic relief to a number of their patients. But the thousands of arthritic sufferers are warned not to pin their entire hopes on this, as it is still in the experimental field and much more research must be done.

Cortisone, which promised so much to arthritis sufferers, is hardly heard about today. Many of those who had this expensive treatment are right back where they started.

In experimental laboratories, arthritis has been produced in animals by depriving them of vitamin C over a period of weeks and then injecting bacteria into them. The bacteria were carried throughout the body and lodged in the small joints first; there the body tried desperately to stop the infection by depositing calcium all around it. Pain and swelling developed, and arthritic stiffness followed. *On the other hand, where animals had been on a balanced diet with optimum amounts of vitamin C, the injected bacteria did not enter the blood stream but caused an abscess to form at the point of injection.* When the abscess broke, the dangerous bacteria were drained away and there was no arthritis. The lesson to be learned from this is: Do not tolerate any infection anywhere in the body. Consult your doctor immediately.

Our Look Younger, Live Longer program is the best possible insurance against conditions that might lead to arthritis. Do use maximum amounts of vitamin C daily. Get plenty of protective proteins, especially lean meats, cheese, and yogurt. Use only whole-grain breads and cereals, and eat generous amounts of fruits and vegetables. Calcium should never be restricted as it was in old-fashioned incomplete diets.

I cannot accept defeatism in regard to even so serious a problem as arthritis. As with so many other ailments, we can at the very least stop its progress. I have known many cases in which arthritic patients have overcome many of their difficulties by means of nutrition and exercise.

One of the most encouraging cases I know of is a middle-aged English woman who was almost totally crippled with arthritis. At the Royal Free Hospital in London, she was put on the Bircher-Benner diet (composed chiefly of fresh vegetables and vegetable juices). She was also given physical therapy, including heat treatments and daily exercise of the joints, as well as the usual medical treatment. With two months of treatment, most of her joints were once again movable and she was able to walk out of the hospital with only the aid of a cane. The case was so remarkable that they made a movie of it—a complete week-to-week record of progress. The movie can be seen at the hospital.

A second encouraging report I would like to pass on to you comes from Dr. William Brady of Beverly Hills, California, in his book *An 80-Year-Old Doctor's Secrets of Positive Health* (Prentice-Hall). He notes the confusion in terms used to denote disturbances of the various joints and settles on the term *rheumatiz* for a serious arthritic condition. This degeneration of joint tissues, he says, is due to nutritional deficiency throughout the years, chiefly a lack of vitamins B and D and iodine. If you or any of your family suffer from arthritis, I suggest that you read Dr. Brady's book. For an optimum supply of vitamins B and D, he recommends cod liver oil, whole wheat and wheat kernels, at least 1½ pints of milk a day, B complex and other food supplements, plus iodine from seaweed. Many reports from those who have followed these suggestions show that they have gone back to a normal life—even to scrubbing floors!

Bee Venom for Arthritis and Rheumatism

In the Balkan countries there is a saying, "If you want to live a long, healthy life, you should become a beekeeper; raise your own honey and eat it as it comes from the wax comb."

Now there is new excitement in Europe. It has been discovered that beekeepers never suffer from rheumatism or crippling arthritis. Not because they eat a lot of honey, but because they are stung frequently by their bees. It seems that the bee venom contains a natural anti-arthritic, anti-rheumatic agent, and this simple remedy is actually helping thousands of rheumatism and arthritis sufferers.

In Russia and Czechoslovakia, to this day, the afflicted flock in droves to their nearest apiaries to be stung by the bees. As a nutritionist I have always been interested in honey. It is a Wonder Food and should be used instead of the empty white sugar. But I didn't become interested in bee venom until I read a book by Dr. B.

Beck, in which he gave a quotation from the Koran: "From their bellies [the bees] comes a liquor which is medicine for man."

Today bee venom therapy is successfully used in England, Germany, and Switzerland, but it is no longer necessary to submit to painful bee stings. Bee venom has made bee-keeping a lucrative business. The venom is carefully taken from the bees and put in capsules under the most sanitary conditions. European doctors say that bee venom injections give very little discomfort. I am happy to report that American doctors are now becoming interested in this therapy. For the first time, bee-venom therapy is explained in the English language. Dr. Joseph Broadman, a New York physician, has been so successful with this therapy that he has written an interesting book, *Bee Venom*, published by Putnam. Dr. Broadman, a conscientious and serious physician, believes that he finally has found a key to the salvation of the many sufferers from rheumatism and arthritis. Best of all, says Dr. Broadman, any doctor can learn to use this method, and he is willing to teach your doctor how to use this therapy. I hope to report more about bee-venom therapy from time to time in my Newsletter. In the meantime, I suggest that all those interested in the subject of rheumatism and arthritis read this fascinating book.

MENOPAUSE

Some women find menopause as free from difficulty as was the experience of puberty. They are aware only that the ovaries become less active and cease to bring about the conditions necessary to conception. And few indeed are the women over forty who wish to continue bearing children.

Other women, a majority perhaps, experience difficulties all the way from "merely annoying" to serious nervous and bodily upsets. Frequently it is sheer fear of the unknown, fear that can be set at rest through talks with a physician or psychologist. Equally as frequently, it may be a glandular imbalance, which indicates hormone treatment by a physician.

It is my belief that the truly healthy woman—in mind and body—finds her menopause quite uncomplicated. There is no denying the fact that a well-balanced, vitality diet is a great contributor to health of mind and body. Deficiencies bring about a variety of disruptions in the mechanisms of the body, many of which contribute to nervous upset and accentuate the fears of menopause. While a well-balanced diet is always of the utmost importance, it becomes even more necessary under the stresses of menopause. The inclusion of foods extra rich in B vitamins, calcium, and iron is most advisable. Brewers' yeast, wheat germ, yogurt, and molasses all can be used with profit. Some gynecologists recommend vitamin E to relieve menopause symptoms.

According to Dr. N. R. Kavinoky, from 10 to 25 milligrams of vitamin E give relief from hot flashes, backache, and excessive menstrual flow. And a dosage of 50 to 100 milligrams of vitamin E daily also minimizes high blood pressure and muscle pains.

Before leaving the subject let me remark about some general attitudes that prevail and may cause needless concern.

For the healthy woman, sexual desire does not end with the end of the reproductive functions. It can continue indefinitely, and with adjustment to the menopause she can embark upon a new life that is satisfactory and harmonious. Moreover, freed from the fear of unwanted pregnancy and other problems of menstruation, the well-adjusted and healthy woman is pleased to have her energies freed for the many other interests and activities of life.

All too often, both men and women mistakenly believe that a woman's capacity for sexual feeling disappears after the menopause. They quite fail to realize that her sexual feelings come from many sources which are in no way affected by decreased ovarian activity. Contrary to their mistaken beliefs, a woman's sexual enjoyment may be greatly increased after menopause.

Loving and being loved is the fundamental human experience, essential to the formation of character and a positive attitude toward life. Sex is both spiritual and physical; from a mutual exchange of affection emerge tenderness and security which bring health and harmony and enhance the total personality. Longevity statistics indicate conclusively that older people who are happily married have the best chance of achieving a healthy long life.

If false sex education has given you latent hangovers of guilt, or if the constrictive influence of possessive parents has created a problem, have no hesitation in discussing such problems fully and openly with a doctor or psychiatrist, and be guided accordingly. Know that thousands upon thousands of other humans have had such troubles and have overcome them. Know also that sex is a natural and normal function, that it can be one of life's greatest blessings for both men and women.

It is my conviction that much of the bugaboo of menopausal troubles could be dispelled if our overcivilized diets gave way to planned nutritional diets. The forethought of an adequate diet, begun with our first spoonful of food, would obviate the need for afterthought in our later years.

You Can Feed Your Glands

Let us get down to cases. The glands of the body must draw their substance from the food we eat. Moreover, since they represent highly specialized tissues, dietary deficiencies can produce profound changes in them. While nutritional and medical sciences combined have not as yet been able to give us a complete picture of all the interrelationships between diet and the glands, certain specific ones have been clearly defined.

We know that the thyroid gland exerts its effect directly on the metabolic rate. When the gland is overactive, the metabolism is increased; when underactive, it is lowered. In animals overactive thyroid causes loss of weight, interrupted sexual cycles, liver damage, disorders of the heart and vascular system, and a fall in liver glycogen. These symptoms can be relieved through the use of B vitamins, found in brewers' yeast and liver. Thiamine administration is accompanied by beneficial effects in some cases of exophthalmic goiter. Thus the *symptoms* of hyperthyroidism really are symptoms of vitamin deficiency, the deficiency being caused by the elevated metabolic rate. Dr. Roger Williams and his colleagues point out that there is a real possibility that the thyroid and other glands have a marked influence on vitamin metabolism, particularly in regard to absorption and excretion. The parathyroid glands can profoundly affect the state of calcium in the body.

In animals with a pantothenic acid (a B vitamin) deficiency, a section of the adrenal glands develops changes that cause the hair to turn gray. If the glands are removed from such animals, either the graying of the hair is prevented or the color is restored. If after the glands have been removed, desoxycorticosterone is administered, the hair turns gray! Desoxycorticosterone is only one of many similar hormones secreted by the adrenal cortex. A pantothenic acid deficiency has definitely been shown to affect the adrenals adversely. Many authorities believe that a certain abnormal "steroid" produced by the adrenal cortex may play a role in cancer and mental diseases. This shows a distinct relationship between diet and an endocrine gland; there is no reason to suspect that such a relationship is unique to a single gland.

Vitamins A and E long have been identified with sexual and reproductive functions, and more recent knowledge has included many of the B vitamins in the same category. Deficiencies of B vitamins affect the production of sperm and ovum, the mating urge, and the entire sexual cycle, embryonic development, lactation, and the maternal instinct (all functions which fall under the control of the endocrine glands). Dr. R. Hertz links failures of these functions to the direct part played by the B vitamins in the maintenance of general health, which is another way of saying general nutrition. As it is the quality of the diet that determines nutrition, diet must supply the B vitamins.

The liver truly is a great workshop of the body. A list of its functions is almost unbelievable. But the one that is of special interest to us here is that of maintaining the balance between the hormones that stimulate the sex glands. The adrenals secrete both androgenic and estrogenic hormones (substances which stimulate male and female characteristics, respectively), in one and the same individual. The liver maintains the balance between the two by inactivating excesses of either hormone.

It has been shown that in laboratory animals deficiencies of B vitamins, notably thiamine and riboflavin, cause the liver to fail in the inactivation of estrogens but not androgens. On this basis the Drs. Biskind have reported successful use of B vitamin therapy in cases of premenstrual tension, excessive menstrual flow, morbid discharges, and cystic breasts.

Williams and his colleagues point to cases of greatly enlarged breasts among many male prisoners of war in the Orient, which always were accompanied by a serious condition of malnutrition.

The endocrine glands have been a subject of widely publicized research because their malfunction can produce profound and sometimes bizarre changes in the body. They have been proved to be subject to the state of our nutrition. A vital diet, well balanced in all of its nutritive factors, with special emphasis on vitamins, is basic to their health and proper functions.

The Pituitary Gland

Weighing only six-tenths of a gram, it is located just back of the nose and beneath the brain; but small as it is, the pituitary has been termed the "director" of the entire "glandular symphony." This tiny gland manufactures ten or more hormones which are tremendously important in their effect on every other gland in the body. One of its hormones directs the growth of bones and tissues; through its sex hormone it directs sex stimulation and the activities of the ovaries. It controls the thyroid gland and the insulin-producing gland (the pancreas).

One condition of malfunction of the pituitary gland appears to be manifested as a fatty deposit around the chest and abdomen, in a girdle-like fashion. Men take on female characteristics and women become somewhat masculine. The external genitalia of the male appear to become smaller—so-called fatty degeneration. That this girdle-like fat is not necessarily true obesity has been shown by Drs. Freyberg, Barker, Newburgh, and Coller.

In the pituitary case they report on, a boy of 19 years, there was accompanying obesity, with apparent disappearance of the external genitalia. The weight was reduced to normal, by restricted calories in the usual way. Also, the genitalia reappeared, and in normal size; there had been no fatty degeneration. However, on attaining normal weight, the shape of the body remained the same; the girdle of "fat" had merely shrunk in proportion to the rest of the body. It was not due to fat itself but to a deformity in the *shape* of the body. The deformity resulted from decalcification of the skeleton, which is common in Cushing's disease. The spine had so thinned that it had collapsed forward, elevating the ribs until they were horizontal, causing the girdle-like shape of the body. The calcium metabolism probably was disturbed indirectly by the pituitary, through its effect on the parathyroids.

When the pituitary gland does not function properly, it adversely affects the ovaries and brings about premature menopause. It is interesting to note that whereas underfunction of the pituitary produces an earlier menopause, the underfunctioning of the thyroid causes a later-than-normal menopause.

The Thyroid Gland

This gland lies in the foreground of the throat, astride the windpipe, and has been called the "watchman" between the physical and mental body. The thyroid secretes a liquid which is constantly poured into the blood stream and carried to all parts of the body. Removal or disability of the thyroid can turn a youthful person into an old one. Dr. G. W. Crile, who has done much research with the thyroid, discovered that it secretes hormones which give the body much of its verve and virility.

A weak or lazy thyroid can made the sex glands lazy, and an overactive thyroid overstimulates the sex glands. The great Don Juans you read about are the overactive thyroid type, and the indifferent lovers usually have a lazy thyroid.

One of the functions of the thyroid is that of controlling the body's metabolism. An underactive thyroid lowers the basal rate (the rate of energy production that supports the "inner" activities of the body). It does this through the hormone thyroxin, which it secretes into the blood. A deficiency of thyroxin reduces the need for calories; but if one eats at the required level, one will not become fat, contrary to popular supposition. Drs. MacKay and Sherrell bring this out. I quote from them as follows: "Although it is well known that patients with myxedema (extreme hypothyroidism) are not obese as a rule, the idea persists in the clinical literature that hypothyroidism may be a *cause* for obesity." Dr. W. A. Plummer gives clinical evidence that much of the supposed obesity of myxedema is, in fact, water retention in the body. *One does not have to become fat as a direct result of hypothyroidism, but it is much easier to do so.* The hypothyroid sufferer should seek the counsel of his physician for treatment of this specific condition.

Mental sluggishness, difficulty in remembering, and the constant desire to sleep are typical problems of thyroid starvation. *The thyroid has so many important functions in keeping us slim, trim, and alert, in keeping the hair, nails, and complexion healthy, that it could also be termed the "beauty master" of the body. Not only can wrong diet disturb the balance of this sensitive gland, but the resultant depression, fear, and worry and constant strain can further weaken it.* Fortunately, a great deal is now known about this gland and many difficulties once thought to be incurable now can be permanently corrected.

Adequate iodine is of foremost importance for normal, healthy functioning of the thyroid. Without it, we grow old before our time, are always tired, and wonder whatever became of our usual pep. Without essential iodine, we may find ourselves becoming soft and flabby of flesh; mentally lazy, and unable to take much interest in anything; lapsing into the blues; and never feeling warm enough, especially in the hands and feet.

Dr. Russell Wilder of the Mayo Foundation has found that when human volunteers do not get sufficient vitamin B_1, the thyroid gland becomes less active and the basal metabolism drops far below normal. The condition was not corrected by giving thyroid extract; it was corrected by giving vitamin B_1 without any thyroid. Probably thousands of people who now take thyroid extract would be helped far more by following a diet rich in all the B vitamins.

Here, then, are the essential foods for a well-balanced, smoothly functioning thyroid. First-class proteins: meat, eggs, cheese, and fortified milk. Abundant iodine: shrimps, oysters, salmon, radishes, tomatoes, watercress, sea greens, and iodized vegetable salt. All the B vitamins, which are richly contained in brewers' yeast, yogurt, wheat germ, and dark molasses. And for the rest of your long life, season all foods with iodized salt, preferably iodized vegetable salt.

The Parathyroid Glands

These are tiny oval glands located at each side of the thyroid, so small that the average number (4) have a total weight of about half a gram. Our chief interest in the parathyroids is the fact that they regulate the bodily supply of calcium, distributing it throughout the body, and, when necessary, extracting it from one place to supply another—"robbing Peter to pay Paul." If the calcium level in the blood stream decreases, it may cause painful cramps and spasms. Serious deficiencies or an imbalance of calcium and phosphorus are associated with neurotic conditions; adequate calcium is essential to keeping the nerves free from irritation as well as to the building of strong healthy bones and teeth.

The Adrenals

There are two of these glands, weighing only half an ounce, and located one atop each kidney like little caps. The adrenals produce the hormone *adrenalin,* which is poured into the blood stream in time of danger or strong emotional upheaval, to brace us for action or to sustain shock. A deficiency of adrenalin causes slowed-down reactions. The adrenal glands appear to have power to affect certain toxins, and have been termed "the glands of survival." While much remains to be learned about these glands, it has been found that nicotine, lead, and other chemicals can cause them great damage, and that an unbalanced diet is definitely injurious. It is also suspected that malfunctioning of these glands plays a part in graying of the hair.

The cortex of the adrenal glands recently has become a focal point of considerable scientific interest. Cortisone, one of the hormones it secretes, has been shown to be of extraordinary clinical value in the treatment of rheumatoid arthritis, rheumatic fever, bronchial asthma, inflammatory diseases of the skin and eye, and Addison's disease, which is manifested by a bronze coloration of the skin and is due to changes in the adrenal cortex.

Here we may mention that the pituitary gland secretes a hormone (known as the adrenocortropic hormone) that affects the adrenals and is also of considerable therapeutic interest. This hormone is better known as *ACTH.* It has been isolated and used in cases of deficiency; but while it promised much, the results have been disappointing.

The adrenal cortex secretes a variety of steroid substances, some of which are affected by injury to the cortex, as apparently occurs with pantothenic acid (a B vitamin) deficiency, in the matter of graying hair; and there is reason to believe that some of the abnormal steroids may play a role in cancer and mental diseases.

The Pancreas

As is well known, this gland manufactures the hormone we call insulin, whose chief purpose is to help the body utilize and store sugar, or glycogen. When the pancreas becomes damaged and no longer secretes insulin, sugar is lost in the urine; and we have diabetes. This vital gland, which is several inches long, lies across the middle of the abdominal cavity. In addition to the production of insulin, it pours enzymes into the upper intestine for the digestion of proteins, fats, sugars, and starches.

While the exact cause, or causes, of diabetes is not entirely known, there is reason to believe that the overeating of sugars overworks the pancreas, and after years of such abuse it finally slows down the production of insulin. (See discussion of diabetes on page 138.)

The Sex Glands

"Yet all were lacking if sex were lacking," said Walt Whitman, and one cannot deny the importance of a well-regulated and controlled sex life. Most people, however, do not realize that the sex glands also have other functions and purposes. According to the famous Dr. Steinach, both the male and female sex glands have two distinctly different functions; they produce internal as well as external secretions. The external secretion, as we all know, produces human offspring, whereas the internal secretion revitalizes your own body. It is continuation of this inner revitalization which becomes so important to us in later life, since it perpetuates our own vitality and well-being. Dr. Steinach created a furor in Vienna (and all over the world) by applying this principle to aging men. The famous Steinach operation—a relatively simple procedure for men—consists in tying up the vas deferens duct to prevent ejaculation of secretions, and thus diverting them to increasing the bodily vigor. This simple operation takes about twenty minutes, and Dr. Adolph Lorenz has testified openly to its beneficial effects. However, as this is quite controversial, if you have further interest in it I suggest consulting your own physician.

Our chief interest here is in how to keep the sex glands healthy via the most reliable and most permanent way—sound nutrition. A basically well-balanced diet is the first step toward improvement of the general health, hence that of all glands. When nutritional deficiencies have been overcome, improved health and vigor will be reflected in greater virility and normal libido. Remember that first-class proteins, as well as vitamins A, C, E, and all the B vitamins (especially pantothenic acid, para-aminobenzoic acid, and folic acid) are imperative.

When the ovaries do not function properly, a type of fat is deposited on the breasts and upper thighs, usually at middle age. While glandular therapy can be of great help in such cases, a common-sense reducing diet is necessary to get rid of the fat.

In men, fear and worry may be the worst troublemakers in preventing normal sexual functioning, especially in later years. And such fears and worries may be brought on by a lack of B vitamins as much as by a man's own erroneous beliefs concerning sex. How often, and how wrongly, the man views an active sex life as the symbol of youth. Medical records show that libido, the ability to have intercourse, and the production of living semen sometimes are sustained up to a very great age, and that frustration will create all the unpleasant neurotic symptoms of any forced abstinence. Actually, the need for sexual outlet is an individual matter depending entirely upon the make-up of each individual person. No standard patterns can be set up for what might be called normal or average sex activity for all.

Sexual emotion depends upon the amount of internal secretions delivered to the blood by the gonads. These in turn must depend upon the amount of nutrients available to maintain the health of the ovaries and testicles. People who have lived on inadequate or starvation diets (as did those in concentration camps) invariably report that sex interest quickly and completely disappeared.

Animals maintained on diets low in protein, or inadequate in any of the essential amino acids, show so little sex interest that mating soon ceases. On a high protein diet, restoration of sexual potency and the resumption of mating quickly take place. The importance of a diet adequate in all nutrients in maintaining sexual potency cannot be overemphasized. A lack of the amino acid arginine causes sterility in male animals. In experiments with young men it was shown that inadequate arginine, over a period of only one week, resulted in a marked decrease in sperm production.

The studies of Reynolds and Macomber showed that calcium deficiency had the same effect as that of protein starvation. Too little vitamin A can cause in animals a marked reduction in fertility, disturbed sexual behavior, and, in severe cases, complete loss of libido.

I believe that, with our ever-increasing understanding of the glands and their vital secretions, we are about to enter the "Hormone Age," and I predict that the day is not distant when diets rich in hormone-producing vitamins, to protect our life-giving and life-sustaining glands against depletion and disease, will be the general rule rather than the exception.

The Niehans Cellular Therapy

A great deal of publicity has recently been given to the Niehans treatment. This cellular therapy is quite popular throughout Europe, although today it is relatively unknown to the average person in the United States. I believe the Niehans cellular therapy has great promise for people who want to keep their tissues young.

After reading all the French and German reports on this treatment, I had the pleasure of meeting Dr. Paul Niehans in Paris. He is an amazing-looking man, full of enthusiasm—especially for his treatment. It consists basically of *Frisch Zellen,* fresh living cells taken from unborn animals, usually lambs or calves. These tissues are ground up and added to a saline solution to make a scrum. The secret lies in the fact that the tissues are only twenty minutes from the unborn animal to the injection in the human patient.

Perhaps the best-known person among those to benefit from this treatment was Pope Pius XII, on whom it worked miracles. Other people who have taken this treatment are Winston Churchill, Bernard Baruch, Somerset Maugham, Charlie Chaplin, Bob Cummings, the ever-young Gloria Swanson, and two of Hollywood's columnists, known for their verve and vitality, Cobina Wright and Hedda Hopper—and over 40,000 other important people.

At the clinic *La Prairie* in Switzerland, Dr. Niehans' visitors include many physicians who come to learn more about his therapy. Although Dr. Niehans has worked in this field for thirty years, American doctors say more research is needed before cellular therapy will be used in America. One of the problems relating to the treatment is the fact that live tissues are not always immediately available; and, because of the painstaking care in the preparation of these *Frisch Zellen,* the treatment of necessity is still expensive.

One of the latest accomplishments of Dr. Niehans' research is the injection of young cells of pancreas tissue for diabetics. This offers great hope that many diabetics may be freed from the inconvenience of daily insulin injections. Certain specific pancreatic cells which Dr. Niehans has succeeded in separating may achieve lasting results. For more specific and detailed information, I recommend that you read Dr. Niehans' own book, *Introduction to Cellular Therapy* (Cooper Square Publishers, 59 Fourth Avenue, New York City).

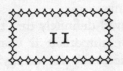

II

Fight Fatigue with Relaxation and Exercise

FATIGUE

Constant fatigue is not normal at any age. I believe that much
of it is caused by dietary deficiencies, and extensive scientific experiments (both with animals and human volunteers) have shown
this to be so.

At the famous Mayo Clinic, several young women who volun-
teered for experimental studies deprived themselves of fresh vegetables and protein foods such as milk, eggs, and meat. They put
themselves on a diet of devitalized starches, cooked-to-death vegetables, white bread, white sugar, and gooey pastries. (A typical
Old Ladies' Home diet!) Before long, these once-energetic and
good-natured young women found themselves listless, jumpy, tense,
and irritable enough to scratch out one another's eyes. And it ran
in a vicious circle. The more tired they felt, the more they ate, in
an effort to recapture their accustomed energy. But the more of
their devitalized diet they ate, the more tired and listless they became.

Fatigue is a deadly enemy in our busy lives, one that we must
wipe out, right from the start. Forty years ago I discovered that
people who eat enough of the good protein foods, good breads, and
only natural sugars, never complain of being tired. The tired ones

were those who ate white breads, over-refined cereals, and lots of white sugar and cola drinks.

Now it has been proved definitely that these empty foods have been robbed of the ever-important B vitamins, especially of B_1 (thiamine) which is necessary for energy. *An abundance of B vitamins is most important in outwitting fatigue; they provide the spark which releases energy from the foods we eat,* much as a match furnishes the necessary spark for the wood in your fireplace.

In my classes I am constantly bombarded with questions about fatigue and how to prevent it. A type of fatigue, especially in older people, is often caused by inadequate amounts of protein foods. Proteins, as we know, contain the amino acids essential to the many enzymes of the body. It is amazing how many older people still eat only small portions of protein foods daily, in spite of the fact that, more than any other foods, proteins are necessary for body repair at all ages. Stop and check your protein intake for the last 48 hours, right now. (See page 27 for list of protein foods.) If you have eaten less than 60 grams a day, you can probably help that tired feeling disappear quickly by increasing your protein intake to 80 or 100 grams until all tiredness is gone.

Still another (usually temporary) fatigue problem is caused by a decrease, or sudden drop, in the blood sugar. You can bring this on when you do not eat a good breakfast. Many women have complained of this fatigue which came on while they were so busy shopping for bargains that they forgot all about eating. You can prevent it by taking time to eat-for-energy. A stop at the soda fountain for a lean milk shake will help you out of that slump.

Many of my students are strenuous people, busy, important, highly paid, indispensable. These men and women refuse to be tired. They cannot afford tension. Their lives require a full, steady flow of energy all day, every day.

For such men and women, my Look Younger, Live Longer program is basic. It is as much a part of their thinking as their political views or their professional vocabularies. When they think of food, they know that a good breakfast is of greatest importance. For the rest of the meals they think in terms of lean broiled or roasted meats, short-cooked vegetables, crisp salad bowls, eggs, cheese, fruit, and fortified milk or yogurt every day. Wheat germ, brewers' yeast, and honey are stocked on their household shelves as regularly as salt, herbs, and vinegar. So are tablets and capsules with extra vitamins and minerals. These are used so there can be no possible deficiency of any important nutrient. Many of my important students have acquired the habit of eating intelligently at mealtime and between meals. The latter are small snack-meals of vitality boosters such as cheese and crackers and fortified milk drinks, which ward off energy letdowns, irritability, and nervous tension. (See page 78.) The wise ones have learned from experience that there are just two secrets for living and working at a sustained pace, without strain, without overdoing, without knowing the meaning of fatigue. Their million dollar secrets are: a high-vitality diet and the art of relaxation—the same secrets we taught the maharajah who couldn't sleep.

The Million Dollar Secret of Relaxation

Unless you are able to "let go" and relax, all the extra vitamins and minerals will not do you much good. Our Look Younger, Live Longer program, with its balanced, superbly nutritious high-vitality diet, can gradually establish for you a state of healthily balanced nerves to cope with life's ups and downs. But it is also necessary that you learn how not to *waste* energy by learning the art of banishing tension.

One of my friends, a delightful woman in her late sixties, who has long enjoyed agelessness and who is a very busy and successful artist, summed up the point for me in a few brief sentences. She said, "Tension is tiredness. Relaxation is youthfulness. Or you might put it another way: tension is ugliness, relaxation is beauty."

Who would be better qualified to define beauty than an artist? I think we can take her word for it. Relax. Remove the hectic tensions from your face and it will become tranquil, more harmonious and attractive, no matter what your age. Relax your body and it will serve you better, no matter what your age or figure. The men and women of all ages who are "naturally attractive" are not always those whom Nature has endowed with good looks; they may be far from it. They are the ones you like to be with, the people who never make you uneasy because they are so completely at ease themselves. Every man or woman who is truly great has learned this art of being at ease with himself and others; he is a normal, healthy, warm human being. I do not like to be in the presence of tense, twitchy individuals, regardless of their name or fame. To me, they seem immature; they have not learned the first law of successful living—to relax.

If I can make *you* relax and stay relaxed for the rest of your life, I will have given you one of life's greatest treasures. My hope is to get you excited enough about relaxing so that you will make it a part of your life.

When you first learn the art of relaxation it is best to be alone. There should be no tension anywhere in your body. For complete comfort, you might buy some small pillows. These should be placed under the neck, the elbows, and the knees.

I believe one of Winston Churchill's million dollar secrets is the ability to relax completely. No matter where he is, he retires every afternoon to his private room to relax, to let go, to forget the stresses and strains of his hectic career. He lies on his bed, with a little pillow under each arm, and relaxes so completely that he falls asleep. No one, not even his wife, is allowed to disturb him during his afternoon relaxing period. You too can learn to relax this way from head to foot.

Lie comfortably on a couch or bed. Let your imagination help you. Make believe you are floating on a cloud, or that you are a rag doll with entirely loose and floppy joints. Be the branch of a bush blowing in the wind, or seaweed in the ocean going back and forth with the waves. Think of anything which helps you to let go, so that your muscles become loose and free.

I find it best to start with the feet. First, turn each foot a few times to loosen it up; then think of your feet as being very loose, of dangling like two tassels. Now relax the calves and thighs. You might flex them a couple of times, or shake each leg a bit—then let your legs lie heavy, heavy as lead. *Think* of your legs, and your feet, as utterly relaxed—no tension, no tightness, anywhere. Make believe they are made of cement, that you could not possibly move either of them even a little bit.

Now, take a few breaths, deep as possible. Breathe gently and make your exhalations longer than your inhalations. Feel your body sink into the bed. Banish every thought of tension and tautness. Next, tense your arms; stretch them as long as you can. Tense your fingers, spread them apart, make them as rigid as you can. Now, make tight and hard fists, as though you were boxing.

Now, relax the muscles of your hands and arms, and let them drop heavily by your sides. Your hands and arms should now be as relaxed as sleeping kittens. Now comes the neck, the part of the body that shows so much tension, and is so susceptible to it. Roll your head from side to side a few times, as though you were saying, No! No! No! You will probably find several kinks in your neck. Now, make believe your head is unbearably heavy, and then let it sink deep into the pillow—assume that the neck has no power to move it.

The eyes are next, and it is very important that you learn how to relax them. This can be accomplished in many ways. First of all, squeeze the eyes a few times by just closing them tightly. Now open and close them a few more times, but lightly, delicately, loosely. If you are still tense and nervous, the eyelids will quiver. So keep on letting go, breathe calmly until the eyes don't quiver and flutter. With the eyes closed, make believe that the muscles that control the eyeballs are loose, very loose, and completely relaxed— let go of all tightness and tension here, too. Banish the idea. Perish the thought. Think loose.

There are other methods. I find the one of Dr. David Harold Fink, of Beverly Hills, very useful. This California physician tells you to lie undressed in a completely relaxed position and to talk to your arms, telling them to let go, to talk to your legs and feet. In fact, he says, talking to the different parts of the body is the best way to learn to relax. Then there is Dr. Jacobson of Chicago, who teaches progressive relaxation and believes that if you can relax the muscles of the eyes you can stop worry.

This head-to-toe relaxation will do you good any time of the day, but it is ideal when done just before going to sleep. It has helped many insomniacs to overcome their tensions and sleeplessness. The whole relaxing procedure takes between five and ten minutes. Do it at least once a day. But if you are weary, and really anxious to conquer the strains and tensions of life, do it two or three times a day, until you have learned to prevent tightness and tension. Even then, though, do it each night before going to sleep. For when you sleep in a relaxed and peaceful attitude, you will wake up refreshed, with added strength and energy for the new day.

Yes, I believe that better eating and conscious relaxation will help you put an end to exhaustion and unhappy, tense living.

Now, I can hear some of you readers say, but I cannot always lie down and relax when my calendar is filled with important and urgent appointments. And my answer is, the more appointments you have and the more valuable a human being you are, the more important it is for you to relax—believe me, you will *last* longer, and you will be worth more—and while you do last, you will be more human and more efficient.

Instant Relaxation for a V.I.P.

Psychiatrists tell us that the more strenuous and humdrum our jobs are, the more it is necessary to escape "the monotony." In just a few minutes of relaxation you can, with the aid of your imagination, escape to any beautiful and calm spot—woods—shore—flying above the clouds.

Here is a simple way, and a quick one, for relaxing and relieving yourself of nervous tension during the day. It is my favorite method when I am on television (which is perhaps the most killing of all work) or when I am on a lecture tour. It only takes a few moments and is most helpful. Open your nearest window, sit at your desk, and sit straight. Close your eyes and keep them closed. Now, breathe as deeply and as slowly as you can. Remember to breathe in through the nose and to exhale through the mouth, slowly, slowly, and as long as you comfortably can. Hum the letter "U" as you exhale, but not so loudly that your secretary will think you are going berserk. While you hum—and it is not necessary to do it loudly—and breathe slowly and peacefully, allow yourself to escape for a few moments. Use your imagination, and think of your favorite pastime—fishing in a brook—lying under a blooming apple tree—floating in the Mediterranean; think of anything and everything that brings you happy, peaceful, and calm memories.

This letting go, this breathing deeply and slowly, plus a few happy thoughts, can refresh you miraculously. I am anxious to pass this million dollar secret on to you, Mr. Executive. Make it one of yours. If you tell me you don't have time to relax, let your secretary type these words on a card and place it on your desk where you will be constantly reminded:

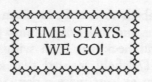

THE MAGIC YOGA SLANT FROM INDIA

The ageless Lady Mendl was famous for standing on her head when she was 80. The Great Om, a yogi from India, had promised her a long and youthful life if she stood on her head for three minutes each day. There were other famous headstanders in the twenties, too, such as Ina Claire, Anne Morgan, Blanche Yurka, Greta Garbo, and Leopold Stokowski. I learned to do the headstand under the tutelage of Miss Garbo, and there is no question of its efficacy; nothing stops the constant downward pull of the face and abdominal muscles so quickly as this upside-down position. But I also discovered that some of my students who practiced the headstand did damage to their necks and backs. I was glad when another yogi introduced the *Magic Yoga Slant,* which is so easy to do; anyone, regardless of age, can lie in this comfortable position. Many of my students, especially in California, have installed what they call the Beauty Slant, a wooden or plastic board with the foot end raised 12 to 15 inches. (It should never be higher, or the position becomes uncomfortable.) At this elevated angle, you can obtain all the benefits of the headstand without the possibility of injury. It is actually the laziest and most effective way of stopping the downward pull of gravity. Lady Mendl was full of praise for this Yoga Slant, and used it constantly in place of her headstand until her 94th birthday.

Make Your Own Yoga Slant

All you need is a solid board, one and a half feet wide and six feet long (a little longer if you are very tall). You simply raise the foot end of the board to a low chair or attach two legs to the foot end, not higher than 12 to 15 inches. For more comfort, you can pad the board with a thin sheet of foam rubber and cover it with canvas or plastic. On expensive and sophisticated beautyfarms, the Yoga Slant boards are in every room as well as clustered around the swimming pool. The lovely and ageless Ann Delafield, who was director of the Elizabeth Arden Beautyfarm, says that this Yoga Slant brings the spine and inner organs into proper alignment and lifts falling faces and necklines from within, via your own red blood stream. Ann Delafield insisted that all beautyfarm guests take the Beauty Slant at least twice a day, 15 minutes during the afternoon and 15 minutes before retiring. Serious yoga experts believe that reversing the downward pull of the body, for a few minutes each day, forces the blood into the vital centers of the body. While such a statement may seem exaggerated to scientists of the Western world, the fact remains that, when the feet are higher than the head, the pull of gravity on the body fluids is reversed.

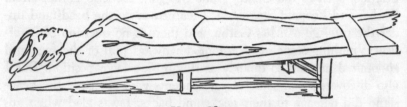

Yoga Slant
The magic angle—feet 12 inches above floor

In the Yoga Slant position, the spine straightens out and the back flattens itself. Muscles which ordinarily are somewhat tense, even in easy standing or sitting, are relaxed and at ease. The feet and legs, freed from their customary burden and the force of gravity, have a chance to release accumulated congestions in the blood stream and tissues, and thereby reduce the possibility of swollen limbs and strained blood vessels. Sagging abdominal muscles get a lift, and the blood flows more freely to the muscles of the chin, throat, and cheeks, helping to maintain their firmness. The complexion, hair, and scalp benefit from this increased blood circulation. It is because the Yoga Slant is such an aid to beauty that it is often called the *Beauty Slant.*

In this position the brain also is rested and cleared. In fact, Dr. Donald Laird, of Colgate University, says that the brain functions 14 percent better when the head is lower than the feet.

Take the Yoga Slant for fifteen minutes, twice a day. Take it whenever you can—on arising, before retiring, or best of all when you come home tired from work.

I know an important woman executive who has made it her daily habit to come home, undress, and take a short nap on her

Yoga Slant board before dinner. Awakening, she consciously relaxes her eyes. Then she lies in a tub filled with warm water, scented with bath oil. In the bath, she continues to relax—shoulder blades, calves, feet—and does the Stomach Lift ten or fifteen times.

Then, refreshed and rejuvenated, she is ready to dress for dinner and an evening of entertaining or being entertained. She is full of humor and vitality, her eyes are bright and sparkling and she needs no glasses—and she is past sixty years of age. She tells me that her before-dinner relaxation also assures her of deep, sound sleep.

MIDRIFF FLATTENER—THE STOMACH LIFT

Lying completely relaxed in the Yoga Slant position, draw in your stomach as you count one. (Continue breathing naturally while doing this exercise.) Draw your stomach in and up, farther, on the count of two. On the count of three, you draw it in close to your spine, which is pressed flat against the board. Try to hold this position to the count of ten. Then relax. Repeat the exercise as often as you wish.

I call this exercise the Stomach Lift. In the years when people were flocking to Munich to learn it at Dr. Bauer's famous clinic, it was called the *Bauchgymnastik* or "belly gymnastic."

Do the Stomach Lift wherever you happen to be. Make a habit of it. On the beach, in the bathtub, when you are riding in an elevator, waiting for a bus, standing in line at a ticket window. Do it under the hair dryer, in a hotel lobby, sitting through a dull movie short.

Do the Stomach Lift for the rest of your long life, and save your waistline permanently. With it, you will save your posture, grace, self-confidence, and well-being. You will be saved from sagging shoulders, middle-age spread, "jelly belly," face and throat wrinkles, bulges and rigidity. Why? Because you will have a strong, permanent "muscular corset" supporting the center of all the vital processes of your body.

Dr. Erich A. Mueller, after ten years of research, has come up with a related discovery that should be exciting to many busy people—especially men who dislike exercise. He found that one intense muscular contraction, the maximum possible, held for only seconds, and performed just once a day, will rapidly strengthen the muscle. His research shows that the one maximum contraction, performed once a day, makes the muscle 6 percent stronger in one week, 66 percent stronger in 11 weeks. These quick muscle-tensing exercises have become very popular in England, Germany and Italy.

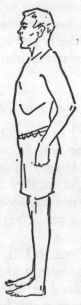

The Stomach Lift
Try one intense muscular contraction once a day

Good health depends upon abdominal firmness; this region is the center of absorption, assimilation, and elimination. Energy and emotional health also depend on it. Behind the stomach lies what is known as the "abdominal brain," a sympathetic nerve apparatus connected with all the other abdominal organs. It is not for nothing that we speak admiringly of a person who has "good guts," and when we say good guts, we mean firm guts.

And finally you can do the Stomach Lift and be saved forever from the nagging voice of conscience telling you that you must do exercises. Of course, you can also do a "daily dozen," turn cartwheels, work out with a punching bag or rowing machine. However, I do not recommend strenuous exercise for older people. To Look Younger, Live Longer, you do not need it. You can be free of all that, for the rest of your long life. The Stomach Lift is one of the best of all my million dollar secrets I have to give you—the exercise to end all other setting-up exercises.

Master the Stomach Lift and, when you walk, you will keep your stomach flat without effort. Take long steps when you walk, feel the good, rewarding "pull" in the muscles of your legs and buttocks, feel your shoulders go up, your neck straighten to carry your head proudly. Imagine that you are a movie heroine walking down a long corridor toward the dramatic climax of the story, or a model on the runway at a fashion show. Or a dignitary crossing the platform of a huge amphitheater to receive the decoration of the Legion of Honor.

EXERCISE

Rediscover Your Favorite Sport

If you have a favorite sport, one that you have allowed to slip out of your life in recent years, go back to it. You are fortunate to possess an active skill on which you can draw; it is like money in an old savings account that you had forgotten about. Do not be discouraged if your skill has become a bit rusty and your muscles protest at first. No one ever forgets how to swim, dance, ski, bicycle, ice-skate, play tennis, or swing a golf club. Your body remembers; only give it a chance, and start slowly!

And give it the energy of your high-vitality diet to draw on. You will soon feel again the exhilaration you used to enjoy. Even if you are not, and perhaps never have been, a champion, what of it? The muscular joy (see page 406) of using your body will keep you happy at your sport.

Swimming is, as you know, one of the most joyous exercises. If you are at all skilled in the water, I urge you to seek out a pool in your locality and begin to swim regularly, all year 'round. But I do mean swim. Just dunking yourself in the water will be fun, but not really enough fun for real muscular joy. Swim your one, two, or three steady laps across or around the pool. Speed is not important.

Swim, ride, walk, dance—enjoy whatever you like, but *enjoy* it.

Just Seven Minutes a Day

For the apartment-dweller and the other millions of people who do not have much opportunity to pursue their favorite sports, just seven minutes a day spent doing simple rhythmic exercises can do wonders.

Here is some cheerful news about exercise: It does not have to be a long, complicated, strenuous routine. All the men and women who have told me how they successfully made exercise a part of their daily lives have confirmed my own experience. A few well-chosen, basic, *simple* exercises make the best routine. They can be gone through in a few minutes as part of the getting up, bathing, and dressing ritual that begins your day.

I have studied countless exercise routines—American, European, and Oriental—for every country has its favorites. The best ones have been developed out of natural body movements and do not demand a contortionist's or an acrobat's abilities. Let me give you seven basic exercises. You can do them well and thoroughly in no more than seven minutes of your day, and they will keep you trim and fit all your life. Remember, we exercise not only to keep slim; we exercise because it helps us to feel so much better.

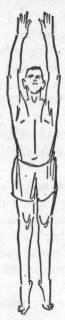

Stretch . . .

1. *Stretch:* Rise up on your toes, arms up; with your hands try to touch the ceiling. Drop arms. Relax. Do ten times.

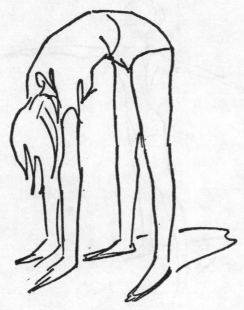

Bend . . .

   2. *Bend:* Down, down, from the waist, hands reaching for the floor. Stretch, stretch, until you can touch the flour with the palms of your hands. Each time bend down as far as you can comfortably —but don't overdo. The best vitalizing exercise and cure for backache. Do ten times.

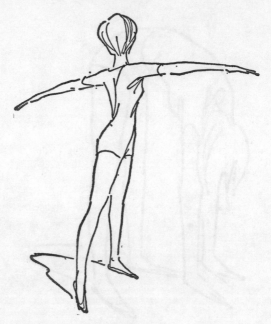

Twist . . .

3. *Torso twist:* With arms outstretched to the sides, reach to the left, to the right; twist at the waist and reach backward to the left, then to the right. Back and forth. A wonderful, easy way to keep your waistline. Do ten times.

4. *Hip roll:* With hands on hips, rotate the middle, holding shoulders still, first to the left, then to the right. Do ten times slowly in each direction.

5. *Bicycle:* Lie on the floor on your back, legs up; pedal slowly and rhythmically. The more you breathe, the better it feels. Do for two minutes, then relax. This helps to counteract varicose veins.

6. *Stomach lift:* Pull your abdominal muscles in, hard, harder. Hold tight for about thirty seconds or until muscles quiver, then relax. Do at least once a day, but regularly. (See also page 175.)

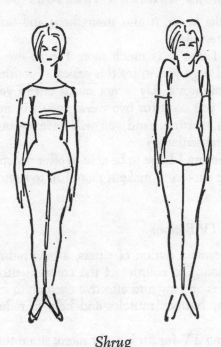

Shrug

7. *Shoulder shrug:* Important for neck, face, and scalp. Lift the shoulders to the ears and hold for ten seconds. Relax. Repeat ten times.

Now shake yourself all over, take a few deep breaths, and off to your shower or tub. You have done your muscle work for the day. Any other exercise, sport, or physical work you do will be so much gravy. Try to make these easy, lazy twists and stretches a daily fun habit.

Every one of these seven exercises has its particular as well as its general value for your health and good looks. The stomach lift explains itself; you can reduce several inches in just a few weeks. But you must do it regularly. The bicycling and hip roll take care of circulation in the legs and middle. The stretches, bends, and twists do wonders in loosening spinal and torso tensions. Those large muscles across your back and ribs contract by reflex, without your conscious effort; in your sedentary life, they are in tension most of the time. The same is true of the shoulder shrug, which loosens tension in the neck, face, and scalp and creates revitalizing circulation to the brain; it also strengthens and firms the muscles that hold the chest high.

I have found that it is much more fun to exercise with good snappy music. I urge you to try this easiest of routines for just two weeks; seven minutes a day is not much out of your busy life. I promise you, if you do it for two weeks, you will never give it up. The results are amazing. And you will have learned to transform pain into sheer muscular joy.

In the near future I hope to be able to offer my students a record of music I have chosen to make it more fun to stretch, bend, twist, and shrug.

Rock-a-way for TV Bottom

Since we became a nation of sitters, a new nuisance has arisen called TV Bottom. To counteract the constant sitting in front of television, here is an easy and effective exercise to strengthen those large and flabby buttock muscles and help to reduce an oversize *derrière*.

After watching TV for an hour or more, sit on the floor, pull up your knees, take hold of your ankles on the outside, and rock-rock-rock like a little rocking horse; swing back and forth. You will feel the buttock muscles getting a terrific squeezing, your whole circula-

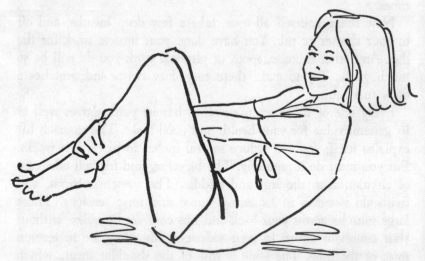

Rocking back and forth is the best antidote for TV bottom

tion is pepped up, and, what's important, you will discover that rocking is fun!

Sexercises

That's what Bonnie Prudden, a woman who has the courage to speak her own mind and a member of the President's Fitness Committee, calls exercises that improve circulation and make you feel good all over. She believes that a healthy body is basic to marital happiness. For a complete program of building and slimming techniques, plus her fabulous Sexercises (first aid for ailing marriages) read her book: *How to Keep Fit after Thirty*, published by Random House.

WALK AND LIVE LONGER

One of my favorite muscular joys is walking. Let me introduce you to a distinguished and rapidly growing society: the walkers. They are anonymous, unorganized, without a constitution or by-laws. Some have a favorite daily walk, some will walk anywhere, any time. Your true walker will automatically find walking opportunities wherever he or she may be.

Most people will do almost anything to avoid walking, but there are exceptions—and they are exceptional people. Greta Garbo for years walked on the beaches and hills of Hollywood; it kept her going during her strenuous Hollywood days. Lynn Fontanne, one of the most enduringly beautiful women, walks over the rolling hills on her Wisconsin farm. Marlene Dietrich, famous for her young legs, is a walker; even in New York she takes long walks in the park, sometimes with her grandchildren. Ingrid Bergman is another woman who walks, whether she is in Hollywood, Rome, or Paris, often with her children. I could go on endlessly with this list.

Be Sociable, Take a Walk!

Most walkers are sociable people who would like company if they could find it. A few years ago I discovered that a walking companion is not easy to find. Most of my friends would gladly come to my dinners, adorn my parties, drink any number of cocktails, soft or hard, and stay up until any hour; but few would go walking with me. I began to think that walking, like dieting, is a solo performance.

Then, one season in Paris, I made a contrary discovery. It was a particularly busy season. The popular magazine *Paris-Match* had given my work so much publicity that it seemed as though everyone wanted an appointment with me. I was beginning to feel like a prisoner in my office at No. 4, Rue Faubourg Saint Honoré, when an idea struck me. The Bois de Boulogne was not far. I began asking the people who wanted to see me to walk in the park with me.

They were surprised, to put it mildly, but they were too polite to refuse. And I discovered some expert walkers among my friends, and converted some to the society. Maurice Chevalier needed no introduction to walking; we took long walks down the Champs Elysée to the park. King Peter and Queen Alexandra were also confirmed walkers; we walked for miles in the woods of Versailles. Lovely Martine Carol, who had helped me sign autographs for enthusiastic fans, confessed that she loved walking in the Bois. When she got home she felt wonderfully relaxed, and her skin, as she put it, was "blooming."

We Need More Pleasant Walks

Perhaps you think I'm going overboard about walking, but I'm not. Walking preserves health and lengthens life. A New York physician said bluntly that half the patients in his waiting room could cure themselves of what ailed them if they would spend an hour walking every day. Walking cures tensions, insomnia, chronic fatigue, and a host of minor physical and mental complaints that drag down the spirit and body and take the joy out of living. Walking—free striding, free-swinging, rhythmic, unhurried and unharried walking—is the perfect aid to digestion, elimination, circulation, relaxation of body, mind, and spirit.

The next time you feel low, go out for a walk. Put on your most comfortable shoes. (See also page 213.) Walk with your head up, take long steps, let your arms swing freely and easily, and deepen your breathing. Keep a good rhythm—not necessarily fast, but steady. See how your mood changes, how the dark color of your thoughts becomes gradually brighter. Your low spirits will not accompany you very far on a good walk. Psychologists remind us again and again that the mind cannot remain depressed when the body is in motion.

Believe me, walking does do all this for you; and furthermore, it is a very special pleasure. Why do you suppose so many intelligent, gifted people, who could choose any recreation they like, enjoy walking? Because it is truly a sheer muscular joy.

SLEEP

Deep, sound sleep is a gift from heaven, and if you have it, give thanks, for nothing is as rejuvenating as a good night's rest. I hope that you are not in the habit of taking barbiturates. Figures show that more than 6,000,000 people in the United States are unwise enough to shorten their lives by taking these so-called "sleeping pills." Do not worry about sleeping; the more you worry, the more sleepless you become. It is a vicious circle that you create for yourself.

I know one famous movie star who worried all day long about not sleeping at night. She not only worried about it, but she talked about it endlessly. When night came, of course she could not sleep. I have no doubt that insomnia very often is caused by the *fear* of not sleeping. I have been able to help thousands (including the famous movie star) to acquire deep, sound sleep by teaching them to relax and by insisting on a diet rich in the foods which help to relax tense muscles and nerves.

Many food factors contribute to the relaxation that is necessary for sound sleep. The three most important, however, appear to be calcium, vitamin D, and vitamin B₆.

Vitamin B₆ seems to have a sedative effect on the nerves. It has even been used in the treatment of St. Vitus dance and palsy, with some apparent effect. In any case, it does seem to be essential to a healthy nervous system. Although some lesser-known vitamins of the B family have not as yet been definitely identified with specific deficiency diseases, they do seem to play a role in many deficiency conditions. For example, many of the nervous symptoms that remain after treatment with thiamine, riboflavin, and niacin respond rapidly to the administration of B₆. But B₆ is not found in many common foods. It is removed during the refining of grains, and is not added to "enriched" flour. To get adequate amounts of vitamin B₆ you must eat such foods as wheat germ, brewers' yeast, molasses, and liver—not occasionally, but often.

A lack of calcium can also be responsible for much sleeplessness. Every person, regardless of age, should get 1 gram of calcium daily. This can be obtained most easily from a quart of milk. This may be skim milk, buttermilk, or yogurt; the choice depends on your weight and on your own preference. Since calcium dissolves in acid, "soured" milks, such as buttermilk and yogurt, which contain lactic acid, supply calcium in a form more quickly and completely absorbed into the blood. Those milk drinks that have been advertised as conducive to sound sleep depend primarily on the calcium in the milk you make them with; it helps the nerves to relax and thus promotes sleep.

Although calcium is abundant in dairy products, it is found in very few other foods. Green leafy vegetables, for example, have calcium; but it is in an insoluble form that cannot pass into the blood. But a tablespoon of dark molasses supplies as much calcium as does half a glass of milk. A cup of hot milk with 2 teaspoons of the darkest molasses you can find is still one of my favorite "sleep cocktails." All meat dishes prepared with bone should include a little lemon, vinegar, tomato juice, yogurt, or cooking wine to help dissolve calcium from the bone and make it available. Many primitive peoples, such as Eskimos, get their entire calcium supply from eating bones.

Here in the United States some baby foods are now fortified with very fine bone flour. Let's hope that bone flour fortification soon will also be applied to foods for adults. Dr. Henry C. Sherman of Columbia University repeatedly stated that the need for calcium in adults does not decrease and the intake should be kept high.

Calcium cannot be efficiently absorbed and utilized without vitamin D. And vitamin D is found in only a few foods—vitamin D milk, certain fish, and that rare delicacy caviar. The best source is sunshine. If it is impossible for you to have a half-hour sunbath daily, get your vitamin D by taking cod-liver oil. (It comes in capsule form.)

Fresh skim milk fortified with dry skim milk powder also insures a rich supply of calcium. However, where a calcium deficiency is of long standing, nutritionists recommend calcium tablets with vitamin D. When the body is brought into positive calcium balance, the ability to sleep readily and soundly should follow.

Calcium tablets must never be considered a substitute for milk. The person whose health is so below par that he suffers from insomnia also needs the protein, vitamins, and minerals that dairy products supply; deficiencies do not occur singly.

For restful sleep, base your menus on this sample:

Breakfast: fruit or fruit juice; egg or whole-grain cereal with wheat germ; whole-wheat toast; milk or Swiss coffee—half hot coffee, half hot milk

Midmorning: buttermilk, yogurt, or skim milk flavored with molasses or cinnamon; plus 2 calcium tablets

Luncheon: fruit or vegetable salad with cottage cheese; milk, buttermilk, or yogurt; junket or custard

Midafternoon: a tablespoon of brewers' yeast stirred into tomato juice; plus 2 calcium tablets

Dinner: vegetable espresso or fruit cocktail; meat or broiled liver; 1 or 2 short-cooked vegetables; milk, buttermilk, or yogurt; fresh fruit or cheese with whole-wheat crackers

Before Retiring: hot milk drink, yogurt, or cheese and whole-wheat crackers; plus 2 calcium tablets

---

DEEP SLEEP NITE CAP

1 tbsp. powdered skim milk
2 tsp. molasses or honey
1 tsp. brewers' yeast
Stir into cup of warm milk and sip slowly.

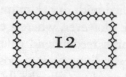

12

Keep Your Body Young

The heart is vastly too important to risk even the slightest neglect. If you have any symptoms of difficulty with it, rapid pulse or breathing, so-called palpitations, or tendencies toward faintness, or if the circulation in your extremities appears to be poor, you should go to your physician for a check-up. Much can be done today if heart conditions are treated early.

Your diet probably needs correcting. In any event, it should contain an abundance of all the B and E vitamins, plus calcium—and you may have to order your life a little differently for a period of time. But I admonish you, here and now, that prevention is vastly better than cure. So much can be done to prevent many conditions of ill health through good nutrition. When I see anyone eating unwisely, I ponder on the tragedy that may be in store for that individual, a tragedy that may be completely unnecessary.

If we plan to live a hundred years, we should do everything in our power to keep the heart and arteries young and the digestion at top performance.

HARDENING OF THE ARTERIES
(ARTERIOSCLEROSIS)

It must be understood that normal blood pressure varies constantly and can become unusually high during strenuous exercise, excitement, or emotional stress. Only in cases where the blood pressure remains abnormally high, year after year, should hardening of the arteries be suspected. Even then it must be remembered that there are people who live long and happy lives in spite of arteriosclerosis.

When the arteries become hard, they lose their elasticity. There is a condition of arteriosclerosis that is caused by an overgrowth on the outer layers, with an accompanying degeneration of the elastic layers. It is known as atherosclerosis, and is caused by faulty utilization of fats and certain substances associated with them, due to vitamin deficiency. When the arteries have become hard in this way, not only do they lose their elasticity, but they become smaller in diameter, ultimately being reduced to inadequate channels. Since the amount of blood in the circulatory system remains the same, the strain on the heart increases as the diameter of the plugged arteries decreases, and the blood pressure rises. You can illustrate this principle with a garden hose, by trying to force the same amount of water through a much smaller hose than would normally be used. Fatalities occur when the coronary arteries become sufficiently reduced in this way.

Until the present time, little could be done to stop this hardening process. Doctors and patients alike said, "Advancing age causes it. It might as well be accepted gracefully." Nowadays, however, the picture is changing. I, myself, have seen intelligent people put a halt to this process of hardening by following a low-fat diet, increasing their vitamin intake, and drinking freely of fresh green and yellow vegetable juices. I am delighted to report that the experimental work of Dr. Lester Morrison and others has been instrumental in finding the cause and developing the prevention and control of atherosclerosis.

In 1947 Dr. J. R. Moreton published his first study of arteriosclerosis. This work pointed to a fatty degeneration of the elastic tissues, which occurred when the fat content of the blood was high. Also, it was shown by Dr. J. W. Gofman that an overgrowth of the outer layer of the arteries occurs, and that it takes place when certain constituents of fats are circulated in the blood, as a result of fat in the diet. Then Drs. Moreton and Necheler demonstrated that when excessive quantities of cholesterol were fed to various animals, arteriosclerosis always followed promptly. And so a disease, a killing disease, was being tracked to its lair.

Now comes the dramatic news. Once the habitat of the "killer" was discovered, we learned how to set about getting him. And that way lay through diet—B vitamins! Drs. Steiner, Morrison, Rossi, Herrman, and others showed that nutritional hardening of the arteries could be prevented and even cured by the use of vitamins that *mobilize* fat, and its associated substances, and also accelerate its assimilation in the body. These three most important vitamins of the B family are choline, inositol, and pyridoxine (vitamin B_6).

We have known for a long time that diseases such as diabetes mellitus, nephrosis, myxedema (a species of dropsy), and a skin disorder called xanthomatosis (which appears as very small patches of connective tissue that has undergone fatty degeneration) all are associated with high blood fat, and frequently are accompanied by hardening of the arteries. Dr. Morrison recently offered evidence when he pointed out that the converse also is true—that in diseases accompanied by low blood fat, such as exophthalmic goiter, arteriosclerosis rarely occurs. Work in the laboratory brings forth more and more evidence. It shows that arteries hardened by excessive fatty matter in the blood display approximately the same composition of fatty matter as that circulating in the blood.

The eating habits of many countries give us further evidence. An examination of the diets of 18 countries shows a much higher occurrence of arteriosclerosis and heart trouble among those that consume a high fat diet.

Percentages of Fats Eaten (in Calories) in Diets of 18 Countries

Japan	8 percent	France	30 percent
South Africa	10	Holland	34
India	12	England	35
Turkey	13	Germany	36
Brazil	17	Switzerland	36
Portugal	19	Sweden	38
Italy	19	Australia	38
Spain	19	Canada	39
Greece	24	U.S.A.	41

One glance at the above list should convince anyone that one reason the U.S.A. leads in circulatory and heart troubles (the No.1

killer) is because we lead the world in excessive fat consumption, especially the hardened and hydrogenated kinds.

Of course there are other causes for the constant mounting of vascular diseases. Man really asked for trouble when he started to denude and refine the Staff of Life—our grains and bread. The throwing away of the wheat and other cereal germs, the richest source of vitamins B and E, parallels the increase in heart difficulties. Vitamins B and E probably lead all the other vitamins in nourishing the heart.

Some may question that there is a rise in arteriosclerosis, and say that it appears to be of greater occurrence because now it is better diagnosed. I refer them to health statistics. Such inquiry cannot stand up in the face of recorded facts.

It has been shown that atherosclerosis (arteriosclerosis caused by the faulty metabolism of fatty substances) can be prevented and cured through the administration of the B vitamins, choline and inositol, either with or without pyridoxine. Little courage is now called for to classify it as a dietary deficiency disease. I am going to ask you now to solemnly promise yourself that from this day forth you will take special pains to see that your diet contains generous amounts of choline and inositol—in fact, all the B vitamins, plus vitamin E, which according to the Doctors Shute in Canada has helped thousands of their patients, when taken regularly in large enough amounts.

Take the precaution of eating wisely, of natural foods, for that is good common sense. But, in being vigilant, do not jump to extremes. Many individuals have consumed normal amounts of fat and lived a long and vital life, with never a touch of arteriosclerosis—perhaps they always ate wisely! If you have the slightest suspicion that to any degree you may be tending toward hardening of the arteries, have an examination made of the state of fatty material in your blood. But be sure to have a reliable examination made.

There is a popular idea that the test depends upon a determination of the total cholesterol in your blood. That is not at all the proper index. It is the state of cholesterol in what is called the "lipoprotein complex" that is the criterion. There is no correlation between the total amount of cholesterol in your blood and the state of the cholesterol in the lipoprotein complex. There are three good tests. That of Dr. John W. Gofman requires rather elaborate apparatus and a team of skilled workers; but I find it the most reliable test, and it is recommended by more and more doctors. If you are at all worried, and wonder whether you are a candidate for a heart attack, I suggest you have your doctor send a sample of your blood directly to the Institute of Medical Physics in Belmont, California. They are a serious and nonprofit organization. After making your blood analysis, they will inform you whether or not you're prone to a heart attack. There also are simpler tests; those of Dr. Morrison and Dr. Killmer can be carried out in any properly equipped clinic.

Once your doctor has confirmed that your blood contains too many lipoproteins, you should be guided in your diet by the following:

1. Go easy on high cholesterol foods; avoid especially hard animal fats and rich cream.
2. Use the golden vegetable oils in place of hard fats for salads and for cooking.
3. Increase your protein intake to 100 grams daily.
4. Cut down on carbohydrates and use only the unrefined variety.
5. Reduce fat to not more than 20 to 25 grams daily and use cold-pressed vegetable oils.
6. To compensate for the vitamin A loss due to omitting animal fat, use other vitamin A and E foods generously.
7. Be sure that the diet supplies ample quantities of vitamin B₆, choline, and inositol. When choline and inositol are taken together they heighten each other's effect; as means of therapy, 3 grams of choline and 1.5 grams of inositol should be taken daily. When therapeutic measures are called for, it is advisable to take these vitamins in the pure form, immediately after meals; your doctor can supply you with these in capsule form.

Even if your physician gives you a clean bill of health as regards atherosclerosis, you should still take precautions. Everyone can profit from a diet which supplies generous quantities of choline, inositol, and pyridoxine. Wheat germ, brewers' yeast, and whole-wheat flour are rich in choline. Egg yolk, which is the richest source, is unfortunately also high in cholesterol. For inositol, heart muscle is the richest source, then brewers' yeast, the whole cereal grains, liver, and milk. Rich sources of pyridoxine are brewers' yeast and rice bran concentrate.

HEART TROUBLE AND THE DIET

The general well-being of your heart depends largely on the food you eat. If that statement startles you, let me tell you why it should not. The muscles of the heart are continuously at work every moment that you live. The energy demanded by the heart is very great, both in amount and in the rate at which it is required. From your diet you must get the food factors—the vitamins—necessary for energy exchanges in the body. As an example, let us take vitamin B_1 deficiency. When the supply of vitamin B_1 is not adequate, many disturbances occur in the utilization of food for the production of energy, and this disturbs many tissues of the body. Nervous tissues are affected because they can utilize only carbohydrates which must be prepared for them by other tissues of the body. The heart muscles are particularly affected because of their high and critical energy demand. Anything that disturbs the fundamental metabolism of the body, as deficiency of most B vitamins does, must in some degree affect the heart. Therefore, I say that unless we select our diets with care, heart disease will remain a scourge.

So many everyday foods do not supply you with a generous amount of B vitamins. Here is where you can turn to the wonder foods for help. One cup of yogurt, two tablespoons of brewers' yeast, one-half cup of wheat germ, and one-half cup of dried skim milk, together give seven times the vitamin B_1, twice the vitamin B_2, and 130 percent of the niacin necessary (on the basis of the dietary allowances of the National Research Council) for a moderately active person.

Not only do you get vitamins B_1, B_2, and niacin, but also choline, inositol, vitamin B_6, pantothenic acid, and other B vitamins too. Natural foods that are particularly rich in any of the B vitamins generally contain virtually the entire B family. That is why

I picked certain foods and called them wonder foods. (See page 33.) We know now that many of the B vitamins work together rather than, as was once thought, in a sharply specific manner. Not all of the accompanying symptoms of the classic niacin deficiency disease, pellagra, are helped by the administration of niacin alone; riboflavin and pantothenic acid also are needed. That is why brewers' yeast achieved such outstanding success in the treatment of pellagra. Moreover, rarely is there a deficiency of only one B vitamin. If you wish, you may take capsules that give you thiamine (vitamin B_1), riboflavin (vitamin B_2), and niacin, even those that add a little pyridoxine (vitamin B_6) and pantothenic acid. But my advice is to also eat the B-vitamin-rich foods such as brewers' yeast and wheat germ. Had this practice been followed, many of us would have obtained choline and inositol in more adequate amounts, and it is more than a probability that there would be less arteriosclerosis. But in our enthusiasm for "pure" vitamins and our tendency to ignore natural products, and because clear-cut deficiency conditions were not identified with the "lesser" B vitamins, we paid them little attention. I am prepared, always, to believe in natural foods, to which man has been adapted for countless generations; if I do no more for my students than passing this secret along to them, I will be well satisfied.

(For a discussion of the role of vitamin E and the heart, see page 54.)

Now let us go back to the subject of the prevention of heart troubles. Intelligent eating is one of the essentials, and unless we take to intelligent eating, I predict that heart troubles will increase. We have discussed hardening of the arteries and shown quite clearly that it can result from a poor diet. Hardened arteries lead to high blood pressure and to heart trouble. A sound, well-balanced diet is fundamental to the well-being of your heart, and intelligent eating is the cornerstone of the Look Younger, Live Longer way of life.

Your heart muscles, like every other muscle in the body, are composed principally of protein. Once it was believed, by physician and layman alike, that with heart trouble one should reduce the proteins in the diet. The opposite is now known to be true. Even in conditions of heart failure, when considerable fluids collect in the tissues, a high-protein and low-salt diet is prescribed.

But once heart trouble has set in, the advice of your physician is essential to a proper diagnosis and plan of treatment best suited to the particular, individual condition. Since I have stressed the importance of vitamins, especially vitamin B, so much you will be interested in what the famous Dr. William Brady, M.D., has to say:

The real heart tonic I recommend can do no harm and may do considerable good not only for the heart and circulation but for the digestion and nerves as well. It is not medicine at all. It is my same old remedy, simply food; food which every child or adult needs to maintain good digestion and good circulation but which few children or adults get in adequate proportions because of our ultrarefined diet. It is vitamin B complex, an optimal, daily ration of it.

"A man is as old as his arteries" is an old and true saying, for hardened arteries lead to heart trouble and all its possible consequences. But nutritional science has pointed a way to keep arteries young through diet. Young arteries, and a heart that is young both physically and emotionally, are essential to the Look Younger, Live Longer way of living. Eat intelligently to keep them young.

VITAMIN P AND YOUR CAPILLARIES

If you want firm gums, strong, supple, and pliant connective tissue, and reasonable freedom from bruising, you should have a generous supply of vitamin C in your diet. Vitamin C is essential to the formation of collagen, the substance that cements the cells together into firm tissues. A lack of vitamin C causes the capillaries to become fragile and bruises to form with only slight injury. All conditions of bruising, however, are not caused by vitamin C deficiency. That was discovered very early in the development of vitamin C. When first the relationship between vitamin C and fragile capillaries was discovered, the hopes of medical men were raised that a cure for the dreaded disease of hemophilia had been found. (This disease recognizes no rank or station. It is hereditary, being transmitted only through the female line, and has afflicted many of the royal families of Europe.) However, those hopes soon were dashed. When the Hungarian scientist Szent-Gyorgyi isolated a factor from peppers that made the capillaries less permeable (able to be passed through), again hopes were raised, and again dashed.

The cause and cure of hemophilia remain elusive to science, but the discovery of Szent-Gyorgyi was not useless. It promises results that were little suspected at the time, when the need for them did not exist—Szent-Gyorgyi's discovery may quite possibly lessen certain effects of atomic bomb explosions! The factor which Szent-Gyorgyi discovered is now known as vitamin P, not because it was first isolated from peppers, but for its effect in decreasing the permeability of the capillaries; it was originally called the antipermeability vitamin.

Capillary fragility and capillary permeability are entirely different. Fragile capillaries are easily ruptured; highly permeable capillaries pass considerably more fluid in a given time than is normal. Although vitamin P is given together with vitamin C in the treatment of scurvy, and appears to aid the progress of the cure, any relationship between these two vitamins is thought to be remote.

Vitamin P belongs to a family of plant substances called the *flavonoids*. They occur in the peel of citrus fruits and in black currants; one active principle, called rutin, occurs in buckwheat. The flavonoids have come in for considerable research recently, and can now be obtained in concentrated form.

Now to return to the profound discovery stemming from Szent-Gyorgyi's original work. Research carried on at a well-known Florida college has led scientists to believe that vitamin P may well prove to be effective protection against secondary irradiation injury following atom bomb explosions. When atom bombs were dropped over Hiroshima and Nagasaki, many of the victims subsequently died of hemorrhage, following exposure to so-called sublethal irradiation intensities. Vitamin P appears to give protection against such hemorrhagic conditions.

Demonstrations with laboratory animals indicate that whereas the mortality rate in exposed animals not receiving vitamin P was 80 percent, the mortality rate in animals identically exposed to irradiation, but previously given vitamin P over a period of time, was only 10 percent.

What this may mean in terms of human life remains to be proved.

Should vitamin P be effective with humans, the lethal range of the atom bomb will become considerably lessened.

Digestive Disturbances

The best insurance of freedom from digestive disturbances is the eating of a sound, well-balanced diet composed of natural, unrefined foods—living foods that have not been destroyed by processing.

The diet must give you proteins that contain the essential amino acids, along with vitamins, especially the B vitamins, needed by the enzymes that digest the food. B vitamins maintain the tone of the digestive tract, the stomach and intestines. You need sound teeth to chew thoroughly the food you eat, and for your teeth's sake you need vitamin C and calcium.

You need hydrochloric acid in your stomach to act with the enzymes in order to digest the proteins completely. People who are addicted to the baking soda "relief," the constant "alkalizers," are making the mistake of helping to produce the very trouble they hope to avoid. Gas pains, more frequently than not, are caused simply by air that has been swallowed. Air swallowing is a pernicious habit. Gum chewing is conducive to air swallowing. Many of us swallow copious quantities of air when we drink beverages; you chronic gas sufferers, try drinking through a straw, and you will be amazed at your freedom from gas.

The crime of crimes is to eat while you are doing something else or while you are under any kind of tension. The stomach works hard on the food you put into it—it has to churn it about and turn it over and over. Nerve tension makes the stomach relatively rigid—spastic. If you want it to work efficiently for you, relax.

Do not discuss annoying subjects at the table. Do not fight with the children. The less attention you pay to them, the better they will eat. Wait until the meal is over and your husband sinks into the comforting lethargy of digestion to tell him about the new hat or fur coat you just bought. Give him a chance to relax; he needs it. And you men, do not discuss business over the luncheon table. Let lunch time be a period of social intercourse with your business associates, relaxed and at ease. You get to know each other better that way and establish a friendlier relationship than by spending the same precious few minutes talking about disturbing business matters. You will live longer and more comfortably for it.

And, Mrs. Housewife, make your family meals seem like social gatherings. Tempt appetites with good food freshly prepared, and with an attractively set and decorated table. At meal times members of your family can get to know each other as interesting people, and can be helpful to one another through quiet, reasonable conversation. Banish worry and contention from your dining room and profit from relaxed meal times.

Eat at your leisure, relaxed and in a contented frame of mind. Eat serenely and slowly. Food bolters deserve indigestion, and fast eating is one crime that almost invariably is promptly punished. Chew your food, divide it very finely, give the stomach juices opportunity to penetrate. When you eat, do not include great volumes of air. Drink slowly; do not gulp. No, this is not Emily Post speaking, but good table manners are good health manners too.

Intestinal Gardening

Some doctors believe that half of humanity's ailments come from the intestinal canal. Metchnikoff, the Russian bacteriologist, was the first to tell the world that within the gastro-intestinal canal there are millions of bacteria, some friendly and some unfriendly. Under the microscope these bacteria look rather like flowers, and that's why we speak of the intestinal flora. It was also Metchnikoff who first discovered that through bad eating habits most people encourage the unfriendly flora and thereby suffer from digestive difficulties, excessive gas, and constipation.

Biochemists were able to prove that certain foods are especially helpful to feed the friendly flora. For successful intestinal gardening, all milk products are recommended; but speedier results are obtained from foods containing the lactobacillus acidophilus and bulgaricus. These are found in fermented acidophilus milk and yogurt, and also in certain kinds of cottage cheese. For those who are unable to use these milk products, whey powder or whey tablets, derived from fermented milk and in cheese-making, are highly recommended. They definitely feed the friendly bacteria and help to make you a successful intestinal gardener.

LAZY ELIMINATION

"A man whose bowels move regularly and normally will live very long," said Herodicus of Selymbria. That observation, made before the Christian era began, holds true to this day. Physicians have long noted that health and longevity are connected with the condition of the alimentary tract. Centenarians, who usually enjoy excellent digestion, often attribute a great deal of their longevity to the healthy functioning of the entire intestinal tract.

Is your elimination lazy—or are you lazy about it? "Obey that impulse" is one of the best possible prescriptions for constipation. Pressure in the rectum is the body's signal to defecate, and the body is very imperious in such matters. It makes a forthright request, even gives you fair warning; if you do not heed it, the body metes out its punishment—constipation. People feel the command, but they do not always obey; they may be reading or just sitting comfortably, or they may be engaged in some task, minor or major, so they put it off. What happens? Precisely this: The rectum being full, a pressure has been exerted on the nerve endings, causing a feeling of the need to defecate. If you put it off, the pressure remains, but the nerve endings become overstimulated; fatigue sets in, and they no longer react. You lose the signal, the urge. You forget it, and constipation results. Had you obeyed the impulse with reasonable promptness when the whole series of connections governing the reactions necessary to defecation were connected up on the body's switchboard and ready to go into action, a normal, comfortable, and satisfying evacuation would have occurred. But there was no response, so all of the connections went dead. Failure to "obey that impulse" is probably responsible for more constipation than any other single cause.

Constipation, sufficiently prolonged, can become chronic and can lead to physical injury to the rectum, ultimately producing hemorrhoids. One of the functions of the colon is to retain water and allow it to be absorbed back into the body. When food wastes remain too long in the colon, they are robbed of much of their water content, and the stools become relatively dry and hard. In that form it is difficult for the normal rhythmic waves of the colon's walls to propel them along toward the exit. Moreover, when they do reach the rectum, they are discharged from the body with difficulty, and mechanical injury frequently results. The entire process is accompanied by a considerable degree of discomfort to the victim, both mental and physical.

Good habits can do much to improve evacuations. Regularity in habits induces regularity in bowel movement. Many conditions of chronic constipation have been relieved through "training." If one creates the conditions conducive to evacuation, regularly, every day, at the same time, preferably on arising in the morning, sooner or later the bowels will respond and continue to do so with most satisfying regularity. Sit comfortably, relax, do not strain, and give the bowels a real chance.

When you first get up in the morning, drink a glass of lukewarm water to which a half teaspoonful of vegetable salt has been added. This drink, on striking the empty stomach, arouses the reflexes and sets peristaltic waves in motion throughout the intestinal canal. If the bowels then are given an opportunity, evacuation generally follows. Moreover, the addition of the salt prevents the water from being absorbed before it reaches the colon where it is useful in maintaining the food wastes in a moist and plastic condition. Patience is required at the start to train the bowels to regularity, but the result is satisfying; you will be rewarded over and over again, for the rest of your long life.

Too many people become addicts of laxatives early in life, partly because of clever advertising and partly because of bad habits and laziness. Children are fed laxatives by intestine-minded mothers from the earliest age. Small wonder, then, that the natural function of bowel movement, which works like a clock *without artificial interference* and is well able to take care of its small disturbances, becomes degenerated in more and more adults.

A daily bowel movement, or even two, is a sign of good intestinal health, and don't let anybody tell you differently. If the diet supplies appreciable quantities of bulkage, derived from vegetables and fruits, there will be more waste reaching the colon, and the movements may be more frequent.

A diet lacking in bulk leaves little for the colon to work on, and the stools become dry, hard, difficult to pass; constipation results. This type of constipation can be quite discomforting. It is the typical constipation of the white flour, refined sugar, meat and potato eater. The introduction of vegetables, fruits, and a daily salad should suffice to rid you of this condition.

The B vitamins are essential for the maintenance of the normal tone of the intestinal tract. The simple inclusion of the wonder foods in the diet will give you a sufficiency of them. But the colon requires a reasonable quantity of bulkage, too. The salad bowl, colored vegetables, and fruits answer that purpose, in addition to giving you a rich supply of vitamins and minerals. There is no substitute for vital eating; hardly a function of the body can be considered fully without reference to it. A man can be only as good as his digestive tract, for he can use only what he takes out of it— and he can take out of it only what he puts into it! Again, we return to the very wellspring of life—the diet.

There are circumstances that can induce temporary constipation, even in the most regular. Then the question arises as to what to do. First, do not jump to the conclusion that you need a laxative. Give Nature a chance; she may correct herself. Mineral oil and products containing it are undesirable. This oil is wholly undigestible, and it robs the intestines of the oil-soluble vitamins A, D, E, and K.

Best Laxative Foods

Food Yeast is a natural laxative because it is so rich in B vitamins. By all means add a teaspoon of good-tasting dry yeast to fruit juice, tomato juice, milk, and other beverages. Use it daily and be generous with it.

Dark Molasses is one of the finest natural laxatives of all times, as our grandmothers knew. Their favorite spring tonic was old-fashioned molasses and sulphur. We no longer need to take this evil-tasting combination; the sulphur we get in young radishes, celery, and green peppers, and the molasses, the darkest you can buy, can be mixed with all sorts of foods and used in place of empty white sugar.

Honey is another natural laxative. It is so mild that pediatricians recommend it for babies. An interesting combination is honey and molasses, half and half; it provides both vitamins and iron. Thousands of my students enthusiastically use this honey-lass combination for all sweetening purposes.

Yogurt, besides being a delicious food, is also helpful in cases of faulty elimination. The bacteria in this cultured milk utilize the sugar in milk and convert it into beneficial lactic acid. Milk sugar also helps to make soft bulky stools which are passed with great facility. The friendly bacteria of yogurt also synthesize the B vitamins so important to good elimination.

Wheat Germ is by far the most valuable of all cereals for its vitamin and protein content, and is also a natural laxative par excellence. When you use the fresh and vital kind, available at your health food store, such "live" wheat germ, sprinkled freely on your morning cereal or into fruit juice, makes a fine self-starter for lazy bowels.

Quick Salt Water Flush. This efficient flush is recommended by Dr. E. V. McCollum of Johns Hopkins, and also by Dr. Victor Heiser, author of *An American Doctor's Odyssey.* Simply add two rounded teaspoons of salt to a quart of very warm water and drink the whole quart on an empty stomach the first thing in the morning. In about thirty minutes a copious flushing will result. Be sure not to eat breakfast until after you have flushed. For a more pleasant-tasting quick flush, many of my students put three level teaspoons of vegetable salt into a quart of very warm water and drink the entire quart. Such a flushing, taken occasionally, is harmless, and thousands swear by it. It should not be taken habitually, however, because the water-soluble vitamins are also flushed away.

Natural Herbs. Following a highly nutritious diet should automatically banish constipation. The ideal way is to get along without any special help. But for those who for some reason are not eating intelligently, and therefore suffer from occasional constipation, instead of synthetic laxatives, pink pills, or oils, I recommend a combination of dried, natural herbs which I discovered in Switzerland. It is as natural a formula as I could find and is made up of 17 crushed herbs. Thousands of pounds of these herbs were formerly imported from Switzerland; but since this formula became such a phenomenal success, it is now made here. So, if you must use a laxative occasionally, try this Swiss formula. It is obtainable at all health and diet shops and drug stores.

Swiss Vinegar-Milk Tonic. For upset stomach or for lack of digestive juices, thousands of Swiss swear by their *Essig-Milch* drink. Cider vinegar or wine vinegar can be used. (In Switzerland they add herbs.) Simply put 1 tablespoon of vinegar into 4 table-spoons of buttermilk or skim milk and drink it down.

Laxative Home Brew. A delightful and very effective laxative tea can be made by brewing a level teaspoon of Swiss Kriss herbs in a large cup of water. Let water come to a boil and add the herbs. Turn off the heat; let stand for three minutes, and strain. Add a teaspoon of honey and a few drops of lemon. (Do not boil, or the tea becomes *too* laxative.) When feeling bloated after eating too much, a cup of this mild laxative tea brings amazing relief.

Strengthen the Abdominal Muscles

For even better results, I suggest you strengthen your inner and outer stomach and intestinal muscles with the laziest and best exercise in the world—the Stomach Lift (see page 175). Doing this muscle-tension exercise two minutes each day can strengthen and flatten a protruding abdomen; and, as the muscles regain their elasticity, lazy elimination becomes a thing of the past.

A generally run-down condition, flaccid muscles, general lack of tone in the intestinal tract are frequently accompanied by constipation. But as the diet is improved, with emphasis on the B vitamins, the general health will in turn be improved and constipation eliminated.

Bear in mind that, in longevity tests, the spriest oldsters are always those who have maintained normal, natural daily elimination. At the St. Louis Clinic, among 200 men and women who had reached the fourscore mark, it was discovered that *all* had normal daily elimination.

And while on the subject of better elimination, I would like to point out that the water closets in our elegant bathrooms belong to antiquity. Our plumbers and anatomists should get together to design a water closet that conforms to human needs. Nothing is so conducive to an easy bowel movement as the squatting position, and I see no reason why the water closet of the future cannot be designed and built so that the squatting position is automatically assumed.

Such a water closet need not be as unattractive as the old-fashioned contraptions in France and Japan (where you *must* squat whether you like to or not). I believe it could be simply and effectively designed to be lower at the back, thus permitting definite elevation of the knees. Until such time as that may be, many wise people have adopted the use of bathroom stools about ten inches high, on which to rest the feet during eliminations. This lifts the knees, bringing the thighs close to the abdominal muscles, and approximates the natural squatting position. I believe that the installation of properly designed water closets, anatomically correct, would be of immense help in banishing constipation.

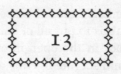

13

Be Happier, Be Healthier

Happiness depends on prevention of the setting up of beachheads by enemies that will make us unhappy. Health requires the prevention of invasion by enemies that will undermine health.

Are you saving your troubles for a rainy day? If so, you will find that it won't rain—it will pour. You won't have a gentle shower of trouble; you'll have a deluge. The best way to have trouble is a little at a time. Space it out. Take it easy. It would be nice if we could have all repairs and corrections attended to at one time, and gotten over, once and for all. But it doesn't work that way.

To be happier and to be healthier, you must be aware of your assets and liabilities. You must look at yourself, you must recognize yourself for what you are, not what you were, or what you would like to be. Candor begins in your own mind. You must cease playing ostrich with yourself. Knowledge, even knowledge of your liabilities, is power.

A physical inventory of your present condition is a *must*.

The point of departure for objectivity and maturity is this very moment.

You have but one body; you will never have another. Do you care for it, do you know it, do you understand it? As you have seen, you are a most miraculous organization of bones, cartilage, muscle, nerves, glands, fluids, organs, and flesh. No one part of your body is independent of any other part. You are a whole, composed of interrelated and interdependent parts.

Now I want you to go on a tour of inspection of your own body. The reason for doing this is to put all of your worries, uncertainties, concerns, and queries out in the open in one place where you can see them, admit them, and act intelligently about them.

Knowledge of your body should give you confidence and make you proud. The chances are that you are worrying about one or two little things, when there are a hundred reasons why you should be happy.

I am not suggesting that you play doctor with yourself. What I do want you to do is to make up your own mind, fairly and fearlessly, as to whether or not there are conditions and circumstances that should be referred to your physician. But I also want you to make a physical inventory of your assets and liabilities. There are little things you can do to increase your efficiency, improve your appearance, enhance your attractiveness. I want you to pass before yourself in review. I want you to do for yourself what every businessman does for his bank, and for his directors and stockholders. You will be on the lookout for habits that could, and possibly should, be improved. You will admit weakness when you come to it. From the top of your head to the tips of your toes, you are going to examine yourself with the fine comb of objectivity.

A SMALL LIST OF MOST IMPORTANT THINGS

Begin with your scalp, your hair, your complexion, your ears, eyes, nose, teeth, tongue. Look at them. Feel them. Think about them. If they satisfy you, if you are happy about them, if they function as nature intended they should, forget them. But if you find cause for concern, take that concern to your family physician. He alone is qualified to help you with any medical problem.

Let me give you a list to go by, and do not try to fool yourself. Don't skip an item. You are not to diagnose causes and prescribe cures; you are to consider conditions; you are to decide if there is anything that should be diagnosed by an expert.

Scalp	Nose
Hair	Mouth
Ears	Teeth
Eyes	Lips

Tongue	Legs
Throat	Knees
Arms	Feet
Hands	Toes
Fingers	Lungs
Chest	Heart
Breasts	Brain
Stomach	Liver
Reproductive organs	Kidneys
Rectum	Intestines

I would now call your attention, briefly but firmly, to certain inevitable and wholly natural circumstances that must be faced. Defecation, urination, menstruation, perspiration, and respiration are all accompanied by odors. Personal hygiene is in large part the constant vigilance of cleanliness that keeps these odors below the threshold of olfactory consciousness. Success is best achieved and insured by the daily bath. We need only recognize that the entire body breathes and, under conditions of exercise, heat, and humidity, perspires, to realize the necessity for keeping outer clothes, as well as underclothes, clean.

Now I can hear you say to yourself, "Is that what Gayelord Hauser calls a self-examination?" The answer is "Yes, it is." But don't jump to the conclusion that this is something you can do in five minutes and forget about. On the contrary, this is something you should do for the rest of your life. Periodically, just as you have regular check-ups with your family physician, so also should you check yourself up to see if your body is serving you the way you want it to, and if you are serving your body the way it needs.

You have two jobs. One is to tend to your body—to feed it, to guard it, to see that it is kept in good repair—to see, even, that it is improved. The second job is to see that your mind is constantly accomplishing more—extracting from the wonderful world in which we live, more happiness.

To maintain and improve our bodies we must eat better, more intelligently, and—as occasion arises—obtain the assistance of a physician. But to obtain the profits of accomplishment, you are on your own. Eternal vigilance and endeavor is the price of happiness. You cannot obtain it with the body alone, or with the mind alone. Happiness is the product of the cooperation of both. The healthy body will give maximum aid to the mind, and the mature mind will give maximum aid to the body. Together, never alone or individually, these will enable your whole self to get somewhere, to do things, to accomplish feats that add up to happiness.

Until the matter of health, though, is reduced to intelligent habit, we must concentrate on it, on our physical selves. And until the matter of maturity is reduced to intelligent habit, we must concentrate on that too, on our mental and psychological selves. But once these habits have been established, once intelligent eating has become an easy habit, once maturity has displaced immaturity, then we can forget about our separate selves and operate as whole humans for the increase of the happiness that comes from accomplishments achieved by bodies and minds operating as a well organized team.

Learn the habits that will make you the happiest possible human being. Once that is done, or once you have established habits that lead in that direction, then a whole new world of pleasure awaits you—the pleasure that comes from the doing of things with the instant and enthusiastic cooperation of both body and mind.

My interest in the human body is not in terms of conditions that should be referred to the best doctors you can obtain, but rather things, concerns, and matters that do not usually come within the domain of medical men. I am interested in happiness and health, in pleasure, beauty, in accomplishment, in the joy that comes from the whole use of the whole body, in those things, big and little, that make for comfort. My interest in the human body has to do with its contribution to the health of the mind, and the happiness of the whole man and woman, to making us more human. We must remember, we must never forget, that a healthy body contributes to a healthy mind, that a mature mind makes a healthier body, and that these two together make for happiness. This is the counterpoint of nature.

What's Normal?

Are you a normally active person? If you are, and you are over the age of twenty-five, then you should be reducing your food intake. According to Dr. Josef Brozek, of the University of Minnesota

Laboratory of Physiological Hygiene, people, beginning at twenty-five, should eat 7½ percent less each decade.

But what is a normally active person?

People, especially nutritionists, talk about activity a great deal, but seldom does anybody do anything about it, or at least anything that would make it possible to define it more accurately or measure it. Presumably, a normally active person is one who expends less energy than an unusually active one, and more than an unusually inactive one. Activity is movement. Inactivity is immobility. But while there is life there is no such thing as complete inactivity. A certain amount of energy is required to run the body even of a completely paralyzed person. On the other hand, the most active person would presumably be one who worked around the clock, without any rest or sleep. Needless to say, such activity would not last very long. Rest is necessary as a restorative and revivifier. But in between complete activity and complete inactivity, presumably half way between, the normally active person will find himself.

He sleeps, say, eight hours a day. He sits down during three daily meals for an average of thirty minutes a meal. He sits down while he works—let us assume an eight-hour working day, or for maybe 75 percent of that time. He sits down, if he is lucky, while he is going to and coming from work—say three quarters of an hour each way. He sits down after dinner, for an hour. Possibly he works in the garden, or around the house, for an hour a day. The rest of the time he is standing or walking. That means that for 5½ hours a day, plus the hour of work at home, say 6½ hours a day, the normally active person is on his feet. The rest of the time he is lying down or is seated. It means he does more sitting than anything else. He is in bed for eight hours. He is in a chair for nine and a half hours. He is on his feet for six and a half hours.

This has been stated another way:

Life is divided into three parts:
One-third on your feet,
One-third in bed, and
One-third on your seat.

BEDS, CHAIRS, AND SHOES

Surely, beds, chairs, and shoes are important things, if for no other reason than that we spend all of our lives in one or the other of them, unless we sometimes go barefoot, as I believe we should do more, especially on our holidays. Going barefoot on a sandy beach or on soft green grass lifts not only one's arches but also one's drooping spirits.

Consider the bed you sleep in, the chairs you sit in, and the shoes you walk and stand in. Don't forget, you spend a third of your life in bed. But when I say *in* it I mean *on* it. Because your bed should not be a *sinker*. Maximum refreshment comes from sleeping on a bed that is soft, but not so soft as to prohibit easy movement. On the other hand, I do not believe your bed should be as hard as a board.

I offer for free a million-dollar idea to the manufacturers of beds: make one with some sort of contraption at the bottom to which the Yoga Slant board can be attached, and make some provision under the bed for storing it when it is not in use. Further, sell beds equipped with Yoga Slant boards—everybody should have one.

And finally, because I am myself one of the tall fellows, I think foot-boards should be done away with. They do little good, serve little purpose except to irk tall people and prevent them from getting a full measure of rest and repose.

Sleep with open windows. And don't forget that better breathing habits, consciously learned, will benefit the whole body while you slumber. If, as Doctors Hofhauer, Schmidt, Douglas, Behr, and Professor Tirala all say, breathing can have curative effects, and they tell of the splendid results they have obtained, then you, by learning to breath better, can be taking a cure while you sleep.

The person who is a success in the business world is still a failure if his eyes do not close when he gets into bed at the end of the day, if his mind does not relax, and his conscious does not give way to his subconscious. This is one of the great tragedies of civilization —that people who work hard, who are good and virtuous and productive, cannot sleep.

Think of the devices that have been invented and are marketed for the exploitation of such unfortunates. There are pills. There are blinders to keep out the light, and stopples for the ears to keep out the noise. There are pillows of various shapes and compositions —pillows of rubber, of kapok, of cotton, of feathers. There are thick pillows and thin ones. There are boards to bolster failing backs. There are patented mattresses and scientific springs. There are sheep to be counted and night-caps to be consumed. There are air-conditioning units, temperature controls, and humidity regulators. There are electric blankets—which should be used only by oldsters who are too feeble to create their own warmth. There are night-clothes that are short, that are long, that have strings around the middle or have elastic bands. There are pullover tops and button-tops. There are hot baths and hot-water bottles. We cannot get along without sleep, but I cannot believe there is any sleep that compares with a natural one. The happy mind and the healthy body will have little use for any of these sleep inducers. But if there is sleep trouble, then I must recommend that you also change to a High Vitality diet, and learn to relax from head to toe (see page 169).

CHAIRS FOR THE HEART AND CHAIRS FOR THE EMOTIONS

I am often asked about contour chairs, and I always say that anything that enables people to obtain necessary rest is good. There can be no question but that these chairs serve a very excellent purpose, but I do wish they were neither so expensive, nor so ugly. (However, you *can* afford a Yoga Slant board, and, personally, I much prefer them.)

We are not only a nation of sitters, we are a nation of spectators. We sit and watch organized sports and entertainment, and we sit and listen to the radio and to speeches. Television, it seems to me, presents a particularly difficult problem. When one goes to a prize fight, or wrestling match, or ball game, one is constantly jumping up and down, squirming, and shouting. One becomes stimulated emotionally, and lets off that emotional steam by par-ticipating, vicariously but still quite actively, in the competition.

But at home, watching television, this letting off of emotional steam is quite lacking. One tends to sit passively and let emotion build up. One stews in his own emotional juices, and this only means that something is bound to happen to you. It would be much better if the family behaved the way the crowd does at the game. They might turn off the set feeling a little tired, but at least they wouldn't go to bed overloaded with powerful chemicals.

By all means watch television, but don't forget to take a good brisk walk after you have seen a particularly exciting contest. The person who doesn't work off his surplus emotional energy is sitting on a powder keg, and sooner or later it will blow up.

And talking of sitting, I would like to know whatever happened to the rocking chair. I shall never forget the first time I saw a rocking chair. I was fascinated by it. In my home in a little town in the Black Forest, I had never seen such a thing. But of course no Europeans knew anything about rocking chairs; they are, you know, an American invention, and a wonderful one. How good it is to sit after dinner, the mother in one and the father in another, rocking away gently while reading, and vigorously while talking. That used to be the standard way of putting a child to sleep. The mother would sit at her spinning wheel, or in her rocking chair, giving the cradle a gentle push with her foot. Such motion is stimulating as well as soothing. It is this principle that is used in connection with oscillating beds that are so beneficial and healthful. We may laugh at the rise of technology and some of the things that it produces, but there are many people in hospitals who can tell you how wonderful a rocking bed can be.

The rocking chair is essentially the same thing, and I would like to start a one-man movement to bring them back. Perhaps President John F. Kennedy has already done this. Certainly the publicizing of the rocking chair in his White House office has stimulated interest in them. I would like to see two rocking chairs in every home, one for Father and one for Mother. They ought to be wonderful for looking at television.

As a matter of fact, though bosses do not like it, the business of putting one's feet on the desk while talking is first rate, as far as the body is concerned. It just seems to be human nature to try and get the feet up in the air, and even women, when they wear slacks, seem to revert to this practice.

But please don't forget that if you sit all day at a desk, and come home tired, the chances are that it is mental and emotional fatigue that has gotten you down, and sitting around for the rest of the evening isn't going to help you much. What you need is a little physical exercise, not more mental and emotional activity. Take a walk. (See page 183.)

Pity Your Poor Feet

Less than twenty years ago, Alan E. Murray had foot trouble. He had corns, calluses, hammer toes, and collapsed metatarsals. He has plaster casts of his feet to prove it. Today, his feet are paragons of perfection, and he will take his shoes and stockings off to prove it. But the shoes that he takes off are most unusual. They are called "space shoes," and people like Arthur Godfrey, Garbo, Lillian Gish, Joe DiMaggio, and Martha Graham, together with 25,000 others, not only wear them, but swear by them. And they cost more than fifty dollars a pair.*

Murray had been a skater, but his feet deteriorated so much he had to give it up. Then he tried to obtain relief and correction. Nothing and no one helped him. So, being the kind of man he is, he set about making a pair of shoes for himself. He believed then, and he now has evidence to prove his point, that just as feet are deformed or distorted by shoes, so can they be corrected by them.

Mr. Murray's theory is to fit the shoes to the feet, not the feet to a space that is available after every concession has been made to the outside form that convention demands. So he fits the inside of the shoe to the foot, and lets the outside come where it may, which makes walking in space shoes like walking on air.

These shoes are expensive. But for those who can afford them, I consider them a highly worthwhile investment in good looks, good health, and good temper.

And here is great news, in tune with our do-it-yourself days: Mr. Murray has now made a do-it-yourself kit. You can make your own, with no special shoemaker's skill, at a fraction of the cost. I urge you to make yourself a pair of space shoes and enjoy this comparatively inexpensive adventure in saving and restoring your feet.

* You may write Mr. Murray at 213 W. 58th Street, New York City.

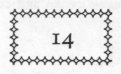

14

Let's Look Ahead

There are three kinds of nutrition: body, mind, and spirit. I would be a poor nutritionist indeed if I set you to eating and thinking in new ways and did not try to get you to look ahead and dream a bit. What shall we dream about? About good food, of course. About intelligent eating. About freedom from fat. Not just for ourselves for the rest of our long lives, but for all people—forever.

WHOLE, NATURAL FOOD

We know that good food means wholesome, natural food. We know that our country, with all its abundance, produces the most denatured, artificial, and over-refined foods of any country in the world. Let us dream of the day when our golden grains will not be denatured in the milling process, when our sugars and fats will not be so over-refined and overpurified that their food value is almost nil, when overcooking and overpeeling will be crimes of the past. And let us implement our dreams by selecting our own food not only for its low-caloric value but also for its health-giving value. And by cooking it as quickly as possible (except some meats, of course). And by making use of all the natural, unprocessed foods we can find and *creating a demand for more*. Do you know, for instance, that there is on the market a small stone mill suitable for home kitchens in which you can grind whole grains into fresh, completely nutritious flour as you need it? Especially if you have a large family to feed, it will pay you in many ways to grind your own flour. Write to the Lee Foundation, Milwaukee, Wisconsin, and ask for information about their little stone mill.

ORGANIC GARDENING

The idea of organic gardening is new to most Americans, but in England thousands of people have learned to produce superior fruits and vegetables even on small plots of land. And wherever a family has an organic garden, their health and well-being are greatly increased.

Here are three good reasons for taking up organic gardening: first, to produce more delicious and nutritious foods for yourself, your family, and friends; second, to avoid foods treated with harmful fertilizers and insecticides; third, to provide yourself a fascinating new occupation which may possibly become a source of income as well.

While health can certainly be improved by selecting for nutritive value such foods as are available, nevertheless, owing to our soil depletion, many of our garden products today lack the vitamins, minerals, and other nutrients they should contain.

Commercial fertilizers supplying phosphorus, nitrogen, and potassium force the growth of vegetables, but fail to furnish seventeen or more other nutrients needed by healthy plants. As these plants are deficient in the missing nutrients, the animals and humans living on such plant foods likewise suffer deficiencies. This chain reaction has resulted in a tremendous increase in diseases among plants, animals, and humans alike, and is exactly the reason why we must fortify our present diets with the vitamins and minerals we *should* but do *not* get from our foods, grown in deficient soil.

The *Journal of the American Medical Association* pointed out that more than 7,000 insecticides now being used for farming purposes are as poisonous to humans as to insects. These harmful substances also kill millions of *valuable* insects needed to combat the crop-destroying ones. Cases of poisoning from sprays left on vegetables are becoming more frequent, and for those with sensitive digestions, I recommend washing sprayed vegetables and fruits in the formula on page 100.

Organic Foods Taste Better

When foods are grown organically, however, not only is their vitamin, mineral, and protein content greatly increased, but their flavor is incredibly superior to that of foods grown on chemically fertilized soil. And for those people who are dubious about the values of organically grown foods, a few samples will convert them —taste alone will win them over. It has been proved beyond doubt by the proponents of organic gardening that healthier plants can be grown; that diseases of plants can be corrected by rebuilding the soil and revitalizing it with natural humus; and that sprays and poisons become unnecessary. And people who have eaten only organically grown foods for a number of years find marked improvement in their health.

You will find organic gardening one of the most exciting and satisfying of occupations. You may start reading up on the subject with mild interest, find that interest mounting with each new discovery, vow you'll not become fanatic on the subject—and quickly become just that.

Browsing through some of the books would surely whet anyone's appetite for gardening. *Harnessing the Earthworm,* by Dr. Thomas J. Barrett, is a fascinating account of how the Nile Valley has sustained the richest soil in the world, even though it has been under constant cultivation for a known span of 6,000 years.

Have you read *Pleasant Valley* and *Malabar Farm,* by Louis Bromfield? Strictly speaking, Bromfield is not an organic gardener, but he can make almost anyone want to buy a farm.

I also recommend Edward H. Faulkner's books, *Plowman's Folly, Uneasy Money,* and *A Second Look.* While you may not agree with all of his arguments, you will surely acquire a great respect for the moisture-holding power of organic material stirred into the soil.

Farmers of Forty Centuries, by F. H. King, and all of the writings of Dr. Ehrenfried Pfeiffer, as well as those of Sir Albert Howard and his wife, Louise E. Howard, also are valuable.

To keep my students up to date on all things new in the world of gardening, cooking, homemaking, and the whole field of nutrition in general, I send out a newsletter several times each year.

ORGANIC MARKETS

I am happy to see that organic markets also are springing up here and there, which sell only fruits and vegetables that are organically grown, without poisonous sprays and fertilizers. I have great hopes for such markets. In fact, I hope to see the day when such fruits and vegetables will be generally obtainable and are tagged, "Grown in *certified* soil."

CO-OPERATIVE MARKETS

Let us search out good co-operative markets and create a demand for more of them. Many had their beginnings in post-1929 depression years, when farmers and their wives pooled time, energy, and edibles in an effort to get their crops to the consumer as cheaply and quickly as possible. Starting modestly, these co-operative ventures thrived and grew; the famous Farmers Market in Los Angeles is an example. Its beginning was a small shed; nowadays you can wander about it for hours and still not see all of it. People come from miles around to shop, to drink fresh fruit and vegetable juices (there are some forty varieties to be had), to lunch at tables in the sun on food of every kind and nationality, and to refresh their eyes at the high-piled, colorful stalls. Such markets should be in every city—and will be if you ask for them.

DIET AND HEALTH-FOOD SHOPS

Large chain stores do not sell 100-percent whole-wheat flour and cereals, whole corn meal, and natural sugar, because these foods do not keep indefinitely in storage, as do the refined products. Unrefined foods must be fresh. Some health-food shops have small mills where all whole cereals are freshly ground. Because the incomparable goodness of such 100-percent foods is being more and more widely realized, health-food shops are springing up everywhere. But there is room for thousands more.

If you like and understand just two subjects—food and people—your own health-food shop could be an exciting as well as a profitable adventure for you. But do make it an attractive, *good*-health food shop, not one of those dreary little *ill*-health food places.

Teachers, doctors' wives, ministers' wives, nurses, YWCA workers are especially well adapted to this sort of project. Man and wife combinations are ideal—one can do the counseling and selling, the other the buying.

Many other specialty foods that cannot be obtained in regular stores are sold in health-food shops—such natural foods as uncooked honey, unsulphured molasses, unsprayed dried fruits, fresh wheat germ, wheat-germ oil, brewers' yeast, iodized vegetable salt, powdered milk, soybean flour, peanut flour—staples which sooner or later will be used by all intelligent people. Correctly balanced vitamin and mineral products and calcium tablets have immense sales in these shops; a health bar serving fresh vegetable and fruit juices is an added attraction.

BETTER RESTAURANTS

When you dream of intelligent eating for everyone and then remember how many people do their eating in restaurants, your heart sinks, does it not? You think of typical restaurant fare; you know that wherever you go, whatever the comfort of your surroundings and the size of your check, the menu usually is the same: overgreasy, overcooked, flat-tasting food.

What can we do about American restaurants? I can tell you one thing not to do: Don't blame the chefs. Once in Detroit I addressed an auditorium full of chefs. I wanted to reform them. I had my say and then they had theirs: "Mister, we know what you mean. But, listen. People come into a restaurant and they're forever in a hurry. They want what's ready, and so we've got to keep everything ready. And what do we do when the nice green vegetables get cold? We run hot water over them."

I believe that a golden opportunity is open for the man of vision who will start a coast-to-coast chain of comfortable, medium-priced restaurants where healthful low-caloric food is the specialty —lean roasted and broiled meats, garden-fresh vegetable and fruit salads, short-cooked vegetables prepared to order, whole-grain breads and pastry shells. Don't tell me this would not be a paying venture; it would be, especially if the produce came fresh from nearby farms. Thousands of my students, all over the country, would welcome such an enterprise; and its owner, besides making a fortune, would have the satisfaction of nourishing a group of people who are starving for good food—the American motorists. If you have crossed our big, beautiful country by car, as I have many times, you well know what I mean. With a few exceptions, our roadside eating places are a national disgrace.

While we are about it, let's hope for more open-air restaurants —sidewalk cafés, roof gardens, leisurely eating places in gardens and parks. Let's have teahouses like those in China, coffee cafés where coffee from all over the world is served. In short, let's not only dream but work toward that happy day when Americans will re-discover the joys of sitting together around tables and relaxing, sipping harmless, fragrant, low-caloric beverages and not being forever in a hurry.

VACATION FARMS

Another golden opportunity, I believe, awaits those who will establish moderate-cost guest farms for the growing numbers of people who, for their two to four free weeks a year, would like, instead of eating, drinking, and partying more than usual, to give their harried digestive systems, as well as their harried minds, a real rest. Here the regime would be styled after today's fashionable but expensive beautyfarms—emphasis on lean eating. Plenty of fresh fruit and vegetable juices, lots of good protein, only wholesome carbohydrate. All the food—eggs, poultry, meat—would come right from the farm itself. No chi-chi; no planned entertainment; no enforced sociability; loose, comfortable clothes. No strenuous exercise. Swimming, walking, sunbathing, unambitious fishing, reading, doing nothing. The guests might try their hand at a bit of farming, if they wished, to learn how things grow. It would be certified soil, rich and healthy and free from poisonous chemicals. Such a vacation would be a restoration of body, mind, and soul— a real re-creation.

DOCTORS SPECIALIZING IN OVERWEIGHT

The modern physician is well aware of the health hazard of ten or more pounds of excess weight; he knows the value of weight reduction as preventive medicine. Yet because many doctors still treat reducing in an offhand manner (as though it were a part of the beauty business), the field of weight reduction remains a fertile breeding ground for quackery.

Sound nutritional advice on how to reduce is widely available: abundant proteins, vegetables, vitamin and mineral supplements. Many overweight people can accept this advice and follow it on their own. But many others, especially those who are plagued by well-meaning family and friends, need a good strong hand to uphold them in their reducing program, to cheer and encourage them and boost their morale. The logical person to do this is the family doctor. (P. S. He should be a man who samples his own diets and has licked his own weight problem.) And how about clinics where basal metabolism tests can be taken regularly? They are important in preventive medicine, just as blood pressure checkups are, and chest X rays.

Cornell Obesity Clinic

I cannot say enough in praise of the pioneer work that has been done in the field of overweight (as in the field of nutrition in general) by Cornell University, in Ithaca, New York. Since 1951, the Cornell School of Nutrition has conducted an obesity clinic to help doctors help their patients to lose weight. Doctors in the community refer their overweight patients to the clinic, which is free, provided the patients attend weekly, co-operate, and take the tests. The Cornell reducing plan provides enough good food for health, emotional support, and, when it is needed, psychotherapy. Thousands of overweight people have taken advantage of this opportunity to take tests and receive help. One patient, who lost forty pounds, returned, bringing her sister, also overweight, "because the Cornell doctors did not make me feel ashamed of being fat."

The good effects of a clinic of this kind are inestimable and will reach far into the future. Let us hope that soon there will be more of them, everywhere.

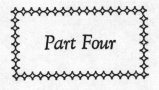

Part Four

YOUR GOOD LOOKS

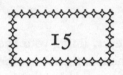

15

Eat and Grow Beautiful

YOUR EYES

A world of the future in which no one will need to wear glasses because mothers will eat a superior diet before children are born was predicted by Dr. Russell Wilder of the famous Mayo Clinic. This is indeed good news. This famous doctor also says that if we apply our *present* knowledge of nutrition, we can delay the development of presbyopia, the kind of far-sightedness that often comes in middle life.

Decide, from today on, to feed your eyes for the rest of your long life. Every body requirement—every vitamin, every mineral, every amino acid—probably plays some part in the health of your eyes. Your best possible vision depends on your blood stream's carrying to your eyes a consistent, steady supply of vitamin A, vitamin B₂ (riboflavin), vitamin C, and vitamin D.

Vitamin A is manufactured in the liver from carotene, the yellow coloring matter found in carrots, apricots, and other yellow foods, and in all green foods such as parsley, spinach, and mustard greens; one generous serving will give you your eyes' daily requirement. Milk will supply riboflavin; citrus fruit juice will furnish vitamin C; eggs, cheese, and plenty of sunshine (and possibly vitamin concentrates) will provide vitamin D.

Do you know why vitamin A is important for your vision? It is an interesting story.

Vitamin A

At the back of your eyes, lining your eyeball like the thin inner skin that lines an egg shell, is the retina, the film of the eye-camera. It is composed of the very special cells of vision. In each eye there are about 137 million of these seeing cells. They are developed from the same tissue that goes to make brain and nerve cells, but they are specialized to respond to light. They are even further specialized among themselves. Some, which are cone-shaped, do all our seeing in bright light, and they also see colors. Others, which are rod-shaped, are for seeing in dim light.

Each kind of cell reacts to light with its own kind of sensitive chemical substance. The cone-shaped cells have special substances that react only to bright light and to light of different wave lengths for the different colors. There is still a great deal the scientists are trying to solve about the differences among the cone cells.

The rod cells have a substance for dim light called visual purple; the cells themselves make this substance out of a special protein plus vitamin A.

Cats see better in the dark than we do, and some human beings see better than others. But if the body is lacking in vitamin A, then the cells cannot make their visual purple. And one result of this lack, the most apparent one, is the inability to see in dim light—night blindness.

The fighter and bomber pilots who flew night runs in World War II were given heavy doses of vitamin A. Long before that, in my first book on beauty and nutrition, *Manger Pour Être Belle*, I told of the experience of thousands of Belgians in World War I who suffered from a mysterious eye affliction, apparently incurable —until spring came and they began to eat fresh green vegetables and butter and cheese and to drink their good rich milk. And then, miraculously, their eyesight recovered! The explanation was that the enemy had confiscated all their fresh foods, and their apparently incurable eye ailment was nothing else but a serious lack of vitamin A.

But the story of vitamin A and the eyes is a great deal older than our two world wars. Five hundred years before Christ, the wise Greek physician Hippocrates recommended raw liver to his patients who had difficulty in seeing at night. Today we know that liver is a rich source of vitamin A.

Vitamin B

When there is a lack of vitamin B_2, or riboflavin, the eyes become bloodshot, itchy, burning; they water frequently, and they are sensitive to light, the condition called photophobia. When these symptoms appear, the recommendation is not only to take riboflavin, but also to increase the whole B group in the diet, just as it occurs in natural foods such as food yeast, wheat germ, and liver.

In my classes I have told the story of a famous motion picture star who suffered for years with burning, bloodshot eyes. She blamed the studio lights, and since she was past her fortieth birthday she also blamed her age. She undertook to follow the nutrition program I recommended, with the same vigor and persistence that made her one of America's most distinguished artists. The results surprised even me. After three months her eyes were clear and beautiful as they had not been for years. The diet that worked this magic was nothing mysterious—simply a diet rich in vitamin A and the entire B complex: vegetable broths, food yeast, liver, milk, all the natural foods that restore health and beauty to hard-working eyes.

Vitamin C

Some exciting studies have been made with vitamin C, in connection with the serious condition of cataract, the clouding of the eye's crystalline lens. Several years ago Dr. Donald T. Atkinson of San Antonio, Texas, found that when he persuaded many of his patients, who habitually lived on salt pork, corn meal, and coffee, to add fresh greens, oranges, and tomatoes to their diet, as well as eggs and other good proteins, the condition improved or the growth of the cataract was arrested.

We do not know just how vitamin C is connected with this serious ailment of the eyes, and anyone suffering with cataract urgently needs the help of an ophthalmologist. But we do know that the eye, and especially its lens, normally contains more vitamin C than any other part of the body except some of the endocrine glands.

And we know that in cataract the vitamin C is conspicuously missing from these tissues.

We also know that vitamin C is crucial to the health of the capillary walls in the body generally, and that a lack of it goes hand in hand with aging of the connective tissues. And if healthy eyes keep up such a high level of vitamin C, there must be a reason!

So let us give them this vitamin in maximum, not minimum, amounts. The body does not store it, and you need to replenish the supply every day. With plenty of vitamin C in your diet, so easily supplied with citrus fruits, green peppers, tomatoes, and the richest of all foods in vitamin C, rose hips, you are feeding your eyes what they themselves take in great quantity from the body's supply.

Vitamin D

Vitamin D is the sunshine vitamin which the body must have to absorb calcium and make good bones and teeth. Now here is a curious fact that came out of two separate experimental studies: A lack of vitamin D and calcium produced nearsightedness in puppies, and the addition of vitamin D to the diet of nearsighted children improved their vision or at least prevented it from getting worse.

Here again the scientist cannot explain exactly how this worked. We do know that a proper balance of calcium in the blood is essential, and that if this balance is disturbed, cramping spasms of muscles, big and small, can occur. Quite possibly, especially in young growing puppies and children, a disturbance in the calcium and vitamin D balance could result in excessive tension of muscles and ligaments, so that the eye fails to accommodate for near vision.

And finally there is good evidence that amblyopia, a general dimming of vision without any apparent defect to account for it, can be a result of general nutritional deficiency. Dr. A. J. Cameron, surgeon at the Royal Eye Hospital in London, found this to be so during the postwar years of austerity diet in England. We can go a step further: In countries of generally poor nutrition—for example, India, and in the Soviet Union during the war years—cataracts appeared at a much earlier age than the average in well-fed countries.

There is still one more point in this feeding of the eyes. It is not enough to take the food into your body. It must also be distributed, and this means good circulation of the blood via exercise.

Gymnastics for the Eyes

Good food, remember, creates a good blood stream, but only exercise can bring that blood stream where it is needed. Attached to your eyeballs are those six fine, silklike little muscles which can be exercised and strengthened like all other muscles of the body. Simple eye drills, which take only a few minutes a day, can greatly improve the looks and function of the eyes. Here are two simple eye drills to keep your eyes young:

1. Turn your head from side to side as if saying an emphatic "no." Do this ten times.

2. Hold your index finger or a pencil about ten inches away from your eyes. Look at its tip, then into the distance. Do this ten times.

Do these two simple eye drills every day; do them especially when you are using your eyes intensely for close work or for reading, and your eyes will serve you better.

How to Relax Tired Eyes

Palming is still the best way to relax tired eyes. This simple method was discovered by Dr. William H. Bates of New York City. It is the same exercise I recommend for relaxing tensions.

Sit in front of a calendar or a picture. Look at it. Now, gently, close your eyes and cover them with your cupped palms. *Be sure not to press on the eyelids.* Rest your arms. Relax. Let go. Breathe slowly and deeply 30, 40, 50 times. As you relax your covered eyes will only see restful gray-black, and as you gradually let go of all tension, your eyes will see a deep dark black. Then open your eyes. Look at the calendar or picture again. You will see it more and more clearly the more you relax. Your eyes and your whole face lose their tension whenever you palm. Do it often.

Another wonderful and lazy way to relax tired eyes is, every once in a while, to look into the distance, just as far as possible. (Remove your glasses, if you are wearing them.) Do this especially when you are on your vacation, for looking at green scenery in the distance is especially beneficial.

Eyeglasses

My students in many lands have made relaxation and these simple eye drills part of their daily living, and many have had remarkable success in keeping their eyes young. Some have succeeded in keeping their eyesight sharp and keen. I actually have met hundreds of men and women who believe that good nutrition, exercise, and the eye relaxation originated by Dr. William Bates have kept their eyes young.

Today there are many teachers of the Bates Method of Eye Relaxation. I have met them in Germany, England, and Switzerland; Mrs. Margaret D. Corbett of Los Angeles, California, an outstanding teacher of the Bates Method, has helped many of our movie stars to strengthen their eyes. I myself have studied these methods and find them valuable for relaxing the eyes. We cannot ignore the successes these eye teachers have with their pupils. The only difficulty I see is that eye exercises and eye relaxation require constant practice and application, for which the great majority of human beings are either too lazy or too busy.

So I definitely do not belong to the school that says: "Throw away your glasses." Unless you are willing to work on your eyes constantly and daily, I suggest that you consult the best eye doctor in your city and let him decide, after a thorough examination, whether or not you need glasses. There are few things so damaging to a person's looks as a straining, squinting effort to see. It is not only detrimental to the eyes, but the tissues around the eyes become a mass of fine, squinting lines. Along with the muscles of the eyes, your whole face and even the muscles of your neck and shoulders become tense in the struggle to see. The decision should rest entirely with you and your eye doctor. And if you need glasses, wear them boldly and confidently.

Contact Lenses

For actors and actresses and for those who frequently appear before the public, especially if the eyes need help not only for reading but for seeing around the clock, the new types of contact lenses may be a boon. In the past several years there have been improvements that minimize and perhaps eliminate some of the disadvantages of these plastic lenses that fit directly over the eye.

Formerly, contact lenses were fitted to cover the entire front of the eyeball, but today they can be made to fit only the seeing part of the eye. Recently, two Boston specialists, Doctors Donald R. Korb and Morton Shaw, found that they could make these tiny lenses with a pinpoint hole through which the cornea can, so to speak, breathe. Through this opening the heat of the cornea can escape and air and fluids can circulate to keep the eye comfortable.

Whether contact lenses are for you is a very personal question. Some swear by them; others still claim they are uncomfortable. Of course, absolute cleanliness is essential for lens wearers to protect against the danger of infection.

New Ways to Hear Better

Most of us are born with more acute hearing than we ever need. Nature starts us out in life with the kind of hearing that primitive man needed to keep alert and alive. Many people keep this acute hearing throughout life; but if in later years the hearing of high tones shades off a bit, there is nothing to worry about. It is a wonder that we retain hearing at all under the constant barrage of loud noises in our modern cities.

Naturally, a thorough check-up by the best ear specialist is the most important thing. In former years, doctors could do very little to prevent or check hearing loss. They removed wax, treated running ears, and dispensed sympathy. Today they can do so much more. Dr. Samuel J. Kopetsky published the clinical studies of 581 cases of different types of deafness and found consistently high levels of cholesterol. He recommended a better diet, low in fat and high in proteins; extra emphasis was put on brewers' yeast, which is high in choline, inositol, and methionine.

Sometimes Surgery Helps

Another approach to correcting deafness is the almost-forgotten science of finger surgery. This was practiced extensively in the early Twenties. The man who had the most outstanding success in correcting deafness was Dr. Curtis H. Muncie of New York City. This doctor discovered that many cases of deafness are due to pressure in the Eustachian tubes. Working with hundreds of patients,

Dr. Muncie learned that the Eustachian tubes are markedly different in deaf people. With his fingers he has been able to restore normal hearing in hundreds of people. Dr. Muncie still practices in his office on Park Avenue in New York, and his son Dr. Douglas Muncie is doing the same simple and successful bloodless operation in his office in Miami, Florida.

More good news! There is a simple surgical operation that has helped thousands who were hard of hearing because of a hardening of the earbone (otosclerosis). This operation is called "stapes mobilization." The stapes is the important tiny bone in the middle ear. Dr. Samuel Rosen of New York has learned to manipulate it without piercing the eardrum. Since Dr. Rosen reported his first "stapes mobilization" operations, more than 100,000 similar operations have been performed. Those who have had this treatment describe it as being about as painful as having a tooth extracted. Any ear surgeon can ascertain whether your hearing difficulty is due to otosclerosis; if so, you should avail yourself of this "stapes mobilization," which requires only one day of hospital care. Many have called this a surgical miracle.

Steps to Take

If you have a hearing loss serious enough to be a handicap, by all means do something about it to prevent further deterioration. There are at least 15,000,000 people in the United States who are hard of hearing. In addition to these 15,000,000 who are known to be hard of hearing, there are probably 5,000,000 more who are hard of hearing and will not acknowledge it—people who are going through life always misunderstanding a little, always feeling a little misunderstood, wasting valuable nervous, emotional, and creative energy trying to keep secret what everybody already knows.

If you are hard of hearing, face it with courage, patience, and a wide-open mind. Courage, because impaired hearing is one of the most difficult of all the handicaps to live with. Patience, because there is no easy cure for impaired hearing. An open mind, because impaired hearing is now gaining the widespread attention of top doctors, educators, and electronic engineers. Today, whatever your type or degree of hearing loss may be, you may be sure that otologists, audiologists, speech and speech-reading experts, and hearing aid manufacturers are working on your special problems. That is why I urge you to face this handicap with an open mind and to have endless curiosity about:

Diet in relation to hearing
Relaxation in relation to hearing
New medical techniques
Hearing aids
Auditory training

Relaxation is of the utmost importance to you. Modern living is geared to auditory stimuli, to the sound of the doorbell, the telephone, the radio, the automobile horn, the public address system. People with faulty hearing live in a constant state of tension which is reflected in the strained expression on their faces, the rigidity of their muscles—especially the muscles of the neck and back. They strain their eyes to compensate for their ears, and, since the nerves governing the eye muscles are centered at the back of the brain, they are likely to find their impairment literally as well as figuratively "a pain in the neck."

If you are hard of hearing, face the fact that you need more rest than a normally hearing person, and see that you get it. Make relaxation your hobby. You will find deep-breathing exercises particularly valuable; I am told that hard-of-hearing people are likely to be shallow breathers, even to hold their breaths, unconsciously, in their effort to "pay attention." I am also told that they are likely to be so busy paying attention at the table that they swallow their food without chewing it. Relax—at meals, in conversation, everywhere.

Have a check-up once a year with the best ear specialist in your community, either in his private office or in his hospital clinic. Discuss with your doctor whatever new medical techniques you read or hear about; perhaps some of them may help you. The fenestration operation which has been developed by Dr. Julius Lempert in New York City is proving successful in a large percentage of carefully selected cases of otosclerosis. This incredibly delicate operation consists of making a new window into the inner ear and keeping this window open for the reception of sound. Write to your State Medical Society for information.

Keep Posted on New Developments

As I have said, research in the field of hearing is steadily going forward. Follow this research. But do not be gullible. There is a vast difference between being gullible and having a hopeful point of view and an open mind.

Explore everything mechanical, also, by all means. If a test of your hearing on your doctor's audiometer shows a loss of 30 decibels (units of hearing) in the better ear, you need a hearing aid. Get it even if you have to beg or borrow the money. It will take ten years off your age. I have seen that happen repeatedly. A hearing aid can be one of the best Look Younger recipes I know of. A Live Longer recipe, too. I recently heard of an elderly gentleman who was so inspired by the possibilities of renewed living, with a hearing aid, that he exclaimed, "I want a *good* hearing aid, because I'm going to use it for a *long* time and I don't mind paying a lot of money for something I can use a long while." He was ninety-five years old.

A good way to keep an informed, open mind is through the American Hearing Society, which has its headquarters in Washington, D. C., and over 100 local chapters throughout the country. Through this organization you can learn how and where to get speech reading and speech training. You can explore the exciting new field of Auditory Training which holds out hope for better hearing with and without a hearing aid. Auditory Training centers are being established in many cities, and research in this new field is going forward at a number of universities, including the University of Southern California where the Phipps Bone Conduction Unit was developed a few years ago. It is said that this instrument can stimulate the hearing organs and, even in cases where impairment is extensive, restore their function to some degree. A new method of improving the use of residual hearing by means of scientifically made phonograph recordings is also being widely and successfully experimented with.

Impaired hearing can stem from many causes. It can be congenital, or result from infections or accidents. If your diet ever becomes grossly deficient, and remains that way long enough, impaired hearing could follow. The various specialized tissues of the ear, and the nerves that receive and transmit the stimulus of sound, like all other tissues and nerves in the body, require proteins, vitamins, and minerals for their integrity. For the rest of your long life be sure to eat for a sound body—each and every part of it.

YOUR TEETH

There will always be some controversy about the exact role played by diet in the soundness of the teeth, but I have no doubt that the food we eat, or fail to eat, profoundly affects them. There are records upon records of peoples living in primitive regions on diets of fish, game, whole grains, vegetables, and fruit who have the soundest of teeth. When our civilization touches them, and the native diet is abandoned in favor of highly milled flour, white sugar, and colas, the new generations develop unsound teeth, highly subject to infection and decay.

How to Feed Your Teeth

Besides the best external care, the health and looks of your teeth depend on good solid nutrition. The teeth, hard and inert as they seem, are alive. They build themselves and renew themselves with the materials that you give them. Their materials come, as to all other parts of the body, in the blood stream. Like plants, the teeth take their nutrition through their roots. Tiny branches carry these precious molecules of building material through the living core of the tooth, the pulp within its casing of hard enamel, and the cells take what they need for their health.

"If the repair materials supplied to the blood by our daily food is second or third rate, the teeth are rebuilt with shoddy material that deteriorates as surely as a shoddy piece of cloth in a suit deteriorates," says Dr. Fred D. Miller in his very fine book, *Open Door to Health,* a book which I highly recommend to parents.

One of the most widely known facts about the teeth is that they need calcium. The teeth are composed of the hardest substance in the body, calcium phosphate, which is also the hard material of the bones. But here are some curious facts that few people know:

A lack of vitamin A can lead to decay of that hard substance. And a lack of vitamin D means that no matter how rich in calcium your diet may be, the body is unable to absorb and use it, and the badly needed tooth-building material will never get to the teeth at all.

Vitamin C is essential to the production of collagen, the connective tissue that provides the framework for the dentine or bony structure of the teeth. And the bone of your jaw, in which each tooth is implanted, needs its proper supply of calcium and phosphorus like any other bone.

Fluorine and Tooth Decay

All over the United States there is great controversy about fluoridation of our drinking water for the protection of our teeth, and people become very emotional and violent on the subject. I personally believe it is always safest to follow the concepts of old Mother Nature and eat plenty of fish and seafood of every kind. These gifts of nature provide us with the right kind of fluorine to protect our teeth. Sicilians usually have excellent teeth, probably because a large part of their diet comes from the sea.

Bone Flour and Good Teeth

Where tooth decay is rampant, many dentists now recommend the addition of fine bone flour, a rich source of calcium, phosphorus, and fluorine in food form.

Here's an interesting experiment by the Swedish dentist, Dr. Alfred Aslander, of Stockholm, which he carried out with his own children.

He and his wife both had very bad teeth, and he was determined to give his own children a better start. Incidentally, he thought he might prove that although poor teeth may be inherited, an unfortunate heredity could be corrected. And he did prove just that. He prescribed finely ground bone flour to be added to the family's orange juice. The result is that this foresighted father's lucky children have grown up with beautiful, sturdy teeth which will probably last them all their lives long.

When the teeth of over a thousand children were inspected in a school in Stockholm, there were only four children with perfect teeth; and whose children do you suppose they were? They were the children of Dr. and Mrs. Aslander.

There is a booklet describing Dr. Aslander's bone-meal method, with pictures of his handsome children displaying perfect teeth. I believe this booklet should be of tremendous interest to dentists and parents. For a copy of "Tooth Formation in the Light of Plant Nutrition," write to the Royal Institute of Technology, Division of Agriculture, Stockholm, Sweden, and enclose one dollar.

Analysis of Bone Flour

	Percent		Percent
Sodium oxide	.46	Lead oxide	.005
Potassium oxide	.20	Zinc oxide	.018
Calcium oxide	30.52	Chlorine	.22
Magnesium oxide	.73	Phosphoric oxide	22.52
Barium oxide	.001	Boron oxide	trace
Copper oxide	.0005	Fluorine	.043
Iron oxide	.004	Iodine	.00002
Manganese oxide	.0014	Sulfur	.25

All the large packing houses now make very fine bone flour from veal and young beef bones. Many dentists prescribe such bone flour tablets, with vitamin D for better absorption, to their patients. They feel that these tablets, added to a good diet, provide a better and less expensive way to combat tooth decay than the fluoridation of water.

Exercise Your Teeth

And here is another almost forgotten fact. Your teeth and gums need *exercise:* exercise to strengthen the surrounding tissue and to stimulate the circulation for gums and teeth. This is essential to the health of all living tissue and your mouth and teeth are no exception.

How does one exercise the teeth? No doubt your dentist told you, when you were still a youngster, how to massage your gums vigorously with your brush, and I hope you still do it conscientiously. Another way to stimulate the circulation of gums and teeth is simply to do what your teeth were meant to do: CHEW!

Chewing your food well not only helps your digestion (and your weight); it also brings the blood stream to gums and teeth, and incidentally it brings the cleansing, germ-killing saliva to them as well. By chewing, I mean chewing good solid food like whole-grain bread or toast, raw vegetables such as celery and carrot sticks or any of your own favorites.

Munching a handful of firm, nutritious seeds not only exercises the teeth but also gives them real nourishment. Try them, all kinds, fresh or light toasted, including sunflower and pumpkin and other melon seeds, plain or salted.

Cosmetic Dentistry

If your teeth are already in trouble, then you cannot chew raw or other solid foods; and the first and best thing for you to do is to find the best dentist in your city.

If you have lost some teeth, he can skillfully replace them for you; and if you need a whole denture, a modern dentist can adjust your bite and give you chewing comfort. Cosmetic dentistry has made tremendous advances; today no one needs to know that your teeth are artificial, thanks to a Swiss dentist who introduced new artificial teeth that look transparent and alive.

Today, especially in the United States, dentistry has developed splendid solutions to repair the damage done by neglect or inadequate dentistry performed in the past. Teeth may be sturdy and still be unbeautiful if they are crooked, badly spaced, or discolored. I urge you to look into this new kind of dentistry, which combines beautification with skillful engineering that saves teeth for many years and improves your appearance, too.

This is the system of capping the teeth with porcelain jackets lined with platinum alloy. Missing teeth are replaced; broken or injured teeth, badly discolored or misshapen teeth are given a coat of glistening, natural-looking porcelain, shaped to make a beautiful mouth and also to give you a sturdy, comfortable bite.

It is an expensive kind of dentistry. But automobiles and air conditioners and big shiny refrigerators are also expensive. I believe the improvement to your looks, in teeth that truly need this kind of dentistry, is worth more than some highly advertised appliances of modern living.

Infected Teeth

A so-called "dead" tooth is a misnomer, because if proper root-canal therapy has been done, with the nerve removed and the canal thoroughly cleaned and filled, the tooth is actually *pulpless*, not dead. It is "dead" only if the surrounding areas of the socket, jawbone, and gums have no nerves. Pulpless teeth, if properly treated, may last for many years. However, if there is any infection at the base of a root, whether the tooth has a live nerve or is pulp-less, have it attended to at once. Even if you have no pain, the in-fection may be there—it will show up on an X-ray photograph, which you should have made by your dentist if there is any reason to suspect trouble.

I myself have always considered infected teeth a serious threat to our Look Younger, Live Longer program. Seemingly minor in-fections can be carried to all parts of the body and cause trouble when we least expect it, especially the heart and joints.

I shall never forget the near-chaos that one such tooth caused the international celebrity, Lady Mendl. She had just flown over to America and was my guest in Beverly Hills, California, when she received a wire from Colonel McCormick in Chicago. The *Chicago Tribune* was holding its first American Fashion Show and Colonel McCormick wanted Lady Mendl to judge it. I urged Lady Mendl to go. I wanted to see Chicago again, and I wanted Chicago to see Lady Mendl. This truly remarkable woman was a dear friend and faithful student of nutrition, and I was very proud of her.

We flew to Chicago and were greeted with pomp and splendor by Colonel McCormick. Batteries of photographers and reporters rushed to greet the fabulous Elsie de Wolfe Mendl. The *Chicago Tribune's* beautiful auditorium was packed with people. A special "throne" had been erected for Lady Mendl in the center of magnifi-cent stage settings. The lights went on, the curtain rolled up, and Lady Mendl was being presented to the audience as the interna-tionally famous authority on style and beauty.

At this moment, the unforeseen happened; one of Lady Mendl's knees stiffened and refused to work. For one long minute we all stood helplessly, with bated breath. But, as usual, Elsie de Wolfe Mendl accomplished the impossible. Somehow, as though nothing at all were wrong, she walked proudly and erectly across the stage and climbed to her "throne." No one in that vast audience knew or suspected that for the next two and a half hours the fabulous Lady Mendl was in intense pain because of *one tooth*.

As soon as the show was over we flew back to Beverly Hills. Needless to say, that tooth was not just "pulled"; it was neatly and efficiently extracted, the socket scraped, and every possible trace of infection removed. And there was no further trouble in the knee.

If you have decayed and infected teeth I would recommend that you go to the best dental surgeon in your vicinity (borrow the money if necessary) and have all sources of dental infection removed. Healthy teeth and jaws are a must in your Live Longer program. The modern dentist, with all the aids of medical science at his finger tips, works quickly and efficiently and with little or no pain.

Pyorrhea

Pyorrhea is an infectious disease of the bony sockets of the teeth. If left untreated it can cause much destruction to the jaw bone— so much that even on extraction of teeth, which generally is necessary, the fitting of artificial dentures becomes difficult. Pyorrhea requires the promptest kind of treatment by a dentist. The occurrence of pyorrhea is an indication of considerable neglect. (It should not be confused with gingivitis, in which only the gums are involved and which can be treated much more simply.)

Among native races on completely adequate diets, such as those studied by Sir Robert McCarrison, of England, and the late Dr. Weston A. Price, of the United States, pyorrhea is unknown. I believe that future generations, living on adequate diets, will continue to brush their teeth not to prevent decay—they will not have tooth decay—but because they like the idea of a clean mouth. In the meantime, remember that a balanced diet rich in large amounts of calcium and vitamins A, C, and D can and will help you keep sound teeth for the rest of your long life.

Your Hair

The war against gray hair and baldness is an exciting one in which, little by little, the enemies are being pushed back. For many years I have been following experiments in research laboratories all over the United States, some of which have shown remarkable results in restoring hair color and improving hair quantity on laboratory animals. I have also witnessed much human experimentation among my students, some of whom have achieved remarkable results.

I have no doubt that one day the battle for hair that stays thick and healthy and retains its natural color will be won. And I firmly believe that it will be won in the field of nutrition.

Hungry Hair Needs Nourishment

If you have hair you "can't do a thing with," nine times out of ten it first of all needs more body, and for this it needs feeding from the inside. Contrary to what you may have heard, there is nothing known to scientists which can in any way, shape, or form feed your hair from the *outside*. Dr. Irwin Lubowe, the famous dermatologist of New York's Flower-Fifth Avenue Hospital, says: "If the diet is unbalanced, particularly if there is an excessive intake of carbohydrates and animal fats, the sebaceous glands are adversely affected."

There is one way to correct a multitude of hair troubles, and that is to replace empty starches and sugars, cakes, candies, soda pops, and nutritionless cereals with foods that will nourish your hair. Most important are the first-class proteins like lean meat, fish, eggs, cottage cheese. Use only whole grains, good breads, fruit juices, and honey. Cut to a minimum all animal fats with the exception of butter. But be generous with the golden vegetable oils. You have a wide choice to fit your taste and pocketbook: sunflower oil, sesame oil, soya oil, wheat-germ oil, corn oil, olive oil, and many others. These oils make tasty salad dressings. Use them singly or mix them in a salad dressing. (See page 480.) Cook with these oils and bake with them, and if your hair is especially dry and mousey, take a tablespoonful of oil every day. You will find that these natural golden oils taste sweet and fresh.

Exercise Your Hair

If your hair is excessively oily and dank, it tells the nutritionist that something has gone wrong with the little sebaceous glands in the scalp. That is why, first of all, the animal fats should be cut down and replaced by vegetable oils. Excessively oily hair also shows a lack of "exercise." Brushing is one of the million-dollar secrets of healthier and more beautiful hair.

Obviously, there are some scalp and hair conditions which are medical problems and should be handled only by a dermatologist. If you have a problem like an infected scalp, or if your hair comes out in bunches, do not waste your money on tonics and salves, but get the best professional help.

There are also some hair problems which can be caused by poor thyroid function. Some years ago, in our Great Lakes region in the Middle West, the farmers complained that they were having trouble growing wool on their sheep. This is one of the areas in the world where iodine is lacking in the soil; Switzerland is another such area. When the farmers added an iodine ration to their animals' feed, the animals responded with good healthy fleece. Unfortunately, growing hair for human beings is a much more complicated affair, but it is always wise to make use of the iodine-rich foods or at least use salt that has been iodized.

What goes on inside your head, believe it or not, can also affect your hair. Stresses and strains can definitely interfere with the circulation in the scalp and so can constant worry affect the health of your hair. Obviously this is where the art of relaxation comes in.

A famous New York dermatologist tells his patients that the surest way to have a good head of hair is to choose parents with good hair. No doubt he has a point. Heredity has a good deal to do with good hair; but I insist, and I have thousands of students to prove it, that it is not heredity we should blame for many defects. We inherit not only the traits but also the cookbooks and eating habits of our parents.

Think for a moment: How different is your diet today from the way your parents ate? Have you taken advantage of the scientific advances in nutrition that have been made in the last 10 years?

The Chinese Have Good Hair

Our bad eating habits are more often at fault than our inheritance. Let me give you an example. The Chinese people in general have handsome, thick, black hair as long as they stick to their native diet. They rarely suffer from baldness and their hair keeps its blue-black color until late in life. Inheritance? No doubt, but it is also true that the Chinese cuisine is very high in minerals and many B vitamins. They eat quantities of soybeans and soy sauce and a great variety of vegetables, and their diet is rich in first-class proteins such as fish and sea food. They also consume quantities of iodine-rich sea greens of all kinds. The Chinese never overcook their vegetables, they never throw away the cooking water, and their cooking fat is golden vegetable oil, rich with the unsaturated fatty acids. You never find hardened fat in a Chinese household.

Sicilians Have Good Hair

The Italian people, and especially the people of Sicily, where I spend a good deal of my time in summer, also have thick, black, curly hair. I have many Sicilian women neighbors who still have beautiful black hair at the age of seventy. No doubt inheritance plays a part, but listen to this: The Sicilians practically live on the foods coming from the sea. They eat quantities of clams, mussels, and other shellfish fresh out of the ocean, and also quantities of fish, broiled, boiled, or roasted over wood fires. They also eat vegetables coming from the sea. One of their favorites, Spaghetti del Mare, a sea green that looks like spaghetti, they eat both fresh and dried. And, of course, Sicily also produces some of the finest olive oil in the world. This is their only source of fat, and, as with the Chinese, you find no hardened fat in a Sicilian kitchen.

Natural Hair Color

The Chinese and Sicilian diets are both rich in B vitamins. I am convinced that the vitamins of the B complex are important for the health, beauty, and even the color of the hair. Scientists have been able to prove in animal experiments that there are three so-called anti-gray hair factors. They are called pantothenic acid, para-amino-benzoic acid, and folic acid. In animal experiments there have been definite successes, but with human beings the results have not been satisfactory. Some of my students have reported that with large amounts of the three anti-gray hair factors, their hair did get darker. Many others found that diet had no effect on the color of their hair, but their hair became healthier and more vigorous.

Your Skin

Your skin is not just an inert covering like the glove you put on your hand. It is a living organ, as truly as your lungs or kidneys. As an organ the skin has two main functions. It is first of all the body's protective covering, its shield against the outer environment. And secondly, it is the body's principal mechanism for maintaining that steady temperature of 98.6 degrees Fahrenheit in which all our cells and body systems are adapted to function. If the skin fails in this task, the body becomes gravely ill. In health and in illness, the skin is one of the hardest working of the body's organs.

Think of it, the skin covering your body weighs about seven pounds. It has an area of about nineteen square feet. It is made up of living, busily working cells, and every inch of it is supplied with delicate, responsive nerves that keep your body and mind informed about your environment, whether it is hot or cold, wet or dry, soft or hard, agreeable or disagreeable.

This outer covering of your body looks fragile, but actually it is tough and amazingly resistant. It can withstand much punishment from nature. It heals and renews itself, day in and day out. It makes spectacular recoveries from disease and accident.

Your skin is your body's protection against dirt and foreign invaders of every kind. It is a barrier to the billions of germs and viruses in the air and on every surface that we touch. It lets none of these pass into the body; at worst, they may penetrate into the outer layers or pores of the skin itself and set up local infection there, but the skin must be wounded or damaged before it will let anything get into even its own deeper layers. But remember that this same barrier keeps out creams and lotions with which you may be attempting to feed the skin itself.

How Your Skin Is Nourished

Always remember that the skin needs nourishment and that nourishment comes only from within. I have been teaching this principle of Eat and Grow Beautiful in many languages for many years, and each year science adds some new confirmation of its truth. There is no part of the body that can thrive without good nutrition, and there is no part of the body that derives more glow-ing beauty from good nutrition than the skin.

Let me tell you how remarkably your skin is made, so that you will carry a picture of it in your mind. It is thin on some parts of the body and thicker on others, as on the palms and soles; but even where it is only one thirty-second of an inch in depth, it is made up of four separate layers.

The outer layer of cells, the epidermis, is the one you see. This layer is constantly flaking and rubbing off. But that need not worry you, for it is forever being renewed from underneath. Under it is always a fresh layer, growing from the buds of living cells below. Interlaced through these growing layers are the capillaries of the skin's own circulatory system. These tiny blood vessels are of a special design, unlike capillaries elsewhere in the body. They are shaped like hairpin loops, each one curving up and down again, carrying the nutritious blood to the cells in every layer of your skin.

And your skin is being newly made every day, *every hour*, by the growing layer of skin cells below. Those cells, which you do not see, can make a finer, healthier skin for you, but only if you give them the materials to work with. Those materials can come only through the blood, flowing up and down the tiny capillary loops, in and out among the cell layers of your skin.

New Skin for Old

What are these life-giving elements?

First, our old friends, the proteins, building blocks out of which new cells are made. And these must be the whole, complete pro-teins, containing all the essential amino acids for the healthy new protoplasm.

Then, the full list of essential minerals, especially iron which gives your blood its power to carry a full load of oxygen. Your skin cells need a constant supply of oxygen so that the well-oxygenated red blood, flowing through those capillaries close to the surface, can give your skin its live, glowing radiance.

Finally come the vitamins: vitamin A to preserve smooth tex-ture and avoid drying and roughness; all the members of the B family of vitamins, to keep the skin youthful and firm, to prevent excessive oiliness, to keep the color clear and free from ugly pigmentation; and vitamin C for elasticity and also for resistance to infection.

None of these can be fed to the skin from the outside, out of jars. These are nature's own foundation, supplied from within to the growing layers for a healthy complexion. See how simple and familiar they are.

More Complexion Secrets

On my lecture tours, where do you suppose I have found the most radiant and glowing complexions? In Holland, Denmark, Sweden, and Norway, those lands where women cherish their fresh supplies of milk and cheese, of greens from their gardens and fish from the seas that lap those shores on nearly every side. The fish and sea food, which the Scandinavians eat so plentifully, are rich in iodine, essential to the thyroid gland; when the thyroid is functioning inadequately, the skin can become coarse, thickened, and dry.

Skin specialists have been paying increasing attention to the role of vitamin A in skin health. Dr. Erno Laszlo, the famous New York City skin specialist, insists on a high intake of vitamin A, especially for dry skin. I have reports from women the world over who found vitamin A a benefaction for dry, rough, lifeless-looking skin. Since there is a possibility of overdosage with this vitamin when it is taken in other forms than food, your physician should prescribe and supervise any special vitamin A therapy of more than 50,000 International Units a day.

Skin blemished with blackheads and whiteheads, and with that affliction of many adolescents, *acne vulgaris*, is often the result of vitamin A deficiency. In severe cases, doctors administer high doses of vitamin A, not in oil, but in water-soluble capsules. They also insist on cutting down on animal fats, chocolates, pastries, and sweets of all kinds.

B Vitamins and the Skin

It may surprise you that the B vitamins are specific skin vitamins. All the B group play a part in keeping the skin youthful. Vitamin B_2, riboflavin, when liberally added to the diet, has been known to help clear those disfiguring brown blemishes, the so-called "liver spots."

Long ago I began to teach the value of food yeast as one of the most potent natural sources of the B complex vitamins. Just one or two tablespoons of this wholesome food, added every day to fruit or vegetable juices, can bring a new, alive beauty to the skin.

You need never worry about taking too much of the B vitamins; there is no such thing as an overdose, whether taken in natural foods or as a food supplement in capsules. A deficiency is not easy to discover, and it is better to be sure. Among the symptoms of B deficiency are dryness, redness, or pigmented irritations of the skin.

One of this country's most celebrated internists, Dr. Harold Thomas Hyman, who was for many years professor of pharmacology at Columbia University, writes in his book for physicians, *Treatment in Internal Medicine,* on dealing with severe deficiencies: "It is wise to provide the patient with blanket coverage of the entire B spectrum, particularly since there are no known risks attendant on overdoses of whole vitamin B complex or of its constituent parts."

Skin Beauty from the Outside

I have referred many times to the brilliant results of correcting skin conditions with unsaturated fatty acids and the remarkable effect they have on fine lines and wrinkles. These fatty acids (called polyunsaturates), which are found in all vegetable oils, were used both internally and externally, with excellent results.

I want you to think of your skin in a way that might never occur to you: from the inside, as part of the wonderful interweaving of all the parts of the body. I want you to think of your skin as dependent upon the same healthful nutrition as every other part of your body, with some special nutrients that are specifically valuable for your skin. First, you must feed it from the inside.

Second comes protection from the outside. Your skin is your body's shelter. Like the outer walls of your home, your skin is directly exposed to the physical environment. It lives in heat and cold, in wet and dry climates. It copes with sharp changes of temperature, with too little sunshine or too much, with wind, soot, industrial fumes, fog and smog, dust and smoke. Your skin lives an outer as well as an inner life.

Wind and water can wear away stone, and the sun can peel and crack a painted wall or a leather chair. The skin is living tissue, and it can defend itself against the elements far better than these inert substances. But the environment takes its toll all the same. Too much sun makes the skin lined and leathery, too much cold and wind cracks and roughens it, and too much water makes it first puffy and then wrinkled.

Dryness, the Skin's Enemy Number One

Even when we protect our skin from the harshest environment, as most of us are ordinarily able to do, there is one continuous threat to its outer surface of cells. That is dryness. More women complain of dry skin than of any other skin condition.

The skin has its own protective mechanism against drying. All over its surface are millions of tiny glands, the sebaceous or oil glands. There are more oil glands in the face and scalp, fewer on the throat and fewest on the hands. These tiny glands spread a thin invisible coating of natural oil that helps to protect the skin against losing its moisture too rapidly.

To living tissue, moisture is even more vital than food. A man can go without food for many days and survive; he will perish of thirst long before he starves. What is true of the body as a whole is also true of each cell. It must have water in order to carry on its life processes.

Your skin is exposed to sun and wind outdoors, and even more to the dry warm air of our winter heating systems. It is constantly losing moisture, in spite of its self-oiling system of sebaceous glands.

Protection of Natural Oils

People of the ancient world, 3000 years ago, used to oil their bodies. So did our own American Indians; they rubbed their bodies from top to toe with bear grease. The first Europeans who came to these shores were apparently not too repelled by the odor of this primitive cosmetic to observe its advantages. They wrote home that this was a good way to protect the skin against insects and dirt and also to keep it from becoming chapped in cold weather. Some historians give credit to the Indians for the revival of cold cream, which had been forgotten since Roman times. The Romans made their cold cream out of the natural organic oils, which were the only oils they knew. Only in the last century were these, unfortunately, replaced by mineral oils, which are drying to the skin.

We can learn wisdom from the ancients, and from the peoples who lived close to nature, like our own Indians. Today we are very insistent on keeping the skin clean; Americans definitely believe that cleanliness is next to godliness. Yet, each time you scrub, you wash off not only dirt and germs, but also the natural oils that protect your skin. Soap, even the gentlest, dissolves these oils away. Detergents do it even more thoroughly.

There are some dermatologists who believe we use too much soap on our bodies. They urge that we should rub and scrub the skin more to keep up its circulation and clear the pores of waste. They do not recommend daily soapings which wash away all the natural protective oils.

The wise old Greeks did not use soap. They did not have it. The Romans learned the art of soap-making from barbarian tribes they conquered in central Europe. The Greeks, who always gave their bodies loving care, cleansed the skin by oiling it with their own sweet oils, then scraped off the oil together with the scruff of dead cells. They had a special toilet tool for the purpose, a scraper, which the Romans also used in their famous baths. All the excess oil and dead skin were scraped away. After this daily "skin peel," a thin film remained on the body or was absorbed into the outermost layer of the skin, and this helped to conserve the skin's own moisture and keep the surface unbelievably supple and smooth.

And this is the true value of our fine creams, oils, and lotions today. They cannot nourish the skin, because the skin cannot absorb nourishment from the outside. But like the fine oils that the Greeks rubbed on their bodies and scraped away, the creams and lotions first cleanse and smooth the outer skin and then protect it from drying.

Skin and the Sun

Today our standard of beauty does not exclude a healthy, golden tan—far from it! We also know that in the sun the skin manufactures vitamin D for the whole body, and that water, air, and sunshine and the healthy exercise of the body out of doors are nature's best and finest beautifying agents.

But unless you want your skin to become tough and leathery and aged, do not overdo the sunbathing. Southern women, even today, protect their skins from too much sun. The erring sisters are usually Northerners, escapees from bleak winter, who try to soak up enough sunshine in a few weeks of a Southern vacation to last for months of sunless weather at home. Some California women, too, carry their sun worship to an extreme.

English women are famous for their lovely complexions. So are many chic San Franciscans. In London and in San Francisco the moist air is an ally of women in keeping the skin beautiful. By contrast, an Arab scholar a thousand years ago observed that women who lived in the desert had withered, wrinkled faces before they were thirty.

So be wise. Take your sun, but take it in safe doses, gradually, and know when your skin has had enough. Too dark a tan is unattractive, but a sunburn is unforgivable. Sunburn, like any other kind of burn, destroys skin cells. It is an actual wound to the body.

Sophisticated Sunbathing

No one deliberately courts a sunburn, but there are some situations in which you may not realize the intensity of the sun's rays. Be especially cautious in the mountains, at the seashore, and wherever there is a reflecting surface such as snow, beach, water, or light-colored surroundings, for then you are getting a double exposure, twice the sunlight in half the time. When you sunbathe, move about, change your position frequently, and never, never go to sleep.

One of the sun's benefits to your skin is that it draws the blood to the surface cells, a skin exercise that takes place without your having to do a thing, like massage. But for the same reason, be careful not to sunbathe for an hour or more after eating, any more than you would engage in strenuous exercise, because the sun, like exercise, draws the blood away from your digestive organs.

When you sunbathe it is always wise to give your skin the protection of a light natural oil cover. Swiss mountaineers use a combination of oil and quinine to prevent burning in the brilliant sun of their snowcapped heights.

Today the chemists have developed many kinds of protective oils and creams that filter some of the sun's rays. They are helpful to the fair-skinned, and for those features such as the nose and forehead which may get more than their share of the sun.

In Sicily if you want to sunbathe, your Sicilian friends will hand you a cup filled with half olive oil and half vinegar. It is an old recipe, and as good as any suntan lotion you can buy. The oil intensifies the sun's rays and helps you to tan more quickly, while the vinegar protects your skin against burning. Lotions are helpful, but the best protection against overdoing is to use your watch and time your exposure. Then you can be certain of getting just the right amount that will bring a golden glow of vitality to your skin, along with a golden tan. (See also page 261.)

Your Lines and Wrinkles Tell a Story

There are exactly fifty-five muscles in your face; with these muscles you express all your feelings. The muscles are "wired" with nerves and these nerves are connected with your brain and are related, therefore, to every part of your body. Everything you think, everything you do, everything you eat—pleasant or unpleasant, healthy or unhealthy—eventually shows up in your face. Each habit, good or bad, brings into play certain sets of the fifty-five muscles and produces folds, lines, and wrinkles. It would be impossible to make a wrinkle all at once; you must tense and pull muscles fiercely every day for years before wrinkles become noticeable, conspicuous, and permanent.

A famous plastic surgeon says that lines and wrinkles are an index to personality. Stubborn, self-willed people who are set in their ways press their lips together tightly until they have deep wrinkles on the upper lip. The earliest wrinkles appear around the eyes. These are not necessarily due to age; they may be mirth or laughing lines. Wrinkles between the eyes, especially if they are deep, indicate excessive determination; they are often found in homemakers who are overly efficient or in people who drive themselves in some other way.

It is the daily overuse of the same facial muscles that forms lines and wrinkles in the skin. This explains why certain occupations and professions produce the same kinds of lines and wrinkles. Have you noticed that many speakers, lawyers, and actors have deep lines in the middle of the cheek, going all the way down to the chin? A forceful business executive often has a few wrinkles directly under his nose. Dressmakers, secretaries, and others whose jobs necessitate pushing the chin down often have an extra roll or double chin. People who have been ill or have suffered a great deal frequently have very fine wrinkles all over the face. Unbalanced reducing diets also can cause lines and wrinkles. By no means are *all* lines caused by age. By no means are all lines undesirable. Some lines are desirable. How often you see a person who has been plain become increasingly attractive with age. And how often you see a mature person with a baby-smooth face, and sense that this is a person who is superficial and wanting in feeling.

Do not worry about character lines and fine wrinkles. Just be sure that they are in the right places and that they have an upward, not a downward, slant.

LEARN ABOUT PSYCHOCOSMETICS

Years ago the well-known surgeon Dr. Frank Slaughter announced that it is impossible to put "beautiful skins on unhappy faces." Cosmeticians the world over complain about women coming for beauty treatments tense, nervous, and so rigid that their creams and lotions and treatments can do precious little good. All the external treatments offered by the most glamorous beauty salons can do very little to help a tense and cranky face. Yet just one happy emotion that makes you smile, lifts up the corners of your mouth, and brings forth an inner shine, is what really makes a woman beautiful—and it costs nothing in time or money.

In France and Germany, the new science of *Psychocosmetics* is gaining momentum. It teaches that only thirteen facial muscles are required to create a happy uplifted look, but all fifty-five muscles are required for a depressed and cranky appearance. The modern psychocosmetician then says: "Why waste all that energy to look unhappy and depressed?" Naturally, people should not become pallid Pollyannas; life brings to all of us some dark moments that may make us look sad and depressed momentarily. But never should an intelligent person permit himself to live habitually in a climate of discontent, because your habitual emotional climate is registered on your face. If your habit of mind is hopeful and outgoing, the muscles of your face pull upward; if your inner life habitually is a sunny one, your face reflects its brightness.

Give yourself a few moments of psychocosmetic treatment. It is the most natural and effective of all beauty treatments. Its origin is from mighty Mother Nature, the wellspring of all good and enduring things. Even though cream, paint, and powder may fail, psychocosmetic treatments, rightly used, will always help. True beauty comes from within; and no matter how many birthdays you have had, if the face radiates an inner beauty, all the joys of life are yours. If you have lost the ability to rest and to rid yourself of all vexing thoughts, with will power you can regain it.

The psychocosmetic treatment begins with face control in front of the mirror. First, bend your head backward, then bend it slowly forward until your chin touches your chest. Relax the lower jaw. Start shaking your head—at first gently, then more and more firmly. While doing so, expel little humming sounds, increasing, decreasing. This relaxation of the face may last several seconds to three minutes, depending on your comfort.

Now look in the mirror. Place your hands gently on your cheeks and close your eyes, bending your head back as far as possible. Remain in this position a few seconds. Then, have another look in the mirror. Now it is time to send little impulses to your facial muscles. In this, the psychocosmetic treatment resembles autogenic training and autosuggestion. For hand in hand with the relaxation of your features goes the brightening of your facial expression through orders you give to yourself: "Life is beautiful—I am happy—The corners of my mouth rise—I smile—No wrinkles in my forehead." Later you extend these orders to the position of your body: "I stand erect—I can cope with any situation—I am strong—My chin up—I am conscious of my powers."

Remember that optimism is the best cosmetic.

After one of my "Look Younger, Live Longer" classes in London, one of my students presented me with the following charming poem:

IT SHOWS ON YOUR FACE

You don't have to tell how you live each day;
You don't have to say if you work or you play;
A tried true barometer serves in its place,
However you live, it will show on your face.

The hate, the deceit, you may bear in your heart
Will not stay inside where it first got its start
For the skin and the blood are a thin veil of lace
What you wear in your heart, you wear on your face.

If your life is unselfish, if for others you live,
For not what you get, but how much you give;
If you live close to God, in His infinite grace,
You don't have to tell it, it shows on your face.

THREE WAYS TO LIFT YOUR FACE

Look at your face honestly, open-mindedly, or as one student expressed it, "I look at myself as my dearest enemy would." What do you see? A too-full face, perhaps, with jowls along the once-piquant jawline; perhaps a double chin. There is no need to put up with this distortion.

You can get rid of heavy jowls and that extra chin with this new gymnastic recommended by the famous German dermatologist, Dr. Hans Weyhbrecht in Stuttgart. Oil the face and throat. Sit high and straight in front of a mirror. Push your chin forward as far as it will go. Now push your lower lip forward à la Maurice Chevalier. Stay in this position and turn your head slowly to the

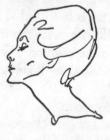   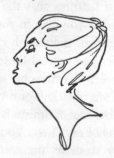

Head up . . .   *. . . lip forward*

left, then slowly to the right. This brings all the weakened muscles of the throat and jaw into play. The more you push forward with your lip and the more you tighten these muscles, the sooner you will establish a firm throat and neckline. Do it daily, twelve times left and twelve times right. This takes only about sixty seconds.

How does your mouth look in your mirror? I hope the corners go up and not down. If your mouth droops, investigate your upper teeth. If some are missing, have them replaced at once. Nothing can give you such an unhappy look as missing teeth. If your teeth are in order and the corners of the mouth are down, then perhaps your spirits need lifting as well.

Disappointments, sadness, constant worry, all register, especially around the mouth. All of us have our share of disappointments, but why advertise it? In the meantime, cheer up! Remember, if you do your best each day you can also expect the best.

Now this is how you can pull up the corners of your mouth so that they will stay up: Put both hands on your cheeks, and hold the cheek muscles tight. Now draw your mouth as far to the right as it will go, then as far to the left. Be sure to hold your cheek muscles tight. Just exercising and pulling the mouth left and right will do you no good. It is the muscular left and right pull, against the cheeks you are holding with both hands, which can do wonders for weakened muscles around the mouth. Do this twelve times toward the left and twelve times toward the right. Dr. Rudolf Drobil, the well-known Viennese physician, teaches this scientific face-lifting-via-exercise and insists that unless you give your facial muscles resistance, facial gymnastics are a waste of time. Dr. Drobil, in his book, *Gesichts-Gymnastik*, says that before considering plastic surgery, first strengthen your facial musculature via his face gymnastics; then if the face lift is still desired, it will be twice as lasting.

If you are too busy or just too lazy to do these three-minute facial gymnastics, do as Ann Delafield taught thousands of women in the New York Success School: Lie down on your Yoga Slant board and let the law of gravity pull your muscles upward and flood their cells with your own nourishing, reviving blood while you rest. You can actually feel and see the lifting up of the entire face.

Don't Let the Light Go Out

Every once in a while I meet a woman who proudly, almost boastfully, announces that she has never in all of her life used any make-up of any kind whatsoever. And usually, as I look at her, I think to myself, "Sister, you look it!" I have never seen a woman whose appearance could not be improved by wise use of make-up. It was not very long ago that make-up was associated with easy virtue, but, fortunately, that is all now in the past. The art of make-up is as old as the oldest civilizations. Cleopatra highlighted her features, and I have seen, in ancient Indian temple-paintings, figures of women whose lips, eyes, and brows were all accentuated very delicately and exquisitely. Every female face has some good features and milady's job is to highlight the good and de-emphasize the nose that is too large or the chin that is too small, etc.

I do not at all agree with the beauticians who say that soap should not be used on the face. I think that soap is as necessary for the face as it is for any other part of the skin. Healthy skin is clean skin, and there is but one way to clean it. Having cleaned it, though, the first law is to oil it, to use the proper lotions to keep it soft.

When those women tell me that they have never used make-up, I tell them that I think it is impolite for anybody not to look as attractive as possible. (See also page 263.) No one has any right at all to go around looking unattractive and unhappy. It is as natural, I think, for women to enhance their features as it is for birds and animals to preen and clean themselves. Just as we need food for the body, so do we need food for the spirit, and the confidence and satisfaction that comes from knowing one looks well is the best food the spirit can get. Let us fortify the food for the spirit as we fortify the food for the body. I know of a woman whose house was bombed in London during the blitz, and when they finally dug her out of the rubble the first thing she did was to reach for her lipstick.

We cannot really be very happy when we don't think we look well. So, don't be afraid to do things with your lashes, your brows, your lips. Why be a shrub when you can be a flower?

AGELESS BEAUTY

There is no country in the world that places so high a price on beauty as America. And there is no place in America where beauty is so richly rewarded as Hollywood. Yes, we Americans worship beauty, and our American women are the most beautiful in the world. There can be no question of that. But have you ever noticed that the traffic, in and out of Hollywood, is terrific? Yesterday's beauty, often enough, is gone and forgotten tomorrow. We worship beauty, and Hollywood pays a high price for it; but it is a transient kind of beauty, as a rule. These beauties, by and large, are annuals, not perennials.

But there are a few beauties who stay. These are the ones, the Garbos, the Swansons, the Goddards, the Dietrichs, whose beauty is more than that of form and face. These are the ones whose beauty is *enhanced* by time. To them, time has done a beautiful and wonderful thing: It has increased their charm, their skill, their ability to convey emotion. *This* is the great beauty, the beauty of fullness, not the shallow beauty of a fragile flower, sweet and perfect at the short moment of its opening.

If beauty is only skin-deep, then it must be that one is only talking about skin-beauty. But the beauty of character, the grace of a beautiful person, grows, as it did in the incomparable Bernhardt and Eleonora Duse, with every moment and hour. These beauties are the perennials of Hollywood, of Broadway, of the world stage. To my mind it is this beauty of character that made Eleanor Roosevelt beloved by so many. This is why I felt that Lady Mendl was one of the most interesting of women.

It is this inward force, this pressure from the vitality within, that distinguishes people. It was the sense of this *élan,* this vital power, that made the sculpture of Rodin so real, so great. Vitality is a force that presses for escape. It makes the body *alive.* It gives it that dynamic symmetry which constitutes the greatest appeal that man's eye can discern or enjoy.

How can you obtain this force, this beauty? I believe it comes from enjoyment and appreciation. It certainly does not come from fear, or from weakness. There is nothing more beautiful than health and happiness; *these* are the cosmetics of permanent beauty. From this comes color and grace, and charm and dignity.

The most beautiful women I know are not beautiful because of showy clothes or *striking* make-up. They are beautiful because of the force and power that emanates from within. They have sublimated the superficial, and have accentuated the positive. And, need I add, the most beautiful women I know are intelligent about their food. To be beautiful, they must care for their bodies from within, which is the only place from which the spirit can be fed.

There is too much imitation, it seems to me. When the gracious Jacqueline Kennedy began to make the frequent public appearances required of our First Lady, thousands of women copied the "Jackie Kennedy Look." The real Jacqueline Kennedy is a beautiful woman. But most of the imitation "Jackies" dissolved their own personalities to become pale copies of the real person. True beauty is the enhancement of one's own personal characteristics. Wear the style of clothing that is most becoming to *you*. Let your hair frame your face in a way that brings out *your* best features. Make the most of the real *you*. Then, amplify yourself with the beauty of a healthy body and a happy mind. Do this, and your beauty will grow and grow, and never wither and fade. This is the million dollar secret of beautiful women all over the world.

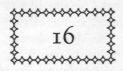

16

Other Ways to Look Younger

BATHS FOR MANY PURPOSES

"Water contains great healing power," said Father Kneipp, and today in Woerishofen, Bavaria, this inspired priest's "water cure" attracts thousands of people from all over the world. There you may see a group of men and women wading knee-deep in the cool fresh streams. According to Father Kneipp's theory, the fresh "alive" water brings better circulation to the feet and legs and the organs of the abdominal region. You may also see another group holding their arms, up to their shoulders, in cool running water in pine wood troughs, to create better circulation for the upper part of the body, especially the heart and lungs.

You will find the scientific counterpart of Father Kneipp's "water cure" in many of our modern hospitals where hydrotherapy (water therapy), given in tubs, tanks, pools, and specially designed showers, is a standard procedure in overcoming the effects of many diseases and disabling accidents.

Whether or not we agree that water has healing power, we do know that it is a marvelous medium for pepping up lazy circulation when applied to the feet, face, or entire body. And we know that better circulation means a better blood supply, a better blood stream rich in all the bodily nutrients, bringing good wherever it flows.

It is for this reason that I would like to establish a new "Order of the Bath," a new interest in the efficacy of water. Not just the Saturday night soak or the daily shower, but many other baths which can be of great value in our Look Younger, Live Longer program. No people are so ideally equipped for modern bathing as we Americans with our modern bathrooms. With a little ingenuity and practice you can use your bathroom for all sorts of refreshing and youthifying baths. There are two schools of the bath: tub devotees and shower addicts. Since it is easier to relax in the tub, I shall emphasize tub baths.

The Alternating Bath

My favorite bath, which thousands of my students also have enjoyed, is the Wechsel-Bad or alternating bath. I recommend this highly, especially to those whose circulation needs stimulating or those who get one cold after another.

Simply lie and relax to your heart's content in a tub of pleasantly warm water. Put a small rubber pillow under your head, if you like. Do your relaxing exercises or the Stomach Lift. (There is definite additional benefit from exercises done under warm water.) If your skin is dry, make doubly sure that the water is not too hot. Add a teaspoon of fine bath oil. You can soap and scrub while you are soaking. Use a good super-fatted toilet soap.

After you are clean and relaxed (and this is important) let half the warm water run out. As the warm water runs away, turn on the cold water full force. Then lie back, and with both hands mix the cold water with the remaining warm water. Keep mixing, while the water gets cooler and cooler and cooler. In three minutes your whole body will tingle and glow. You will feel refreshed and *not at all cold*. Have one of those immense bath towels ready and wrap yourself in it. Rub yourself dry, or, if you have the time, wrap the towel around you, go to bed and cover up; and relax, relax, let go of all your real or imaginary burdens.

A Sitz Bath for Adam

Hot baths are wonderfully comforting and relaxing. Take them whenever you are tense, tired, and out of sorts. But remember that it is cool to cold water which peps you up. At the famous water *kurort* in Woerishofen in Bavaria, they call this bath the "youth bath" because the increased circulation to the vital centers helps to keep a man young. They even have special sitz bathtubs.

Here is how the tired husband can get the beneficial effects of plain cold water without a special bathtub: Let the cool water run into the tub until it is about half full. The idea is to concentrate the water as much as possible around the "sitz." Sit in this cool water for three and not more than five minutes with knees drawn up so that only the feet and "sitz" are in the water. The cooler the water, the greater the benefits. Jump out of the tub and rub dry with a coarse bath towel. It is amazing how this sitz bath can refresh you. Thousands of people have thanked me for the benefit they received from this simple five-minute bath. For many men it has taken the place of pink pills, benzedrine, and other stimulants. Take this two or three times a week or whenever you feel the need for a lift.

Another ancient refresher for weary Adams was told to me by a Scandinavian friend; it was handed down from the days of the Vikings. If you haven't the time nor a bathtub for a sitz bath, simply immerse the scrotum in very cold, even ice water, for one or one and a half minutes. It is a quick and simple way of increasing local circulation.

The Herbal Bath

This is especially good for older people. Into pleasantly warm water, put a bundle of your favorite herbs from the garden, or a tablespoonful of pine, eucalyptus, or mint, which are especially relaxing. Be sure that the water is not too hot, and you will find a fifteen-minute herbal soak exceptionally soothing to irritated nerves.

Roman Oil Bath

As early as the year A.D. 212 at the most luxurious of all bath establishments, the Caracalla, the Roman aristocrats had a choice of twenty-five different kinds of baths. The favorite of the ladies was the most expensive one—an oil bath given in a marble bathtub full of pleasantly warm water, precious oils, and perfume. Such baths are having a renaissance here in America, probably because women have learned that the right kind of oil, broken down into millions of fine oil globules by the warm water, moisturizes and smooths dry skin. Here is a million dollar recipe for as luxurious and elegant an oil bath as any Roman ever had:

> 1 cup of corn oil (the Romans used sesame or olive oil)
> 1 tbsp. of any liquid detergent shampoo
> ½ tsp. oil of rose geranium or your favorite perfume

Pour oil, shampoo, and perfume into a bottle. Shake vigorously each time before you use it. The shampoo breaks the oil into millions of fine globules that cling to your seven million open pores. Just two tablespoons of this mixture in a tub of good warm water does wonders for dry skin. And it costs only pennies.

The Sea Bath

Everyone knows that this is wonderful, that it prolongs youthfulness and life. If you live near the ocean, be glad of it and make use of it. Are you afraid of the water? Learn to swim. One of my People, the beloved Annie Laurie, a brilliant San Francisco newspaperwoman, learned to swim at seventy. "What are you afraid of?" a Honolulu fisherman challenged her. "The sea, she is your mother; lie on her and she will caress and carry you." And I am delighted that bathing suits have gotten briefer. The briefer the better, for our sun- and air-starved bodies.

The Dry Bath

In France, where it is very popular, this is called the friction bath. Its value lies in the fact that it is soothing and quieting. You can obtain a coarse bath glove made of twisted wool and horsehair in any of the better drugstores, and it will prove a good investment for one whose nerves need quieting or who wishes to have baby-smooth skin all over.

With the glove on the right hand, proceed gently to massage, with a circular motion, your feet, calves, thighs, abdomen, and as much of the upper body as you can reach. Then change the glove to the left hand and massage the rest of the body. You will be surprised to find how soothing and relaxing this bath can be. In France it is taken before retiring and is proclaimed an excellent remedy for sleeplessness. In hot weather, French people sprinkle a pleasant eau de cologne on the glove which is not only a mild deodorizer but also helps to remove dead, dry skin from the body.

The Air Bath

"Just as fish need water, so man needs air," said Dr. Benedict Lust, a medical doctor who practiced and applied the natural sciences at his Florida sanatorium. In big cities where people live closely together and apartments are small, there is little opportunity to give the body the chance to breathe freely of good fresh air. Yet even busy city people can take air baths at night in the privacy of their bedroom. Fortunately pajamas and nightgowns are becoming thinner, briefer, and more porous. But why not go all the way, and sleep "in the raw"? Try it, the next time you go to bed feeling dead-tired. You will be amazed at how much fresher you feel the next morning.

Try to keep your body surrounded with fresh, crisp air. Take air baths, in the raw, or in the airiest of sleeping garments. Sleep in a well-ventilated bedroom. Wear light, porous clothing. And live outdoors whenever possible.

The Sun Bath

In Switzerland today, sun-bathing is done seriously and scientifically, due to the influence of Dr. Auguste Rollier, a prominent surgeon who fell in love with a nurse suffering with tuberculosis. Determined to cure her, he left his hospital in Bern and took her high up in the Swiss Alps where the sun is at its best. There, with the help of sun baths, he slowly but surely accomplished her cure. Today, up in Leysin in the Swiss Alps, thousands of people come from all over the world to find health, and the Rollier clinic is still accomplishing amazing things.

The Rollier technique of sun-bathing is especially adapted to the Look Younger, Live Longer program because it is gentle and easy to apply. Dr. Rollier absolutely forbids people to take uncontrolled sun baths. When overdone, some of the rays of the sun can be positively dangerous. First of all, that part of the body which is to be exposed to the sun is oiled with a cream that filters out most of the harmful rays. Second, the head is *never* exposed but always covered or shaded. And the duration of the sun bath for older or sickly people is never more than fifteen minutes.

Here is the most important part of the Rollier sun bath technique: only the legs are exposed for the first few days. The upper part of the body is covered with a towel or a shirt. When the legs have a glowing color, then and then only is the upper part of the body exposed. There again, the abdomen and chest are exposed only for fifteen minutes for the first two days. The same procedure is applied to the back and the buttocks.

When the whole body, back and front, is fairly pink and glowing, sun baths can be extended to thirty minutes for three or four days. After that, you can work it up to one hour, but not more; Dr. Rollier has found excessive sun-bathing weakening. At all times, the head should be covered to prevent the possibility of sunstroke.

The best time to take sun baths is around ten o'clock in the morning. The least desirable time is at noon. If you can, go to the seashore and get the combined benefits of sun and water. If you cannot, do manage to let the sun caress your body, not through a window pane, but directly. The sun, like water, has magnificent healing and youthifying power and it is free for the taking. If you cannot go to the beach, why not arrange a small place on your porch or in your bedroom and on sunny days take these short, stimulating, and invigorating Rollier sun baths? Start now, and you too will become an enthusiastic "sun worshipper."

For the rest of your long life, let your bath be not merely a daily habit but a daily ritual. Join the new "Order of the Bath" and get as much as possible out of it, for health's sake as well as for beauty and cleanliness.

Unless your daily schedule requires it, do not take your bath at the same time every day. Try to plan your bath for a time when you have nothing else to do for at least an hour. Follow it, if possible, with fifteen minutes in the Yoga Slant position. (See page 174.) I cannot suggest too often that you invest in a good strong board that does not sag in the middle and is comfortable enough so that you will be able to relax and do the Stomach Lift. Relax, relax. Do the Stomach Lift. One, pull in. Two, pull in more. Three, pull in and flatten still more. Keep the muscles tense for about ten counts, then let go, relax. Do this ten times and know that you are permanently flattening your abdomen, taking inches off your waist, and giving your whole body firmness, youthfulness, and dignity.

Your Make-up

As far back as 500 B.C., wise old Confucius said, "Everything has beauty, but not everyone *sees* it." This is precisely why I urge women to use modern make-up skillfully, creatively, to enhance good points and tone down bad points. Make-up, so used, can take at least ten years from any face; it can boost the morale and give the mature woman the assurance of ageless comeliness. Do not strive for glamour. Instead, strive for symmetry and harmony, for glow rather than glare. The secret of success in make-up is to *underdo* it, so that a natural effect results. Radiance, rather than pink-and-white prettiness, is your aim.

With added years, the skin tends to lose the oiliness of youth; oily creams and powder foundations must be used more liberally and consistently to offset this loss. Determine which of the three basic skin colorings is yours, and have all your cosmetics keyed to your natural coloring. The coloring of the chest and shoulder area will most accurately guide you, as exposure to sun and weather change the coloring of the face. The average American woman's coloring is of the "brownette" type, a neutral beige tone.

Select a foundation cream (it *must* be of the creamy lotion type) which is the color of your skin or a shade darker. Apply it lightly and evenly over the face, throat, neck, and around the ears, using the tips of your fingers to blend it into the skin. Properly applied, it does the same thing a soft veil does: it creates a gentleness, removes harshness, youthifies instantly. Also, it protects and moistens the skin all day long. Wipe off excessive spots with your fingers, always—never with tissues which cause streaking and spoil the blended, natural look.

Your Clothes

Now I am going to lay down the law. After fifty, no bright red. For women, no bright-red hats, dresses, shoes. For men, no bright-red neckties either in solid colors or splashy designs. Why? Because bright red is an emotion. It screams aloud. After fifty, it screams one of three things:

"Look at me; I am old but I don't admit it."

"Look at me; I am old but I can distract your attention from the fact."

"Look at me; I am old but I am really very young at heart."

In short, the person who wears bright red after fifty is saying to the world, "Look at me; I am old."

In the Look Younger, Live Longer program, we are not old. Moreover, we are secure in our agelessness. We wear plenty of bright red, but we wear it inside us, pumping from our hearts, coursing through our arteries, radiating out to our muscles and to the surfaces of our skin from head to foot. The world knows by looking at us that we are youthful. We have nothing to deny, nothing to distract attention from, nothing to prove.

To a lesser degree, be wary of taking refuge in wearing gray, which says, "I am old and I admit it." Use navy blue, black, and white. The smartest women in the world, regardless of age, concentrate on these colors. Use accents of crisp, spotless white with your navy and black. In summer, try wearing all white. Spotless gloves, whether of cotton or the finest kid, are an indispensable accessory.

The well-dressed woman is never "fancy." Neither is she extravagant; her clothes can be few and inexpensive. Countess Bismarck, the fabulous Mona Williams, who for years headed the list of best-dressed women, surprised us all by announcing that her budget for clothes was a comparatively modest one. Line and cut are more important than the material from which the dress is made.

One of my best-dressed friends, the Duchess of Windsor, wears clothes of very simple design. The late Lady Mendl (another of my extremely well-dressed friends) wore a "little girl" dress that became almost a uniform with her. The upper part was loose-fitting with a round neck and three-quarter length sleeves, the full skirt was drawn in at the waist with a cord or a small belt, and there were two little pockets concealed in the folds of the skirt. (And *always,* she wore white gloves.) The Duchess of Windsor wears clothes of similar simplicity and accents them with her beautiful jewels. The last time I saw her we discussed clothes, and she agreed with me that the best-dressed women do not follow "the fashion" but rather stick to the lines and colors that are most becoming to them and make but few concessions to the "style" of the moment. Smart women everywhere adapt their clothes to themselves and never blindly follow any "new" or "old" look.

Your personality is your most precious possession. What you wear, and how you wear it, can be a beautiful expression of your own personality or an unbeautiful imitation of another's. You can be a creative artist in terms of your own personality, and translate the ideal image of yourself into reality. But remember that eccentricity is not chic, and it is not chic to be "too chic."

Make a point of knowing your own figure; the woman with a "perfect" figure is rare indeed. The length of the neck, size of the head, set of the shoulders, size and position of the bust, breadth of shoulders and hips, length of waist and of arms and legs, must be given proportionate consideration in relation to each other.

Be critical about the cut of a garment. Far better one garment of burlap properly cut and fitted, than twenty dresses of the richest fabric poorly designed and put together. Remember that it is not quantity of clothes that makes the well-dressed woman; you can buy dresses by the dozen and still be one of the world's worst-dressed women.

If you can afford to have clothes especially designed for you, then you have no excuse for being dowdy or overdressed. If you plead "can't afford it," I say you have even less excuse, for then you surely cannot afford to waste money on clothing that does not do well by you. Learn something about dress designing and making. Learn about yourself. You can be well dressed economically.

Learn about color and what it can do *to* you or *for* you. What color are your eyes? Your hair? Your skin? These are your guides. Does the color of your clothing distort your self-coloring, or subtly flatter it? Is your present wardrobe a hit-or-miss collection of clashing colors? Snatched-up "bargains" that make no bargain of you? Learn to plan ahead for your purchases. Start with one basically good garment in your best basic color and line. Add harmonious companion pieces as you are able to. Restrict bright colors to accessories that add a small lilting note to the suave harmony of *you*. Beautiful scarves, handkerchiefs, costume jewelry, flowers, discreetly applied, can be inexpensive grace notes expressing the "inner woman."

Avoid, as you would the plague, anything gaudy. Nothing so

quickly stamps the ill-dressed woman as a profusion of attire which screams for attention. On New York's fashionable Fifth Avenue you can see swarms of such misguided females, any day of the week. Clad in a riotous profusion of stuffs, teetering on gaudy slippers, clattering an astonishing load of costume baubles; "over-Saksed," as the punsters put it, to the total loss of their own personalities.

If you are going to live a long life of agelessness, plan an ageless wardrobe. Unsuitable and unbecoming clothing can age your whole appearance. Wisely selected, it can take years off your looks. Strive for *under*statement. Simplicity of line and cut know no age and never go out of style.

I insist that there is no such thing as a "stylish stout." Stoutness is forever unhealthy, unstylish, and unnecessary. If you have allowed yourself to become overweight, get your waistline down again. Flatten it. Strengthen it. Make it your aim in life to keep your muscles so strong and elastic that you can free yourself permanently from that one-piece harness called the corset. Your own natural "muscular corset" is the best of all undergarments.

Give time and thought to discovering your own best style and be true to it for the rest of your long life. It will be suitable to the needs of your way of life, pleasant to look upon, comfortable to wear, and a true expression of your self. It can make you, no matter where or who you are, a well-dressed woman of the world.

As for men, darker suits are the general rule and the most practical for working hours in the city. No need to be somber about it though; there are shades of blue, gray, and brown that are dark enough for wear in a sooty city without having funereal aspects. If you cannot indulge in a large wardrobe, concentrate on navy blue and gray; they are your best colors. And gray flannel slacks with a well-cut tweed jacket can be worn almost any place during the daytime. Insist on a youthful cut. Avoid "off colors" in tans, light blues, greens, or mixtures. I call these bilious colors because they make one look as if he had jaundice.

You may economize on the number of suits you have, but never at the expense of their tailoring. Two expertly tailored suits will give far more satisfaction in long wear and good appearance than will four poorly tailored ones.

Neckties can make or break your claim to being a well-dressed man. I believe hand-painted ties are my pet aversion. They scream, "I am rich, but I do not know what to do with my money." Let discretion be your guide. Plain ties in neutral colors are always in good taste. Small dots, narrow stripes, or small allover patterns in subdued colors take second place. Beware of gaudy, parrot-like colors and screaming patterns; they scream of immaturity. Best of all, wear a maroon, gray, or blue tie with your navy blue suit. Maroon, navy blue, or black ties with your gray flannels. Socks should match your tie and be in solid color. *Always* wear a crisp white handkerchief in your breast pocket and let an inch or so of it show.

White shirts are unquestionably the choice of the best-dressed men; but scrupulously white. However, the growing tendency of American men toward colored shirtings in subdued shades can be a pleasant and practical note, when used with discretion. While frowned upon for after-dark wear in town, this tendency has achieved some standing for daytime attire. Shirt collars are very important. The height and cut of a collar can add to, or subtract from, your age. A higher cut for a thin neck, and a low cut for a plump or normal neck.

Naturally, your problems are few if you have retained a youthful body. If you have permitted yourself to grow fat or have developed a "bay window," start to get rid of it at once. (If Grandma Reynolds did it, you certainly can.) Make the Stomach Lift a daily habit. (See page 175.) In the meantime, you can help matters considerably by wearing one of the elastic abdominal supporters which can be purchased in any drugstore.

Men's clothes, while much more comfortable than they were a few years ago, are still badly in need of reform. The starched white collar, the pointed-toe shoe, and the derby hat are becoming almost nonexistent. In their place we have the more comfortable, collar-attached soft shirts, more comfortable shoes, the comparatively new moccasin, and no hats at all. Our great need, however, is for a glorified coverall, a one-piece garment to take the place of the present coat and trousers. I believe the time is not far off when men will wear clothes resembling those developed by the air force during the war. They are extremely comfortable, practical, and attractive. I am glad to see that in summer and in year-round warm climates, men of all ages are being emancipated from slavery to their heavy suits. Slack suits in light-weight materials and lighter colors are most appropriate for our increasing leisure hours.

For men and women both, I would lay down one final law: whatever you wear, let it be *always* well-pressed, well-brushed, and scrupulously clean.

SUPERFLUOUS HAIR AND MOLES

As the years go by, superfluous hair on the face becomes a real problem for many women. Moles also appear, sometimes covered with hair. In some countries, France, for example, facial hair is not objected to; and I understand that there is a province in Japan where a woman's beauty is judged by the length of her mustache. In this country, however, hair on a woman's upper lip and chin seems unfeminine and unbeautiful and may be the cause of unnecessary mental distress.

A thorough physical checkup is in order in all such cases, with a check on various glandular functions, including a basal metabolism test. If endocrine deficiencies are present, they should be treated. Then, for vanity's sake and for the sake of one's family and friends, have the hair removed. In mild cases depilatory wax is best. For permanent removal the only safe method is electrolysis, which has been used by dermatologists since 1875. This treatment should be given by a trained technician. For such sensitive areas as the face, use of a single needle rather than multiple needles is recommended. Strong hairs are difficult to destroy; often they must be removed more than once. But with patience on the part of the subject and skill on the part of the operator, permanent results can always be obtained, and without scarring. The same operator is equipped to remove moles, but the decision on this should be made by a dermatologist, so consult with one before going ahead with this operation. Unsightly moles should usually be removed, not only for cosmetic but for health reasons. Sometimes a mole will show signs of rapid growth; this condition should always be reported to your doctor.

PLASTIC SURGERY

If there is something about your face that really troubles you, a scar or an ugly feature, or if deep lines and sagging muscles make you look older than your years, consider having the condition corrected by a first-class plastic surgeon. Plastic surgery is an art and a science that has developed fabulously since the end of World War II. Today it is no longer frivolous or vain to have plastic surgery when it is desirable.

In Moscow I went to visit the Medical Cosmetics Institute on Gorki Street. There scars are removed, ears and lips are corrected; a nose is shortened and straightened for 600 rubles.

In Tokyo, at the Jujin Institute, Japanese girls have eyelid surgery to make their eyes look wider and rounder, more like those of the American movie stars they adore. The cost: $8.33. For $13.88 one can have bags under the eyes removed.

But the greatest percentage of this work is done in the United States, England, and France. A good plastic operation is still expensive; but in New York City there is already a clinic, headed by the distinguished Dr. Herbert Conway, at New York Hospital. In Los Angeles, the owner of the famous Abbot Rental Stores will arrange and pay for a plastic operation if the lady in question has a serious beauty defect and is unable to pay. I am sure that foundations will soon spring up all over the world for those who need this work done and are unable to pay for it.

If you have a really troubling facial problem and want to consider plastic surgery, this is my advice: Take the utmost pains to find the best doctor within your reach. Travel to find him, if necessary. Write to the state medical society at your state capital; you will get from them a list of three specialists in your locality. If you live near a large hospital or medical center, ask there for the names of staff surgeons or affiliated surgeons who specialize in plastic surgery. When you have the names of several, find out all you can about them. Consult the doctors themselves and ask, if possible, to see some of their work. Often you will find that these doctors' nurses have had plastic surgery performed and do not hesitate to show the corrections.

In other words, if you are considering plastic surgery, find a first-rate doctor, an artist in his profession. Remember that first-rate doctors never advertise. Remember, also, that first-rate plastic surgery may come high, but is cheap at any price; whereas second-rate work is ruinous, at any price.

For a person who has to make a living and appear before the public, plastic surgery is often a sound solution. This is the advice I have given to people in the middle years who have taken all other measures to keep up their energies and good looks, such as intelligent eating, exercise, and sufficient rest and relaxation.

Here is one of many cases: One of my New York students, who owned her own dress shop for many years, was in her fifties when she suffered business reverses. She lost her shop and all her capital, and was faced with creating a new future for herself. She looked her age, with bags under her eyes and a sagging jaw line; altogether she made a sad appearance for a woman who must go out and seek employment. Even though she was both capable and experienced in her field, and would be an asset to any retail establishment, I knew that no personnel manager would give her the opportunity to prove her abilities. I advised her to investigate plastic surgery before she went looking for a job.

She made doubly sure to perfect her nutrition with extra protein and vitamins. Finally, she entrusted herself to a first-rate plastic surgeon, who performed the operation, removing the under-eye bags and lifting the cheeks and the drooping mouth. I saw her three days after the operation and she looked amazingly well, with only a little black-and-blue evidence under the eyes and very fine red lines showing where the face-lift incisions had been made at the ears. Three weeks later, I could not even see the lines. Just four weeks after the operation she found a position as a buyer in one of the larger New York department stores. She is completely happy with the operation that insured her future livelihood and independence. Needless to say, she realizes that for her skin and muscles to remain firm and her face to keep its attractiveness—as she says, to protect her investment—she needs a high-protein diet and all the required vitamins.

Once when I was lecturing in Denver, a lady who had been one of my students for many years, one of the highest-salaried business women west of the Mississippi, was in my class. She seemed more intent than usual. After the lecture she said to me, "I didn't hear a word you said after your opening sentence about how everybody can live to be one hundred years old. I began thinking about houses."

"Houses?"

She nodded. "Suppose you take a house on a short or an in-definite lease. It's not just what you want, but who cares? Suppose, however, that you take a house on a hundred-year lease. That's different. If it's not what you want, you do something about it."

She looked me squarely in the eye. "I've had a disfiguring nose all my life. I've succeeded in spite of it. But I think I'll be a lot happier and more successful if I have it remodeled. Anyhow, if I'm going to live to be one hundred, I've got time to find out. How do I go about finding a good plastic surgeon in Denver?" My answer, of course, was to consult the local branch of the medical society—and then investigate each doctor (as I mentioned above).

I know many, many instances in which the three following opera-tions in particular have worked wonders for the people who under-went them: the nose plastic, the face lift, and the eye plastic. Here is what you should know about them.

The nose is the most frequent plastic operation—three-to-one compared with any of the others. Straightening and shortening are the simplest repairs; narrowing can also be done within limits. The operation takes about one hour under local anesthetic, and it is best to remain in the hospital for a day or two. There are no scars, because the work is done within the nose; and the improve-ment is permanent.

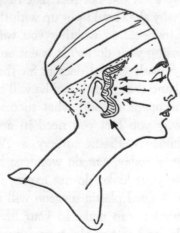

The face lift

The face lift is the second most popular operation and a blessing to many women—men, too—who need to keep a youthful appearance. The operation tightens the loose folds of the neck by pulling the skin upward by incision behind the ears, and tightens cheeks and forehead with another incision within the hairline at the temples. It takes about three hours, under either local or general anesthetic; and the hospital stay is about three days. After two to three weeks, there is almost no sign that an operation has been performed. The improvement lasts five to ten years, depending on how well you take care of your health and your skin. The scars are hardly visible, and can be covered by the hair.

Disfiguring under-eye bagginess and eyelid wrinkles may not be the result of late hours and overindulgence; they can be constitutional. Some faces have a tendency to develop small grape-sized lumps of fat under the eyes, and some skins tend to stretch and wrinkle at the lids. These repairs are two separate operations. Each takes half an hour, under local anesthetic. The hospital stay is one or two days. In a week or ten days the signs of the operation are completely gone. The only scars are thin lines at the eyelid edges, and these can be completely concealed by light make-up.

I was very interested to learn that Lady Mendl had had this operation performed many years ago by the famous Dr. Gillis in London. Lady Mendl was always glad that she did so; she said that she hated puffy eyes, did not feel that they belonged to her, and saw no reason why she should put up with them unnecessarily.

Take your time in deciding whether you want to have plastic surgery and in choosing your doctor. It is not an emergency operation, and you can consult several doctors for their advice. A good surgeon is also kind and thoughtful, and he will advise you whether you really need the operation and what success you can expect. He will ask you why you feel you need it, and you should tell him your reasons honestly. Plastic surgery, as American and English doctors perform it today, can do wonders; but while you can expect it to improve your looks, do not expect it to solve all your other problems too. A good plastic surgeon will not exaggerate the results his reconstruction can make in your life. If your expectations are reasonable, and if you do everything in your power to build up your good looks from within, then your plastic surgery can give added contentment and renewed self-confidence for many years to come.

I believe in plastic surgery. I have seen mature men's lives transformed by simple reshaping of a disfiguring feature. I have seen mature women's morale and earning capacity restored by a face lift. And the psychological effect is often as important as the actual lift. I look forward to the time when the remedying of bodily blemishes and deformities, at all ages, by expert plastic surgeons will be taken as a matter of course, much the same as going to the dentist to have teeth repaired, replaced, or capped. I hope and believe that plastic surgery will soon become a well-regulated therapy, free from hush-hush and free from the unscrupulous practitioners, who thrive in any field that is clouded by moral prejudice and social disapproval.

MORE BEAUTY SECRETS

Herbs, oils, honey, salt, vinegar, milk, yogurt, yeast, and many of the things you now have in your pantry make amazingly helpful health and beauty aids. Here are some formulas and recipes I have gathered in my travels around the world. You can always be sure of the efficacy and purity of these things you prepare with your own hands, and they cost you pennies instead of dollars.

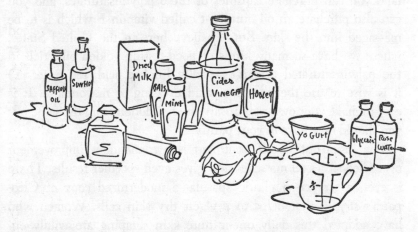

Be your own beauty chemist

Cleopatra's Skin Peeling

It seems that Cleopatra intuitively knew about the importance of polyunsaturates for her skin and complexion. Each day she was anointed and massaged with a combination of sesame and olive oils, heavily scented with musk. After the oils had a chance to soak into the skin, one of Cleopatra's slaves, using a special tool, a *strygil*, scraped off the excess oil; and with the oil the dried up old skin would also come off. These daily mild skin peelings helped to make Cleopatra's complexion famous throughout Egypt.

We know that Cleopatra's mixture of perfumed oils which were massaged into her skin was rich in polyunsaturates and did help to keep her skin young and soft. But German and Swiss doctors today say that in order to stop premature aging and drying of the skin, it is also necessary to use the valuable polyunsaturated oils *internally*. (One German chemist, with a passion for statistics, estimated that the polyunsaturated fat content of a really beautiful woman amounts to about 11 percent of her total volume.) They attack this skin problem in two ways. First, they recommend at least one tablespoonful of vegetable oil to be used daily *internally* (the easy way is in salad dressing) and *externally* the skin should be oiled daily with the same rich polyunsaturated oils. In Switzerland you can purchase capsules of these polyunsaturates, and you can also purchase an oil ointment called vitamin F which is to be massaged into the skin. But I believe here in the United States, where we have so many kinds of good-tasting golden oils, rich in the polyunsaturated acids (especially linoleic acid, see page 32) it is wise to use the oils in a salad dressing or mayonnaise. It is easy to make your own polyunsaturated oil lotion from the same oils you should now have in your pantry.

The inside-outside oil treatment is a tremendous improvement over Cleopatra's oil massages and gives even speedier results. There is even a scraper—a plastic spatula—a modernized copy of Cleopatra's *strygil*, that helps to peel off dry skin cells. Women who have adopted this daily one-minute skin scraping are wildly enthusiastic over their younger-looking skins.

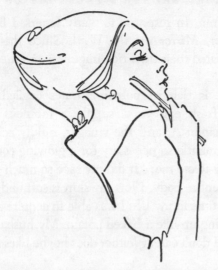

Cleopatra's strygil peels off dead skin

Improving on Cleopatra's Formula

Here is a combination of the world's finest and richest poly-unsaturated oils. No cosmetic externally applied can do more to make the skin softer and younger-looking. It is amazing how dry, wrinkled skin will gratefully soak in this combination of pure and wax-free oils. Modern cosmetic houses already manufacture poly-unsaturated combinations, but it is so easy to make your own. Simply mix in a measuring cup the following clear, natural oils:

3 tbsp. safflower oil	1 tbsp. olive oil
3 tbsp. sesame oil	1 tbsp. wheat germ oil
2 tbsp. sunflower oil	5 drops oil of rose geranium or
2 tbsp. avocado oil	your favorite perfume
2 tbsp. peanut oil	

Seven drops of this combination, applied to your face, will convince you of its efficacy and purity. Use it regularly on face and neck; and if your scalp is dry, rub in a few drops there.

Rich Polyunsaturated Mayonnaise Unguent

This is actually a mayonnaise, but it was prescribed, not for salads, but for the face, by Dr. Leo Kumer of Vienna. Facial mayonnaise has been used by many famous Austrian beauties. Here in America it was the lovely Arlene Dahl who first wrote about it in her beauty column. In response to many letters, I finally gave the recipe in *Mirror, Mirror on the Wall*. Since then many lovely ladies have prepared their own rich unguent; and they are delighted with the results.

This mixture is rich in polyunsaturates (called vitamin F in Europe). The fresh egg yolks supply a fabulous skin softener, lecithin, and vitamin A; and the vinegar, mildly acid, helps to establish the acid mantle so necessary for a glowing complexion. One enthusiastic lady wrote me: "It did my face so much good I decided to use it on my entire body. Now my skin is soft and moist all over, and for the first time in my life I was able to acquire an even golden tan without drying up like a baked potato. My husband says I smell like a salad, but I don't care. Neither does he; he likes salads!"

FACIAL MAYONNAISE UNGUENT

2 fresh egg yolks
½ cup sunflower oil
½ cup sesame oil
1 tbsp. wheat germ oil

1 tbsp. vinegar
2 drops of rose geranium oil
   or your favorite perfume
   (so you won't smell like a
   salad!)

Simply mix the oils in a measuring cup. Put fresh egg yolks in a cold bowl and beat. Add oil, slowly at first; and beat with a rotary beater. Add more oil gradually; and, as the mixture thickens, add vinegar and perfume. Excellent for sunbathing, for dry, rough skin, and for removing make-up.

Help for Scrawny Necks

Warm peanut oil massaged into a lined and scrawny neck gives excellent results. Dr. George Washington Carver, who was responsible for many fine products from the lowly peanut, first learned about the beauty-giving qualities of this inexpensive oil from mothers who reported the results they had using it to massage the skinny legs of children afflicted with polio.

Salon Beauty Mask

One of the most luxurious beauty salons in the world kept this quick complexion pepper-upper as a deep dark secret for many years—and charged fifteen dollars per treatment. Now it is yours to keep—and to make for only a few cents.

> 1 tbsp. of regular toilet lanolin
> 1 scant tsp. Balsam of Peru

Mix in a cup with a teaspoon until smooth and keep it in a jar, tightly covered. Apply this beige mixture over entire face and forehead. *But be careful not to apply it close to the eyes.* Allow to remain for five minutes only (less, the first time you use it). Later you may leave it on a few minutes longer.

This is a fabulous pepper-upper for tired faces. The glow lasts for hours. If you are a blonde with very thin skin, first apply a bit of golden oil or cream and then apply the beige mask over it. Remove mask, with a spatula if you have one, or cleansing tissue. If your face feels too warm, apply a little golden oil. *This is to be used only once a week,* so save it for the night you want to look blooming!

If your throat needs attention, you can use this same circulation treatment on it once a week, but it is best that you do the face and the throat on different days. Apply the beige mixture over throat and under chin; leave it on as long as it feels comfortable (about five minutes). Using the spatula (with upward strokes) also peels

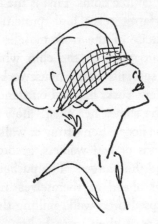

A soft cloth eye-mask relaxes the eyes

off the dead dry skin cells (Cleopatra's secret). Incidentally, keep your throat well oiled at all times, for the skin there has fewer oil cells than the face and shows birthdays first if neglected!

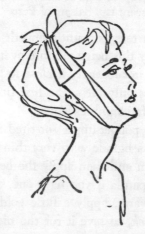

Do-it-yourself chin strap

New Way to Prevent or Correct a Double Chin

Nothing destroys a woman's good looks more than the appearance of a second chin to spoil her youthful neckline. There are three main causes of double chins. First is the lack of protein foods. (That's why beautyfarms serve high protein diets.) The second cause is lack of exercise of the neck muscles. The third cause is the downward-forward push of the chin while reading, writing, walking, working—especially doing housework. Madame Ellene of Vienna, and now New York, has had outstanding success in treating this problem. She shows her clients how to hold the chin always parallel with the floor when sitting or walking.

There are two kinds of bad walkers, according to Madame Ellene: the *pushers* and the *hangers*. The pushers lead with the chin out; they are always ahead of themselves and in a hurry. The hangers have a collapsed tired walk, pulling the neck in and pushing the chin *down* as if they were hiding. Both of these types develop double chins early in life. To break her clients of these bad habits, Madame Ellenc makes an unusual chin strap to be worn at home while working. This band keeps the chin in the right position. For even quicker results, the Viennese beautician, whose own neckline and skin are the best proof of the soundness of her method, insists that her clients place *medicated* cotton pads under the double chin to increase the circulation and bring the blood to the weakened neck muscles.

Here is how you can make Madame Ellene's medicated chin strap in your own home. Buy a package of any good elastic bandage, three inches wide, in any drugstore. Cut a piece long enough to cover your chin and tie on the top of your head. Then soak a cotton square in the medicated solution and apply under chin. Wear for an hour each day.

For the medicated solution, put one tablespoon of hot water into a cup. In it dissolve one-fourth teaspoon of epsom salt. When *thoroughly* dissolved, add one tablespoon glycerin and one teaspoon menthol solution (10 percent). Pour into bottle. Saturate cotton pads with this medicated solution and apply directly under double chin bandage. You will feel a mild, cool stimulation. You will see results the very first time you use this treatment.

How to Stop Forehead Wrinkles

A plastic surgeon in London says he can tell a lot about a person's character by the lines and wrinkles on his face. Significant

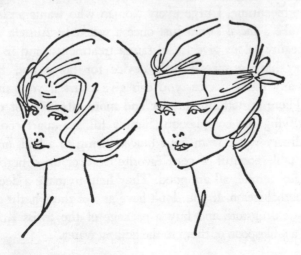

are those vertical lines on the forehead between the eyes; the deeper these are, according to the surgeon, the more intense a person you are—and he says you should learn to relax and not take yourself so seriously. I don't know whether this is always so, but I *do* know that you *can* stop, and even get rid of, heavy forehead wrinkles and lines by *stopping* your habit of frowning. (Frown and the world frowns at you!) To help you stop the habit of frowning and to increase the circulation to those forehead muscles, Madame Ellene recommends that her clients wear a *medicated* elastic headband for an hour each day (while taking a bath or working around the house) until they lose the habit of frowning. This is an adaptation of the chin strap (page 278).

Sensational Facial Sauna

For years the famous sauna bath was the secret of the hardy Finns. Now sauna baths are exported to all parts of the world. In Hollywood it was Bob Hope, Cary Grant, and Jerry Lewis who first raved about the benefits of the Finnish sauna; now several of the stars have their own saunas, most of them imported from Finland at a cost of six to ten thousand dollars. Now they can be purchased in the United States for less money. I predict that sauna baths will some day be used all over the country.

In the meantime, I urge every woman who wants a clean clear skin to take a *facial sauna* just once a week. In Austria and Germany, beauty salons give facial sauna treatments; and in Switzerland they have a special little device for home use. However, without any fancy device, you can give yourself your first facial sauna. There is nothing simpler and more effective for cleansing and purifying the complexion. Simply fill a 2-quart cooking pot with ordinary water from your faucet. Bring to a boil, and add a heaping tablespoonful of your favorite fresh or dried herbs—camomile, anise, fennel, all are good. They help to make a deep, *penetrating* herbal steam. If you don't have any of these herbs on hand, go to your drugstore and buy a package of the Swiss Kriss herbs and add a tablespoon of them to the boiling water.

Now you are ready for your first facial sauna. Place the steaming herbal "witches brew" on your kitchen table. Protect your hair

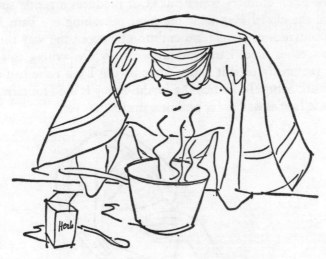

The three-minute sauna facial

with a rubber cap. Cover your head and the pot with a bath towel so no steam escapes on the sides, but it all rises straight up into your face. Start with 3 minutes; later make it 5 minutes. You'll be amazed how this pleasant herbalized steam penetrates deeply and cleanses every pore. This steam is made up of the softest distilled water, free of all chemicals, as soft as rain. It makes the skin unbelievably soft.

The roses in your glowing face after a facial sauna are your own, brought about by your own rushing blood stream. The pearls of perspiration coming from every open pore loosen stale make-up, rancid oils, blackheads, and every bit of dirt. It does all this in just a few minutes. After such a thorough cleansing of the pores, they are wide open; so be sure to close them with very cold water (but not ice). I cannot recommend this facial sauna highly enough. If your skin is troublesome you might take one daily for 3 days; after that, just once a week. Facial saunas can keep your skin beautifully clean! A beautiful skin is a clean skin; for a flawless complexion, your skin needs more *wake up* than *make-up!*

Eye Refresher from Paris

Through my office in Paris I discovered the Hydro-Spray.* When attached to an ordinary water faucet, it produces a gentle spray to massage the closed eyes with the most refreshing eye bath I ever had. Thousands of people are enthusiastic about the way this fine spray refreshes tired, hard-working eyes. While writing this book I have personally used it daily. After its use I felt refreshed and I could work better. In France the Hydro-Spray is used for refreshing the whole face as well as for puffiness under the eyes.

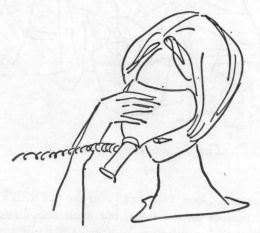

Cool water massage for tired eyes and puffiness

Removing Brown Spots from Hands and Face

The quickest way to get rid of those ugly brown pigmentations, sometimes called liver spots, is to have them planed away by an experienced dermatologist. Even scars and freckles can be planed away with a fast-rotating tool that looks like a dentist's drill.

Another successful and less drastic method is deep-skin peeling. However, it should be done only by a doctor trained in this highly specialized method. It is not painful. After the acid solution is painted on, there is a slight burning. After two or three days the skin gets dark, shrivels off, and with it go the brown spots.

Dr. Jarvis says that many brown spots disappear gradually by rubbing a few drops of castor oil into the brown pigmentation daily.

* Imported by Ellene, 20 E. 67 St., New York, N.Y.

Adelle Davis, a diet authority, attacks these blemishes from the inside. She recommends 100 units of vitamin E to be taken after each meal. She says this method, although slower, is longer lasting.

French Anti-pimple Lotion

This can be a girl's (or boy's) best friend. It was given to me by a French Ambassadress who is famous for her flawless skin. Buy a small bottle of calamine lotion and ask your druggist to put in 1 percent of Phenol. Soak a small bit of cotton in this medicated solution, and press it flat over the pimple; you'll be amazed how quickly it drys up. This treatment also discourages an oncoming pimple.

Salon Blackhead Treatment

One of the simplest and most effective treatments for blackheads (from an exclusive New York salon) is the following: Dissolve 1 tablespoon of ordinary epsom salt in half a cup of very hot water, and add three drops of ordinary iodine. This solution must be kept *hot*; so place the cup with solution in a bowl of *hot* water. Take a strip of absorbent cotton (not too thick) long enough to cover affected area. Saturate the cotton with the mixture and hold firmly in place. To keep maximum heat, cover with dry washcloth. When the cotton has cooled off, dip it again into solution. Apply hot solution three or four times. When finished, blackheads pop out easily. (Don't squeeze by hand; use a blackhead squeezer.)

Some Specific Anti-Gray Hair Factors

In the Gayelord Hauser *Newsletter* I mentioned the many letters I receive from people who tell me that with the changing of their eating habits to a nutritious diet, many surprising things happened. Sometimes even the gray disappears from their hair. Ever since, I have been besieged with requests to tell how these people did it. So here is a résumé of the foods and the vitamins and minerals involved. But I must repeat, it does not work for everybody. However, should your hair color problem be a nutritional one, give this a try. Don't expect results overnight—it is a slow process.

Follow a completely nutritious diet, with extra emphasis on liver of all kinds; eat it twice a week. Use wheat germ, brewers' yeast, yogurt, gelatin, and vegetable oils. All kinds of sea food should be included. Eat only whole-grain breads and cereals. Then, so that there is no possible chance of missing any vitamins or minerals that might help to bring back the color of your hair, let your doctor give you a prescription for the three most important hair recoloring factors, and take them according to his directions:

Para-amino-benzoic acid	100 mg.
Calcium pantothenate	30 mg.
Choline	2 grams

Be patient. It might, and it might not, work for your hair. But in any case you will certainly get all the other benefits from such a nutritious diet.

Russian Wonder Cream

This old-fashioned healing combination contains four of nature's most potent soothing and healing elements for minor irritations, skin troubles, and athlete's foot. Russian soldiers massage this combination into their feet to prevent foot sores. Simply mix in a cup:

4 tsp.	anhydrous lanolin
2 tsp.	cod liver oil
½ tsp.	pure garlic powder
½ tsp.	honey

Beat thoroughly with a fork until the honey-colored mixture turns to a creamy white. Keep it tightly covered in a jar, and use it as necessary.

How to Test Your Cosmetics

If you have the slightest suspicion that some cosmetic is causing an irritation to your eyes, scalp, face, or hands, you should make this simple test. Take a bit of the suspected preparation and press it on a small piece of gauze; tape it to the inside of your upper arm, where the skin is most sensitive. Leave the patch on for 48 hours; then remove it. If there is no red spot or irritation, the preparation is safe; but if there is a red spot and irritation under the patch, then that cosmetic is not for you. Should you be sensitive to many cosmetics, it is best to use only the purest of lotions and oils.

German Wheat-Germ Mask for Sensitive Skins

Place 1 tablespoon of wheat-germ *flour* and 1 tablespoon of yogurt into a cup, and mix until smooth as mayonnaise. Apply this soothing mixture all over face and neck and lie down and relax for 15 minutes. When the preparation is dry, remove with warm water; then rinse with cold water. This mask is very popular in Germany, especially with people who are sensitive to soaps and detergents.

Fragrant Rose Water

You can make your own rose water if you have a rose garden. You need one pound of rose petals, the more fragrant the better, to make a quart of rose water. However, most drugstores sell rose water for about fifty cents for a good-sized bottle. With it you can flavor fruit drinks and compotes; pink grapefruit with a teaspoon of rose water is a happy surprise. But rose water is especially recommended for making delightful cosmetics, as Cleopatra did.

pH Face Astringent

To help re-establish the skin's acid mantle, and to help tighten the skin, apply this face lotion all over your face and neck before applying make-up:

¾ cup rose water	Pinch alum powder
¼ cup witch hazel	¼ tsp. glycerin
1 tsp. honey	½ tsp. spirit of camphor
½ tsp. white vinegar	½ tsp. extract of mint

Mix all in a bottle and shake. Apply with cotton pads.

pH Hand Lotion

This combination is one of the oldest, and still the best, of hand protectors. The skin on our hands has fewer natural oil cells than the skin on our faces and necks; therefore, constant moisturizing is necessary. In this easy-to-make formula you have two of nature's most effective moisturizers: glycerin and honey. The lotion is not sticky. Use it generously. Simply shake together in a bottle:

> ¾ cup rose water
> ¼ cup glycerin
> ¼ tsp. vinegar
> ¼ tsp. honey

Herbal Rinse to Darken Hair

When hair is mousy and lifeless-looking and hard to manage, make this simple hair rinse: Shampoo hair thoroughly with lanolin or oil shampoo and rinse with cosmetic vinegar water (see below). Then put one heaping tablespoon of Swiss Kriss herbs into a pint of water and simmer for 10 minutes. Pour through fine strainer. Apply this herb lotion all over scalp and hair with cotton pad. Do not rinse. (Blondes must never use this herbal lotion. It definitely darkens the hair.)

Cosmetic Vinegar

Dr. Culpepper, a famous English physician, wrote many books. In all of them he was full of praise for vinegar. But long before his day, the old alchemists were concocting vinegar. Some of the early great beauties had their chemists prepare vinegar rinses, vinegar douches, and vinegar bath tonics. To this day you'll find cosmetic vinegar in English herb shops; and in Germany the barbers use a vinegar tonic after shaving. And today vinegar is being made popular in America by Dr. Jarvis' vinegar-honey formula (1 tsp. of honey and 1 tsp. of vinegar in a glass of water).

My interest in vinegar is not only because of its health value, but also because it has many uses as an excellent, inexpensive cosmetic. Many women who have prepared my cosmetic vinegar have written me letters of thanks. They tell me that what they have been able to do for the looks of their hair, hands, and face is almost miraculous. Today we know that skin and scalp, when healthy, exude a mild acid that protects them against infection. Every time you shampoo your hair, every time you wash your face or take a bath, you remove that acid mantle and destroy nature's safeguard. Many scalp and skin troubles, including dry scaly scalp and dry scaly skin, could be halted by protecting the skin and scalp with its natural acid mantle. This is easily done if, after shampooing, washing, or bathing, you use a bit of cosmetic vinegar.

The old-fashioned cosmetic vinegar formula is: Put 2 heaping tablespoonfuls of imported dried peppermint leaves into a pint of water. Let come to a boil, and simmer for 3 minutes. Then pour through a fine strainer. Add the peppermint infusion to a pint of pure cider vinegar.

The quick way to make cosmetic vinegar is to mix a pint of pure cider vinegar with a pint of very hot water, and add half a teaspoonful of oil of peppermint and half a teaspoon of rose geranium. (Never use straight vinegar for cosmetic purposes.)

Either solution can be applied to scalp or face with a bit of cotton; it makes an excellent face tonic. For the bath, especially for dry, itching skin, pour ½ cup cosmetic vinegar into ½ tub of pleasantly warm water.

Milk Pads Sooth Tired Eyes

A charming nurse at the Bay City, Michigan Hospital wants to share this secret. She places cotton pads soaked in plain milk at room temperature over tired and puffy eyes and relaxes for 10 minutes. She has used this many times on her patients and it really puts a sparkle in tired eyes.

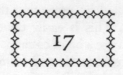

17

Give Yourself One Day a Week

We read in the Bible that the Lord made the world in six days, and on the seventh day, He rested. The Sabbath has become a traditional day of rest, the world over. But how many of us do really observe a day of rest—completely detached from hustle and bustle and habitual routines?

I want to recommend to all wise people—regardless of income, business, family, and friends—that you declare one day of the week YOURday and make it just that. It can become the most important and valuable day of the week to you. Whether you are able to establish it for Saturday, Sunday, or a week day, stake your claim and hold it against all odds. Make it a permanent habit and you will become richer, happier, and healthier for it. If friends and family jeer and scoff, let them; the chances are that after a while they will see what it does for you and stake out THEIRday for themselves.

YOURday is to be one completely detached from the distractions and obligations of other days, both of work and of family. On YOURday you are at no one's beck and call. Don't tell me you cannot possibly do it; the busier you are, the more you need it. The more firmly you establish the habit of YOURday as one freed from anxieties, tensions, cares, and the harassment of "what time is it?" the more easily and efficiently you will find yourself operating throughout the other days of the week. Not for nothing has it been said, "Man does not live by bread alone."

How to Spend YOURday

Some people have become so involved in the hectic rush of existence that they have no clear idea of how to go about using one whole day of freedom from the treadmill. If you are one of these, let me make some suggestions to get you started. We'll take the physical man first, then the inner man—and woman.

No alarm clock to wake you up. On YOURday, wake up naturally, easily, lazy, and relaxed. For once it does not matter what time the bus leaves. Try an oxygen cocktail before arising. Take half a dozen slow, deep breaths—inhale through your nose, exhale through the mouth. Easy does it. Don't hurry out of bed; relax awhile and enjoy the luxury of being relaxed.

Here are some ideas for the day's menus. They are generous.

Breakfast

Ready for breakfast now? Good! Give your digestive system a recuperative lazy day also. Have your favorite fruit juice, or whole fruit. (Remember, the whole fruit is preferable for reducers because it is more slowly digested and provides satisfying bulk for a stomach accustomed to being overloaded.) Treat yourself to Swiss Coffee—a big cup of fresh hot coffee with fortified hot milk, mixed half-and-half, flavored with a teaspoonful of energizing honey. (Of course you use lean skim milk.)

Midmorning

A bracer to keep the energy high: a glass of lean milk, buttermilk, vanilla milk shake, or orange milk shake (page 532).

Luncheon

Now is the time to enjoy a big bowl of salad. Choose either fresh fruits or vegetables with leafy greens, plus four heaping tablespoons of cottage cheese, and sprinkle it with lemon juice and a dash of vegetable salt (and the smallest dash of light dressing, if you must have it). With your salad have one slice of whole-wheat, rye, or protein bread, very lightly buttered. For a beverage, take your choice of Swiss Coffee, buttermilk, or hot tea with lemon and honey.

Midafternoon

Enjoy another refreshing snack, chosen from any *one* of the following: Hot jasmine tea, or mint tea, with honey and lemon. A glass of yogurt flavored with honey. A glass of fresh vegetable juice. A glass of tomato juice spiked with a pinch of herbs and a quarter-section of lemon.

Dinner

Start with something fresh, either a vegetable espresso (page 505) or a generous green salad with light dressing. For the entree, have your choice of: a fluffy omelet; broiled liver sprinkled with parsley; broiled mushrooms; cottage cheese with chives. Add a moderate serving of short-cooked vegetable. Have a light-hearted baked potato flavored with a spoonful of yogurt. Now for dessert: Have a fruit compote made with any small fruits or cut up fruits, of your choice—with honey drizzled over it. For a beverage, choose one of these: demitasse, Swiss Coffee, papaya mint tea, jasmine tea, or buttermilk.

Good Nite Cap

Before retiring, soothe the inner man or woman with a glass of hot lean milk flavored with honey, or molasses, or licorice.

You will find that this one day of extra-lean eating is vastly beneficial to your digestive system, as well as to your mind and emotions.

Now let's think of other ideas for YOURday.

The Relaxing Bath

This is a good day to treat yourself to the most enjoyable and most beneficial sort of bath. Take it any time during the day, except at bedtime. Fill the tub with pleasantly warm water and lie in it limp as a rag doll for ten, fifteen, thirty minutes, or as

long as you like. Try the alternating bath (page 258). Then relax
in the Yoga Slant position (page 173).

Exercise

YOURday is a perfect day to limber up all your body with lazy,
easy exercises. You can make it a really rejuvenating day. You don't
have to dress up and rush out anywhere. No hurry, no worry. Two
or three times during the day, do your favorite exercises, especially
the Stomach Lift (page 175). This is YOURday to set yourself an
example for simple, regular exercise all week.

Sun and Air

Weather permitting, do treat yourself to some sun and air on
YOURday. It's a wonderful time to enjoy sun-bathing and store
up some "sunshine vitamins." Take a brisk walk in the park, to
revitalize the circulation and give your lungs a healthy ration of
good, clean oxygen. Get acquainted with the delights of walking
through woods and fields, with leisure to see and to sense the beauty
of the world you live in.

MENTAL TREATS

If you have been longing for time to putter, read, meditate and
invite the spirit, or to launch some pet project, now is the day to
do so. You know that the only time your conscious mind is un-
occupied is when you are asleep. On YOURday, empty it of
the daily routine, occupy it and refresh it with new thoughts and
things.

You are an oral person, you know. That means you have a keen
appetite for words. You love them: you probably can't get enough
of them, in one form or another. How will you have them served
to you on YOURday? That depends on your individual taste, but
here is the general idea: On YOURday take your words *in the
exact opposite* of the way you get them the rest of the week.

Do you spend much of your time talking to people? Then spend
YOURday talking to as few people as possible. Take your words
in written form—reading, dipping into the dictionary and encyclo-
pedia, cutting and pasting clippings in a scrapbook, writing letters.

Or take your words vocally, aloud. Memorize a favorite poem and recite it aloud to yourself. A well-known lecturer writes me that she spends part of HERday singing. Not that she can sing; she just likes to think she can.

Some professional talkers are gluttons for silence. I am told that one well-known news broadcaster spends HISday like a veritable Trappist monk; he sees no one, turns off the telephone, and eats crossword puzzles alive—complicated ones imported from England. A stage comedian I know spends HISday inventing cryptograms. A university professor has a taste for bird-watching; on HERday she is strictly for the birds. If you have such an appetite for silence, do indulge it on YOURday. Give yourself the greatest treat of all—the joy of sitting still and listening. Listening to what? To your own thoughts and reveries. Meditation, you know, is the nutritional element of the soul: It feeds spiritual strength and power. "Be still," the Bible tells us, "and know that I am God."

Perhaps you live and work alone. If so, on YOURday you will want the opposite of silence. "On MYday," a free-lance writer tells me, "I ride on the bus, sit on park benches, eat in crowded restaurants, smiling at people (with discretion) and starting up casual conversation with anyone and everyone."

This is YOURday to pursue any new project you want to undertake. What is it? Clarinet playing? Languages? How long is it since you browsed through a library or an art gallery or a museum? You are well on your way now toward preventing or eliminating "middle-age spread" of the body. YOURday is the day to take steps against middle-age spread of the mind.

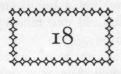

Let's Visit a Beautyfarm

When you arrive at a beautyfarm, you are shown to your bright and airy room. Perhaps there is an Aubusson rug on the floor and a Renoir painting on the wall. After you have unpacked, the staff doctor comes and examines you, unless you have brought a letter from your own doctor saying that you are in good health.

The next morning your breakfast is served to you in bed by an attractive maid; and on your tray, set with very fine silver, very fine linen, and a beautiful flower, will be a bowl of fresh fruit, some scrambled eggs, and one slice of protein toast, plus coffee with hot milk (this is a modern beautyfarm breakfast—the day of coffee and fruit juice is passé). On your tray you will also find your program of activities, your beauty menu for the day.

Right after breakfast you will be asked to put on your exercise suit, a leotard, which the beauty institutes have taken over from the ballet and dance schools. Over this you put your robe, and now you are on your way.

Before your exercise session a nurse or the exercise director—a rather determined woman—will make a record of your measurements. There will be no secrets: the exact weight and measurements will be put down in black and white, and the woman in charge will inform you just what your ideal measurements and weight should be. Then your posture is carefully noted. On California beautyfarms you are asked to walk and they take a film to see you in action. After that a beautician looks over your skin, hair, and nails. Your plus and your minus points are recorded and finally the "work" begins.

One farm has a "beauty barn" where you are pommeled, steamed, oiled, and brushed. After your first workout—about eleven o'clock—you are served a cup of hot broth with an egg yolk, or a fresh vegetable espresso, so that you will not be too hungry by one o'clock. The time before lunch, about an hour, is your own. You can swim in the pool, where you may be given some special underwater gymnastics; some have pools with hot and cold water springs. If you are more than ten pounds overweight, the physical education director will map out a walk for you of two or three miles, according to how much you have to lose. So that you will not feel sorry for yourself, one of the instructors or one of the other guests will accompany you on a lovely country road.

A BEAUTYFARM LUNCHEON

Lunch time is picnic time on a beautyfarm. The managers of a beautyfarm in Palm Springs, California, arrange interesting picnics for their clients. They serve the finest, freshest salads, fortified with the most delicious forms of protein: chicken, lobster, eggs, fish, and gelatin-tongue salads, and always big bowls of lean cottage cheese. There is unlimited choice of salads made with golden oil dressing, but only one piece of high-protein toast, whole-wheat bread, rye bread, or soya muffin is allowed. There is always steaming hot vegetable broth, hot fortified tomato juice, or Swiss broth, which is a great favorite. For dessert there are bowls full of fresh fruit or Lady Mendl compote. Beautyfarm beverages are: clear coffee, Swiss coffee, fortified milk, yogurt, English tea, rose-hip tea, peppermint tea, papaya tea, fresh fruit juices, or vegetable espresso.

After lunch you are glad to retire to your room. You will be tired and you will probably take a nap. Ann Delafield, the dean of physical education, suggests that every woman, before retiring or resting, should take a fifteen-minute refresher on the Beauty Slant and let the law of gravity put her posture into beautiful alignment. This is done on many beautyfarms.

After the noon siesta, you look at your program for the day. The afternoon will be dedicated to more beautifying. There will be fragrant oil of rose geranium baths or herbal facials, hair brushing under the trees, manicures, pedicures. There may be tennis or more swimming. You will be on the move every minute—there is never any time for boredom, and among the ladies there is a splendid spirit of camaraderie; they are all there for the same reason, and the favorite conversation is: how are *your* measurements; how much did you lose? There is also a friendly spirit of competition which makes even reducing easy and more like a game, and of course, the luxurious surroundings, the beautiful service, the lean food, and the absence of family duties are other reasons for the good results.

Besides the tennis courts, swimming pools, nearby golf courses, there are wonderful walks, and it is amazing how gladly women will walk when they have good shoes and good company.

At five o'clock you return to your own room, this time to freshen up. You are expected to change for dinner; the early beauty-farms expected guests to dress, but this is no longer obligatory, they discovered the ladies often were too tired. However, the guests always change from their daytime costumes. Slacks are not permitted in the dining room.

Ever since I introduced vegetable espressos at the Main Chance Beauty Farm, all the other beautyfarms here and abroad have taken advantage of this idea. Cocktails, about half an hour before dinner, consist of foaming glasses of fresh vegetable juices. The most popular combination is carrot, celery, and apple juice. Some of the women are so hungry they drink two glasses right from the spout, and that is all to the good because the natural sugars of the juices raise the blood sugar level, a sure and natural way to prevent overeating at the dinner table.

READY FOR DINNER?

Beautyfarms outdo themselves to give the guests beauty-full and satisfying dinners: broiled livers of all kinds, chicken livers en brochette or parsleyed calves' liver are served several times a week; broiled chicken, broiled lobster tails, lean sirloin steak, are also favorites. There are always two green freshly short-cooked vegetables. The desserts are all delicious, with a choice of fresh fruit sherbet, apricot mousse, exotic fruits, or fruit pies made with thin shells of coconut or wheat germ crust.

The ladies all enjoy one generous portion of everything. For the newcomers with overstretched stomachs there are always trays full of crisp, chilled finger salads made up of fresh bits of raw cauliflower, sliced green and red peppers, radishes, celery hearts, young onions, and green olives. These can be eaten freely without conscience trouble. There is never any difficulty about overeating at beautyfarms. The ladies watch one another and the hostess is usually a dignified woman who keeps a watchful eye on her charges.

After dinner the women gather in the beautiful salon for cards, conversation, and perhaps some fine music. Time never hangs heavy on a well-run beautyfarm. Even the evenings seem to pass too quickly. The women are naturally tired and glad to retire about ten o'clock. There is always a nightcap choice of half a dozen fragrant teas: linden, verbena, licorice, papaya, or hot Swiss broth. And then to dream in your own comfortable room.

This gives you an idea of what it is like to be a guest at one of the luxurious beautyfarms; the service is fabulous, the food superb, the setting is beautiful.

But there should be beautyfarms for all the lovely ladies in the land, not only for millionairesses. And I predict there will be many more in the future. I hope that I can help to speed up the day.

In the meantime, let me assure you that any woman can establish her own miniature beautyfarm right in her own home. You won't be pampered, you won't have your breakfast served in bed, but you also won't have to pay five hundred dollars a week!

Your Own Beautyfarm

It is the easiest thing in the world for you to have a miniature beautyfarm in your own back yard. Even if you have only a small piece of land, you possess the important beautyfarm needs already: sun, soil, air, and water.

To let the sun caress your body, turn a sheltered corner into a suntrap with a sheltering trellis against the wind or prying eyes. If you prefer, you can make or buy an aluminum-coated sun reflector which keeps drafts away and gives a golden tan without harmful chemicals in a few days' time.

Be careful with the sun. Always oil your skin well and follow the sun-exposure schedule faithfully. Begin with no more than twenty minutes and turn from side to side so you will tan evenly.

You will need a Beauty Slant board for your beautyfarm; cover it with plastic to protect it against the elements. You can get double benefits if you do your sunning in the Beauty Slant position and let the law of gravity work for you at the same time. But be careful not to go to sleep in the sun.

For exercise: a hanging bar for you; for your Adam it will be a chinning bar. Get him to put up a punching bag for himself; it is excellent rhythmic exercise for his arms and torso muscles and a first-rate tension releaser.

Iron dumbbells in different weights belong on every beautyfarm. Muscles become firm twice as quickly with these; ten minutes a day strengthens your man's arms, and they are very valuable to you in keeping the bustline high. Five-pound dumbbells are best for him and two-pound dumbbells are best for you.

Add the beauty gift of water to your private beautyfarm. A wonderful investment would be a small swimming pool. I believe there is nothing that can give more pleasure to the whole family. It does not have to be a big expensive one. Investigate the round, oval, and free-form pools. There are companies that install these in one day: they bring the cement ready-mixed and blow it over a steel frame fitted into the excavation. If you say that a pool is too expensive, I say so is a second car. A pool is a much better investment for health and good looks than a second car. If a pool is out of your reach this year, then install an outdoor shower, a great comfort and wonderfully refreshing. Remember, cool water peps you up, warm and hot water relaxes. With a few dollars and a dash of imagination you can make a back yard into your personal beautyfarm.

A Health Spa in Your Own Bathtub

If you can't go to take a cure in the hot springs of Palm Springs, Aix Les Bains, or Carlsbad, you can get some of the same benefits right at home by making your own private mineral bath. You can definitely soak away tension and tiredness, and reduce rheumatism and arthritis-like pains. All you need is lots of hot water and this easy-to-make mixture of medicated minerals:

> 2 cups ordinary epsom salt
>   (magnesium sulphate)
> 1 cup Calgon (best water softener)
> 1 tsp. eucalyptus oil
> 1 tsp. menthol, 10% solution
> 1 tsp. liquid iodine

Place salt and Calgon in a mixing bowl. Add eucalyptus oil, menthol solution, and iodine, and mix with a spoon. This makes a pale yellow mineral bath combination, second to none. (You can double or triple the amounts for future use.) Keep in tightly closed can. Use half a cup to one cup in a tub of pleasantly warm water. Relax and luxuriate for at least fifteen minutes. For complete relaxation and solid comfort, use a small rubber pillow or roll up a towel, place it behind your neck, and lean back.

Your Beautyfarm Kitchen

Any good cook can become a beautyfarm cook.

I will go further: anyone can become a beautyfarm cook if she wants to be one.

Your cooking pots are an important key. Most women use too much water in cooking because the food burns in their ordinary pots. Avoid both the burning and the loss of essential vitamins and minerals by having heavy cooking pots with close-fitting lids that are heavy enough to stay down. You need at least two of these heavy saucepans for your vegetables. In California we use enameled cast-iron pots and lids; in New York we use heavy stainless steel. These pots are a little more expensive than thin light-weight enamel, but they last forever and are a good investment. You will need several appliances to help you save time and valuable nutrients.

A *liquidizer-blender* is used on most beautyfarms. This is a versatile food and beverage machine with a sturdy motor of many speeds. The machine grinds, chops, whips, and even turns nuts and seeds into delicious butters and spreads. The liquidizer is a wonderful avante-garde device.

You need the most *modern juicing machine* to make the important vegetable espressos. (Buy a machine which can't vibrate and is easy to clean.) Every woman in search of a good skin should have a pint of carrot, celery, or apple espresso each day.

A *stainless steel vegetable shredder* is also a good investment. When vegetables are shredded they can be sautéed in five to seven minutes, as the Chinese do. Use a bit of golden oil or a bit of broth.

And every kitchen should have *a set of sharp stainless steel knives* for cutting off all visible fat from all meats. Beautyfarm cookery is lean cookery.

You will also need *a fine stainless steel strainer* to remove fat from the natural juices (fill it with ice cubes and pour the juices over them; the fat will solidify and remain in the strainer).

For making quantities of delicious yogurt you should invest in *a yogurt maker* for making fortified, plain, or fruit-flavored yogurt.

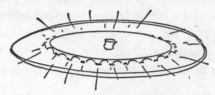

French thermos cover cuts cooking time in half

A special addition to your kitchen are those new *thermos pan covers* from Paris that cut cooking time in half.*

CLEAN OUT YOUR PANTRY

Throw out all the hard, hydrogenated fats, white sugar, and bleached flour. Put in their place the golden oils, whole-grain flours, and natural sugars: honey, brown sugar, and unsulphured molasses. Also try the new sweet licorice and the delicious carob flour.

Always keep a supply of flavorsome herbs and spices of all kinds in your kitchen. By all means use fresh herbs if you have a garden; if not, use the dried ones. But be subtle with them. Beautyfarm cooking requires "a touch of poetry," and spices and herbs can give that poetic touch.

The golden oils all bring their own subtle and agreeable flavors. Try them all, singly or mix two or three varieties and make your own blend.

* Available in diet and health food shops or directly from the importer, Parre-Chef, Distributors, 6821 N. Seville Ave., Milwaukee, Wisc.

And for more flavor and savor, you will want several bottles of wine and cider vinegar to make your own special fragrant herb vinegars, as they do in France. Dr. Jarvis, in his book, *Folk Medicine,* pointed out the many benefits of cider vinegar for your health.

You will always need a supply of lean milk, yogurt, the golden oils, and fresh sweet butter. If possible, use whipped butter; you will need less.

And now for your own cooking skills: You need to learn only how to short-cook your vegetables in a little liquid—two or three tablespoons—so that it is all gone when the vegetable is cooked. For more flavor you can use vegetable or chicken broth. Your heavy cooking pot will conserve the flavor and moisture and prevent burning. Just before serving a fresh vegetable, you add a sprinkle of vegetable salt and a bit of butter; whipped butter looks like hollandaise sauce, and you need very little. You have never tasted more delicious vegetables. And, of course, when you sauté vegetables in golden oil as the Chinese do, you do not need any butter.

Cook with a Low Flame

I can tell a good cook by one sign: the height of the flame under her pot. Always remember, low temperatures give high quality in all cookery: boiling, sautéing, roasting; the simple exception is broiling. But the most important ingredient in beautyfarm cookery is: T.L.C.—Tender Loving Cooking! When the cook cares, the food remains tasty, full of beauty and health-giving goodness; it even looks good when it comes to the table. And that is as it should be. Remember, we also eat with our eyes!

Good food is the everlasting pleasure that never fades. Enjoy your beautyfarm cooking and reap its benefits in health and good looks for you and your loved ones. They say that Frenchmen would rather marry a fine cook than a beautiful girl because the pleasures of good cooking go on long after other passions have diminished.

One more requisite will complete your private beautyfarm. On every beautyfarm there is one wise, inspired man or woman with a strong personality who gently but firmly inspires the guests and the staff with the will to accomplish what they are there to do: to redesign bodies and spirits, both within and without. It used to be said of beautiful Ann Delafield, when she was directing the first Elizabeth Arden farm, that she handled the spoiled ladies with a silken glove and a steel hand. On your private beautyfarm that guiding, inspiring person with the silken glove and the steel hand will have to be *you!*

WE NEED MORE BEAUTYFARMS

The more you become acquainted with the wonders of wise Mother Nature, the more you realize how generous she is with her earthly children. She gives her mightiest gifts—the sun, the soil, the air, the water—to produce the living foods that nourish us. We also know that we can derive great beauty-giving energy directly from the sun, by exposing ourselves intelligently to its healing and soothing rays, and from water in which we bathe and swim. And how comforting the earth itself can be!

You have surely discovered what a happy change it is to walk on soft, springy earth after hard, jolting pavements; to walk in the woods with soft moss underfoot, or just to lie on green grass and smell its fresh fragrance. These are some of nature's priceless gifts, and lucky are the people who still live among trees and grass in fresh air.

Millions of city dwellers, who live far from nature's beauties, look forward to their holidays when they can relax and recharge themselves in the quiet of fields and forests. The wholesome desire to get away from city tensions gave birth to the beautyfarm idea.

Thousands of people have discovered that they come back tired from their holiday; neither their bodies nor their minds have enjoyed a complete change. So many Americans spend their vacations traveling long distances, getting no closer to the countryside than seeing it through a car window, or perhaps from 30,000 feet above in a jet plane.

Only of late have we begun to appreciate the value of getting to the country, preferably to a farm, away from noise and irritations, to eat food that comes directly from the good earth to the table.

This can do wonders, especially for tense and harassed women. Elizabeth Arden was the first to see the possibilities of this idea when she turned her nonpaying Maine farm into a beautyfarm, inviting those who could afford it to come and relax for three or four weeks at a fabulous price. Now there are other beautyfarms and rest resorts springing up all over the world. But they are only a drop in the bucket. There should be beautyfarms in every state.

The women have discovered the beautyfarms first, as they always do in matters pertaining to better looks and health. But the men will follow. I predict that one day soon we shall have VIP farms for men. They cannot come too soon!

BEAUTYFARMS LISTING

Here I present an international list of beautyfarms, spas, and health resorts. For more information, write directly to the addresses given below. For best accommodations, make reservations well in advance.

THE GOLDEN DOOR, Escondido, California. Luxurious and most glamorous of all beautyfarms. Accent on beauty, reducing, and relaxation. Ladies only. Expensive. Address: The Golden Door, Highway 395, Escondido, California.

RANCHO LA PUERTA, Tecate, Mexico, near San Diego, California. Modest ranch-style accommodations. Serious, somewhat cultish regime, with accent on physical and mental fitness. Caters to both men and women. The Rancho produces its own organically grown grapes and features a grape cure. Inexpensive. Address: Rancho La Puerta, Tecate, California.

MAINCHANCE, Mount Vernon, Maine (near Augusta) and MAINCHANCE WEST, Phoenix, Arizona. De luxe establishments with accent on beauty and glamor. Luxurious accommodations. Ladies only. Very expensive! Address: Elizabeth Arden, 691 Fifth Avenue, New York City, attention of Mrs. Versteeg.

LYTTON-BERNARD HEALTH CENTER, Guadalajara, Mexico. Specializing in the Papaya Diet. Many other exotic tropical fruits are served. Ideal year-round climate. Both men and women accepted. Inexpensive. Address: Dr. Lytton-Bernard, P.O. Box 1187, Guadalajara, Mexico.

ANN ROBINSON'S SUNSHINE TERRACE, Croton-on-Hudson, New York (near New York City). Private home atmosphere in a beautiful garden overlooking the Hudson River. Accent on diet for reducing, rest, and relaxation. Ladies only. Moderate prices. Address: Ann Robinson, Croton-on-Hudson, New York.

CLINIQUE DIETETIQUE, Champigny, France. A country house near Paris converted into a well-equipped establishment. Accent on diet, exercise, and physiotherapy. Ladies only. Not expensive by American standards. Address: Clinique Dietetique de Champigny, Champigny, France.

BEAUTY FARM, Knebworth, Hertfordshire, England. About 25 miles north of London. Efficient establishment. All comforts, but not as luxurious as American beautyfarms. Moderate prices. Accent on diet, rest, and relaxation. Caters to both men and women. Address: The Secretary, Beauty Farm, Knebworth, Hertfordshire, England.

BIRCHER-BENNER SANATORIUM, Zurich, Switzerland. Pioneer diet establishment. Home of "Bircher Muesle." Serious, somewhat spartan regime. Beautiful hillside location overlooking the city. Not expensive for Americans. Address: Bircher-Benner Sanatorium, Zurich, Switzerland.

DR. BUCHINGER'S SANATORIUM, Bad Pyrmont, Germany. Ultramodern, semiluxurious establishment specializing in fruit-fasts. Beautiful situation. Excellent staff of doctors, nurses, and therapists. Both men and women accepted. Inexpensive according to American standards. Address: Dr. Buchinger's Sanatorium, Bad Pyrmont, or Uberlingen-Bodensee, Germany.

I hope that with the publication of this book many more new beautyfarms and health farms will spring up everywhere. After investigating, there will be new listings from time to time which I will gladly send to readers via my Newsletter.

Perhaps soon I will be able to settle down in some spot where sun, soil, air, and water are at their best; where modern farmers will supply us with home-grown produce: fresh milk, cheese, meat, grains, fruits, and vegetables, all raised on healthy, rich soil, without harmful sprays and chemicals. I have offers to head beautyfarms everywhere: in California, Florida, Arizona, and Nevada; also from England, from France, in the fertile Dordognes district, and from

Germany, in one of the best sanatoriums specializing in nutrition. When I find an ideal place, I will invite you to join me there.

Luxurious Beauty Cruise

When I first wrote about a floating beautyfarm, letters came back to me from all over. Hundreds of ladies were all ready to go on such a health holiday under my personal supervision. Unfortunately, my lecture tour and the writing of this book made it impossible. But now I have great hopes that the world's first health and beauty cruise will materialize soon.

Starting in New York we plan to go to the Greek Islands, to Italy, and the Riviera. The lucky ladies and gentlemen on this cruise will relax in the sun, swim in the blue water, and eat a planned diet of the most exotic and beauty-full foods each land has to offer, with many picnics and banquets ashore. It will be a great pleasure to show you the ancient beauties of each land: the temples, the statues, the tree on the Island of Cos where Hippocrates sat teaching medicine, and the waters where the thousand ships sailed to recapture Helen of Troy. This will also give me a chance to show you beautiful Taormina where I now have my favorite home, the land of Cyclops and the Pool of the Virgins, where traditionally only virgins could bathe. It will be a dream of delight, with constantly changing scenes and settings and constantly changing cuisine for the rejuvenation of body and spirit.

There will be a capable staff of doctors, dieticians, nurses, masseuses, beauticians, dance and exercise directors, all under my personal supervision with the assistance of the chic Colette Lefort, the director of my Paris office. On this cruise you will meet my friends from many lands; different languages will be spoken and you will have a chance to practice your French, Greek, or Italian. We will be a miniature United Nations, all united to have fun, to relax, to gather happy memories, and to come back slimmer, trimmer, and fit as a fiddle. And this health and beauty holiday will be no more expensive than today's Beautyfarms.

In my next Newsletter (which I gladly send to my new readers), I hope to have more specific information. In the meantime, dream about this happy event and save your money so you'll be aboard on the world's first floating health and beautyfarm.

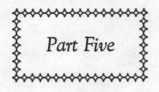

Part Five

YOUR GOOD LIFE

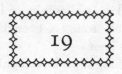

19

You Are What You Think and Feel

A Philosophy of Life

Everyone must have a philosophy of life. Maybe you call it a way of living. I believe they are both the same thing. A philosophy of life is important, essential, because it is a blueprint for all our intellectual and physical activity. It helps us to train our brains to do the things we want to do, and to control our emotions so that we will be happier.

Actually, of course, no man can always do everything he wants to do. But if he has an adequate philosophy of life, he will be happy because of the things he *can* do. And an adequate philosophy of life will help you to channel your energy into productive rather than destructive channels. But in order to arrive at a good philosophy of life one must have values, and these can be obtained only through the exercise of intellectual objectivity.

The world is a changing place. All the things in it are changing all the time. If we have values that are fixed and rigid, or that assume that the world is fixed and rigid, we are not being intellectually objective. We are not being mature. In order to use emotional energy productively we must have energy outlets. An energy outlet, if it is a good one, is a plan for the use of emotion toward a desired end. Emotion will run wild if we are not prepared for it.

The person with a working philosophy of life will be hurt less by the inevitable stresses and strains of everyday, modern life; he will be more elastic, more resilient.

One very important thing must be recognized about your philosophy of life: You must be unselfish. You must recognize that your best guarantee of obtaining the things you want in this world, of exercising your values, is by fighting for the privilege of others to do the same thing, even though their values are not your values.

Being intellectually objective, having good elastic values that are not broken into little pieces every time something goes wrong, and being emotionally stable so that emotion can be controlled and limited, means that you have a philosophy of life, that you are mature, that you are not blown about by the wind of every circumstance. It means also that you are working for the welfare of others as they are working for yours.

I want to recommend a book to you. It contains, I think, the best practical suggestions for a philosophy of life that I have ever seen. But it contains much more; it is a book about managing your mind. In fact that is the title of it: *Managing Your Mind*, by Dr. S. H. Kraines, a wise and experienced psychiatrist, and E. S. Thetford. And the subtitle of this wonderful little book is "You *Can* Change Human Nature."

I cannot recommend this book too highly. It is not a book for sick people, especially. It is a book for people, for all people who have problems and want help in solving them. And that means all of us. Solving problems requires skill. It doesn't make any difference whether they are problems of piano technique or interpretation or of life. The person with skill will do a better job than the person without skill.

And especially in connection with emotional problems, skill is needed, because, as the great doctors of antiquity knew, as the great philosophers have always known, and as medical men and psychologists are now convinced is the case, man is a whole. His mind and his body and his emotions are all interrelated. And a philosophy of life that integrates these aspects of man is one that recognizes the fact that, just as emotion can upset thought, so thought can contain or channel emotion.

Rx Laughter

Laugh and the world laughs with you; laugh and be healthy, advised the Illinois State Medical Society not long ago. Laugh and live long, said the famous Dr. Sara M. Jordan of the Lahey Clinic in Boston.

Why do these people recommend laughter? Because when we are upset emotionally, we are out of balance. And at such moments it is laughter that breaks the strain, snaps the tensions, and quickens the glands to their work.

The whole function of these glands is to keep our inner climate in balance. They work as partners: One set of hormones quickens your heartbeat, another slows it down. One speeds up your metabolism, another tones it down to give your system the rest it needs.

Dr. Jordan says, "There is plenty of evidence that glands like the pituitary, adrenals and others—with their hormonal secretions —exert their beneficent influence in this way."

Good whole-laughter is a respiratory gymnastic. It is good for the organs of the chest. We must have more laughter, and not just the twitching of nervous muscles, but deep-down, hilarious laughter which shakes the whole inner man.

In Paris, there is a school for laughter. It is run by Dr. Vachet of the Paris Institute of Psychology. He gives fabulously successful courses in laughter. He teaches his students, men and women, young and old, to laugh at anything and everything. He gets them to laugh deep, to shake with laughter. Dr. Vachet believes that laughter is a solvent for poisons of the mind, and an exercise for the muscles that make faces pleasant and bodies happy.

When I remark about this during my lectures, my friends often ask me if we do not get enough laughter on radio and television. My answer is No. Neither enough, nor of the right kind. Professional laughter is so often what I call toothpaste laughter—it is squeezed out with considerable effort, it is smooth and neat as a ribbon, and it usually falls flat on the floor, with the comedian doing most of the laughing.

The art of laughter does not depend on slapstick, bad puns, or old chestnuts. Laughter is a physical manifestation of an intellectual reaction. The things to laugh at are all around us. And laughing *at* a thing is not to be construed as scorn or contempt. One laughs because one is entertained—something is funny. Laughter is an expression of pleasure, not of derision. When you laugh you show the world your *happy* side.

Pogo's creator, Walt Kelly, describes laughter as a cleansing lash, and as the benevolent and gentle custodian of the mind. We are all absurd, he suggests, and laughter is the only way absurdities can be revealed as such because they generally hide under the cover of assumed perfection.

Mr. Kelly thinks our laughter is, or has recently been, a little nervous, as though we were a little afraid to exercise it.

Laughter and freedom go together. We must be free to be absurd, if we want to be. But we must also be free to laugh at our absurdities. I think Mr. Kelly has put his finger on the very thing that Dr. Vachet has been teaching for so long. Learn to laugh, and then you cannot help laughing at the things that are laughable. And where there is laughter, there will you find freedom.

Let us have schools of laughter here in America, and all over the world, for that matter. These times cry for more laughter. We have jitters and tensions and strains and stresses enough. Laugh and the world laughs with you! Good humor is a precious instrument of health and happiness.

Garbo Laughs

One day in Hollywood my phone rang, and it was Greta Garbo, asking if she could come for lunch. Now this was when Garbo was the reigning queen of Hollywood, and such a call was almost unheard of. Knowing that Miss Garbo was currently on a strict vegetarian diet, I ordered wild rice burgers, a salad of fresh vegetables, and broiled honeyed grapefruit.

She arrived—a vision of breath-taking beauty, with her long hair and fresh golden complexion.

Miss Garbo had heard of me through her friend Leopold Stokowski, and she came to see me because of her great interest in food. She was at that time following a diet consisting mainly of boiled vegetables and thou-shalt-nots.

In spite of her radiant beauty, this diet had had a marked effect on her vitality; she was suffering from overtiredness and insomnia, and was in danger of serious anemia.

I made it my task to wean her away from strict vegetarianism, and coax her back to intelligent eating—no easy chore with a woman who has a will of steel. Finally she consented to try my suggestions. First of all, of course, I insisted on a balanced diet. The next day, when I stopped by her dressing room at lunchtime, I found that she was having her usual vegetables, in her usual privacy— but this time the vegetables were raw, in a large salad bowl, and well fortified with protein: bits of ham, chicken, cottage cheese, and wheat germ. She had begun the high vitality program, and she quickly regained her energy.

Soon after Miss Garbo began this new way of nutrition, she accepted the leading role in the film *Ninotchka*, widely publicized with the wondrous statement, "Garbo Laughs!" Many people congratulated us both on the "new" Garbo.

The Joy of Participation

A willingness to sit and let others do the thinking and entertaining for us seven days a week, as so many do before the television set, is self-destructive. A willingness to be a passive spectator and let life go by is also self-destructive.

Chronic boredom is an illness, says a distinguished psychosomaticist, Dr. Arnold A. Hutschnecker, in his book, *The Will to Live*.

G. K. Chesterton, a wise and witty man, found that this willingness to be a spectator instead of a participant is "the one main modern defect." He said, "To amuse oneself is a mark of gaiety, vitality, and love of life. To be amused is a mark of melancholy surrender and a potentiality of suicide. The former means that a man's thoughts are attractive, artistic, and satisfying; the latter means that his own thoughts are ugly, unfruitful, and stale."

To let others do our reading, dancing, and playing is like engaging someone to make love for us. It is like requiring the priest or parson to say all our prayers. The human being who has never made love, never prayed, never danced is hardly better than the jellyfish floating in the sea.

The millions of years of life, struggling to achieve a soul, are wasted on such a person. His own fabulous body and the mind that dwells in it are wasted on him.

The "I want to be alone" theory has passed. Don't withdraw. There is no place for hermits in this century. Maintain your radius of acquaintance, and expand it. Join things, help do things that cannot be done alone. There is the P.T.A. There are garden clubs and community improvement groups. If you are lonely, join a walking group, or some bird-watchers, or civilian defense. You will find social groups at the neighborhood center. Other people are lonely, too. Others want to help get things done. Do you belong to a political club or party? Get into the swim. Participate. Show your willingness to do your share. Give some of your time. Any social worker can tell you where you can help. Any minister will have ideas for you. All psychiatrists are full of suggestions about participation. Don't shrink—expand. Don't hide—come out. Society is an organization of volunteers. The warp and woof of your community is made up of people like yourself. Doing things will make you happy. It is an expression of love. It will bring you untold reward.

Today there are clubs almost everywhere for everyone. These are wonderful things. The more people go to them, the less they go to doctors and clinics. I know of one in New York where two hundred people, men and women, gather every week day to swim, dance, look at television, play cards, listen to lectures, discuss current events, weave, make leather goods, go on boat rides or subway picnics, and once a year go away to camp for two weeks. Not one of these people is less than sixty-five, and several are over eighty. Where do they get the time? They make it. And where do they get the energy? They make that, too. It is made on a cooperative basis. Each helps the other be happy. Many of them have learned for the first time what fun life can be, and now they are living to the full, enjoying every second of it. One is the widow of a great conductor. One is the mother of a successful banker. One is the father of a bus driver.

In their discussion groups, they speak all the languages of the earth, but they understand each other. To hear them is a Babel, but a Babel of thrilling experience. You have no idea how young in both looks and behavior these wonderful people are.

How do these clubs get started? People like you get together and say, "Let's start a club." And then people like you find a place, and they dig up the money. They get the managers of movie theaters to give them free tickets for dull times. They get a church to cooperate, and some local businessmen. And the first thing you know, these people have a club that excites them, that stimulates their circulation, that gives them pleasure.

We Need More Vitamin X

The highest attainment of human beings, I firmly believe, is the full love of men and women. This is something that is beyond any *individual*. It can only be achieved through mutuality. Born of attraction, bred in the flames of full passion, heightened by parenthood, and given full force by the whole life of maturity, of understanding of the pleasures and the privileges of life, love is something no man, or woman, can create for himself or herself. But, what horrible things husbands and wives can still do to each other when they get sidetracked or derailed.

Love is anything that one receives that results in the supplementation of one's own capacities with the strength, abilities, encouragement, support, and assets of others who charge no bond, ask no interest, require no mortgage, look for no advantage, and seek no profit. The pleasure of lovers, and their profit, derives from giving, helping, being of assistance, being a means of support, material or spiritual, when people they love can benefit from it or would suffer from lack of it.

M. F. K. Fisher, a discerning woman, with a most articulate palate—she is the famous author of *How to Cook a Wolf*—tells in her *Alphabet for Gourmets* about Xantippe, the wife of Socrates. A shrew, her behavior was such, with pot and pan in the kitchen and at meals, that it may well have been *her* haggling, rather than *his* principles, that encouraged him to accept the cup of hemlock.

Be that as it may, there can be no question but that many wives put emotional poison in their husband's broths. This is by no means as difficult or dangerous as it may sound. The chief ingredient of a poison broth is anger, or dissension, or even petulance. Food should be eaten in the calm of complete happiness, and it should be brewed with love. There is no dish that will not sour with constant nagging. There are no gastric juices that can break down the molecules of animosity. Better fast when love is slow, or has stopped. You wives, you mothers, you makers of the bread of life, stop, look, and listen —make your kitchen a place of love and happiness. Set your table with smiles. Eat with joy. Leaven all your food with love. The loaf so unleavened will be a lump in the stomachs of your loved ones. Reserve your scowls for movie villains, and your anger for the man next door whose incinerator pollutes the air. Take out your ire on the unneighborly generators of noises that unsoothe the nerves. Get mad at the politicians who ignore your mandates. But, for your loved ones, have only sweetness and light. Banter at breakfast. Let dinner take place in an atmosphere of genuine bonhommie.

Are you a book-cook, or are you a creative cook? Your kitchen can be a studio in which you create dishes to build beautiful bodies, or it may be a factory in which you turn out uninspired, tasteless dishes.

Cooking is the art of supplying the body with its many needs and titillating the palate with salivating savors. *Variety* is the spice of life. There is no condiment so powerful as the original dish cooked with imagination and served with that indispensable ingredient of all dishes, *love*.

Fanny Farmer, author of America's most famous cookbook, said, "Cooking may be as much a means of self-expression as any of the arts. No cookbook can provide the spark of genius, but it can serve as a source of inspiration and information."

"This food has been prepared with loving care by Sally Chase." These words appear on the menu of a delightful little restaurant, *Sally Chase's*, on the road between Bethel and Newtown, Connecticut. These words delight me, because I have always thought that love was the most important ingredient of every dish. Sally Chase is Hungarian, and, with her American husband Joe, she runs this charming roadside inn. To it, from miles around, come the natives and the summer residents, the New Yorkers in voluntary and happy exile, for her "out of this world" pot-roasts. It is wonderful to see the best of European culinary practice wedded to the finest of American kitchen art.

Of course, what we all want is a diet to end all diets, a 365-day diet in which every meal is different, in which every meal is better than the one before, in which there is infinite pleasure as well as variety.

I believe there is such a diet. I cannot force you to follow any diet—and I can't eat the food you need for you. But one thing I can tell you about it—I can tell you what the essential ingredient of it is: the anti-ulcer vitamin, the pleasure vitamin, the vitamin of love which I have called "X."

Yes, Vitamin X, the vitamin of love, of peace, and of understanding, makes every meal different, and better. Vitamin X is generated by an intelligent woman who understands the nutritional needs of the human body and the spiritual needs of the human mind. No spiritual hunger can be satisfied by food. No physical hunger can be satisfied by understanding. But the mind in the well-fed body can be left wanting, just as the body of the understanding mind can be left in dire need. Into every dish, if *both* body and mind are to be well fed, must go not only the proper proteins and minerals, but also vitamin X.

THREE HIGHWAYS TO THE MIND

Do you live in a world of vague and general sounds, sights, and smells? Or do you live where the oriole sings, the lilac scents the air, and majestic Grecian columns of Carrara marble form the façade of a museum full of Corot, Rodin and Rembrandt?

Have you ever thought that your eyes, ears, and nose are the three main highways connecting you with the rest of the world? Without them you would live in a Stygian blackness, silent and odorless. No sights would come to your brain, no sounds, no smells. Your happiness depends on more than the maintenance of these wonderful senses, it depends on their training. You should be able to hear more, see more, and smell more—and you can, if you will put your mind to it.

You should see more than a painting, you should see that the painting is a Matisse or a Corot. You should hear more than music, you should hear Beethoven, and an inverted fifth. You should know that that was an oriole, not a warbler, and that this is the odor of jasmine, and that, of lilac.

You should be able to see the beauty of Rodin. Through your

senses the whole world is yours—the past as well as the present. The world of ideas, of sights, of happenings.

For greater happiness, I would like to suggest the habit of visualization. When you refer to a painter or a composer, picture to yourself something you have seen or heard.

Make your mind a museum full of masterpieces, a Carnegie Hall full of visions of Toscanini and the sounds of Beethoven, make it a country garden full of flowers and the scented breezes of summer, make it a hall of fame full of the great people of history, make it a stage on which Shakespeare is re-enacted.

Take at least one picture every time you go to a museum. Transfer the pictures from the Louvre to your own mind. No one will stop you. Have a Cezanne, a Da Vinci, and a Rembrandt all your own. Originals, too.

Now, when you are in a plane high above the clouds, you may spend your time gazing at masterpieces, examining photographs you have taken.

Music is something to remember, not something to recognize. "Oh, yes. I've heard this, but I don't know what it is, or who composed it, or where I heard it." Hang on to some part of every composition you like. Grab a measure and make it yours. Then you will have a little of Beethoven's Fifth in your mind, and you will find that just four notes will evoke many more.

I like flowers. My garden and my home are full of flowers. I have great vases full of riots of color. Every room is scented differently. I have fresh flowers every day. And I recommend that you, too, draw strength from the indulgence of something you love.

My eyes love the color and the form of flowers. My nose loves the subtle odors that emanate from them. Flowers fill my mind with happiness. They displace the too-many dull, drab aspects of life that are about us all the time. They are an escape. When flowers come into my home, a little of the great outdoors comes with them. There are flowers on my bed table so that they may be the last thing I see before closing my eyes, and the first, upon awakening.

My life is bounded by flowers. I memorize flower odors, recalling them at will, as I walk along a crowded, dirty street. Flowers are an important ingredient in the composition of my mental cocktails.

MENTAL COCKTAILS FOR DEEP SLEEP

One of my favorite bedtime soporifics is mental cocktails. I mix them and take them when sleep seems to elude me either at home or abroad.

I prescribe mental cocktails for those moments when you are in need of comfort, inspiration, or a little spiritual boost of some sort. What is a mental cocktail? It is a mixture of the essence of wisdom, beauty, understanding, and love. There are two kinds of mental cocktails—the kind you mix yourself, and those that come already prepared. I like both.

Let me tell you, first, how I make my own, and when and why.

It is midnight. I am lying in my bed in the Grand Hotel in Rome. I have been driving all day. I am tired. Sleep does not come quickly. I have not yet relaxed. Through the window come the many noises of Rome. There are cars, buses, happy people wending their way home. There are a few carts, millions of motor scooters, and bicycles with little auxiliary motors on their front wheels. Rome is in a hurry, and every vehicle has its own ludicrous little toot-toot or peep-peep with which they tell others to get out of the way. And *how* they use them!

So I decide I shall have a mental cocktail. I put my mind to work on it. The ingredients shall come from sensory pleasures and happy remembrances. Yes, this is a strange mixture, but it is not to be drunk with the lips, it is to be taken in through the mind, so don't be surprised at what goes into it.

The ingredients shall be five: some sound, some sight, some taste, some odor, and some feeling. For sound I take the soothing theme of a lullaby, the lullaby from Erminie which I have always loved. For sight I go to the little front room of my home so far away in New York, and from the south wall I take a picture by Renoir, a picture of a peaceful man, an elder, sitting under a tree outside a rural inn-door. For taste, I use the remembrance of tree-ripe peaches as I picked and ate them in Taormina only a few short weeks ago. For odor I add a gardenia from my California garden. And for touch, I add the remembrance of the cool, refreshing waters in which I swam just two days ago—the waters of the Mediterranean.

Into the goblet of my mind, where I mix this cocktail, I have put a jigger of song that soothes me, a dash of a picture I love, for sweetness I put in a trace of that fresh, wonderful peach, now a touch of bouquet of gardenia, and finally a liberal amount of that calming, soothing feeling I get when I rest and relax in the wonderful waters at Taormina, with the sun high above me, giving me warmth and comfort.

Slowly, in my mind I mix these things I love, these things which have always given me such pleasure, things I associate with peace and calm and relaxation. Round and round I stir them, seeing, hearing, tasting, smelling, feeling, as they go. I associate them with me and myself with them. The sounds of Rome die away. The draft is a heavy one, a potent one. It is a wonderful one. Phenobarbitol was never like this.

Try a mental cocktail. I assure you it will give you such rest and sleep as you have not had since childhood. And it will give you sweet dreams, too. At the very least it will keep you occupied in a pleasant pursuit, and keep your mind from things unpleasant.

Prepared mental cocktails, of course, are composed of the things that have been written by the masters of thought and pen. There are few things, either good or bad, that have not happened before. And the world of literature is full of imperishable expressions that have soothed and salved many before you.

To serve you best, I recommend that you get small lightweight volumes that can be held without effort. I have built a small library of such books, and from them I have extracted and written into a little blank volume of my own those words I like best. This is my anthology; there is not another like it in the world. I take it with me wherever I go. I am never without it.

It contains verses and quatrains, paragraphs and aphorisms—those things that have come to mean so much to me. At one time or another, something from the Consolations of Boethius or Aesop's Fables, from Epictetus or Walt Whitman, from Liebman's *Peace of Mind* or Marcus Aurelius, has pleased me, has helped me, has given me comfort or wisdom—so I have taken them out and made them my own.

If you wonder where to look for such things, I would like to recommend a wonderful Bibliography that is very inexpensive. It is called *Good Reading* and is published, for thirty-five cents, by

The New American Library. It is a wonderful little volume, paper-covered. You can probably get it wherever such books are sold. In it you will find 1,250 of the world's best books listed, and described a little, enough so that you can quickly tell if they might interest you. I recommend that you get this book with your next small change. From some of the titles listed in it you can begin to extract your own prepared mental cocktails.

But you need not wait. Tonight when you go to bed you can mix an original mental cocktail composed of sensory recollections that have pleased and comforted you. Try it.

P.S. No hangover from these.

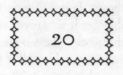

Meet Some of My People

In the course of my life I have met many People. People are my great interest, and many of them are my good friends.

In my lifelong studies, I have discovered that People, whatever their talents, achievements, or position in life, have one thing in common: They make it their habit always to be at their best—to feel their best, look their best, and use their best efforts to make the world better, saner, or happier. In other words, I find that People make it their habit to control themselves and their lives instead of allowing themselves to be controlled and pushed around by circumstances.

Most of my People are in the second half of their lives. It cannot be otherwise. A young person cannot be a Person; he can simply move in that direction, give evidence that one day he will be a Person. Young people can eat intelligently, establish good habits of hygiene, grooming, and dress, establish sound patterns of living, thinking, and behavior. If they do these things, well and good. But they do not know *why* they are doing them; they do not enjoy their self-control. That comes later.

Be glad if you are in the second half of life. As George Bernard Shaw, at ninety-three, said, "Youth is altogether wasted on the young." True self-control comes only with maturity. So does true self-awareness. The young person must conform, be like everyone else, to be happy. The mature person can say to himself, "I am unique. There is no one in the world who is exactly like me," and enjoy this, capitalize on it. He can say, "I love and am loved," and know what he is talking about. It is only in maturity that we have loved enough to understand and evaluate love. The mature person can say, "I am important to myself, to my family, to my community," and know wherein he is important. He can also know wherein he is unimportant; there is the great test of maturity.

Only the mature person, also, can have true self-confidence. In the first half of life, we are finding ourselves, reproducing ourselves, making a living for ourselves and our dependents. In the second half of life, we can confidently appraise ourselves, find out who we are, what we are good for, and what we were put into the world to accomplish. We have enough confidence in our strength to be able to admit and remedy our weaknesses; enough confidence in our education to want to go on learning; enough confidence in our lives to want to go on developing, expanding, *living*.

What are the attributes of youth? They are both plus and minus. The plus attributes are: courage, curiosity, excitement. The minus attributes are: ignorance, egocentricity, overconfidence.

What are the attributes of age? Again, they are both plus and minus. The plus ones: caution, objectivity, wisdom. The minus ones: timidity, intolerance, fear of change.

Check over these attributes, both plus and minus. What do you find? You find that in some respects you are still young; that in some respects you have always been old. *You have been both young and old all of your life.* Now discard all your minuses, both of youth and of age. Make a list of all the plus attributes. Resolve, consciously and deliberately, to rule out all of the minus side and to develop all of the plus side (of both youth and age) for the rest of your long life. This is true maturity.

The French philosopher, Henri Bergson, has said, "To exist is to change, to change is to mature, to mature is to go on creating oneself endlessly."

How Does One Gain Maturity?

Just as some people are lucky enough to inherit good teeth, strong bodies, and superior digestive systems, some people also have the good fortune to be born of happy, well-adjusted parents and to inherit thereby the ingredients for true maturity.

Many others achieve maturity by instinct, often by finding, either in real life or on library shelves, some great friend, teacher, guide, or philosopher with whom they identify themselves, whose life they use as a model for their own lives.

Many others, unfortunately, are neither "born" to maturity, nor do they acquire it. They arrive at the second half of life still woefully immature, still fighting the old battles of their childhood against grownups who ruled or thwarted them; still tense with the insecurity and guilt of their teens; still driven by the ambitions and anxieties of their thirties. These are the "seekers," who run from one thing to another. They are looking for help but have not the maturity nor the wisdom to know what they actually need. Countless such "seekers" have come to my classes, and I believe that by teaching them to strengthen their bodies, especially their nerves, I have been able to help many of them.

However, many of these people need psychiatric help or psychological counseling in order to attain true maturity. I look forward to the day when regular checkups with the family psychiatrist will be as much a matter of course as checkups with the family doctor, dentist, and oculist. Modern life grows more and more complex. There is increasing need for true maturity if, in the course of our long lives, we are to meet serenely the changes, challenges, and anxieties of the atomic era. We need equilibrium and assurance. I agree with that great modern philosopher, Joshua Loth Liebman, that "modern psychology can help normal people to maintain their equilibrium or to regain it." I also agree with Dr. Liebman when he adds that "religion can give both assurance and a spiritual purpose in life."

The famous psychoanalyst, Dr. Carl Jung, in Zurich, Switzerland, once said to me, "In all the thousands who come to me for help, those who have some faith, some religion, get well more quickly."

Truly mature people, wherever you find them, are spiritual people. They may or may not live according to a specific creed or faith; the important thing is that they *have* faith—faith in themselves, in their fellow-men, in the existence of a power, a universal order and purpose which is greater than themselves. This is seldom achieved until the second half of life. Dr. Edward Bortz, a former president of the American Medical Association, tells us that *man reaches physical maturity at 25; emotional maturity at 35; intellectual maturity at 45; but that spiritual maturity comes in the later years.*

If you are falling short of true maturity, finding yourself hampered by impulses, anxieties, depressions which you cannot understand or overcome, even after you have built up your physical health and strength, then by all means consult a psychiatrist or psychologist. Dr. George Lawton, a consulting psychologist, tells us that the aim of such counseling is "to release the individual's potentialities for growth, make him more effective in the use of his energies."

WHOM DO YOU ADMIRE?

Whether or not you need special help, follow the example of those people who have achieved maturity by identification with some mature person whom they admire. Go to your library. Read newspapers, magazines, biographies and autobiographies. Learn to know People, in present-day life and in the pages of history. Find someone whose life story kindles your imagination, someone who resembles yourself in interests, in point of view, in his or her way of attacking a job. Identify yourself with this Person.

I do *not* mean that you should imitate this Person, become a carbon copy, a poseur. Pose is hideous. Identifying oneself with a specific individual, on the other hand, can be constructive. It impresses your subconscious mind with a tendency in the direction of achievement and strength.

Identify yourself with a Person who perhaps shares your handicap. Everyone has a handicap, either real or imaginary. Some are too tall, some too short, some suffer from poor physique, poor vision, poor hearing, shyness, speech defects, poor muscular co-ordination. Some have big noses, big hands, big feet. Some are handicapped by money and social position, and some by being born on the wrong side of the tracks. Some think themselves too ugly, and some think themselves too good-looking. I have met not a few men who suffered acutely from having been called, "Hey, handsome!" all their lives.

Now say to yourself, "I—this person sitting here in this chair —I am a Person. I could do what this similar Person whom I admire has done—

> If I had his talents
> If I had his training
> If I had his opportunities."

Psychologists agree that the majority of people reach middle life without having begun to explore their potentialities. You have talents and capacities for development, of which so far you have only dreamed. Training is yours for the asking, whether you wish to go to college, as my friend Grandma Reynolds did at 60; or, like another 60-year-old student of mine, take a free course in ceramics in the Adult Education Department of your nearest public school. You may not be "discovered" by Hollywood, as Grandma Reynolds was, but you will certainly be discovered by your community.

"You can look the way you want to look, if you want to steadily enough," as my friend Ann Astaire has demonstrated. Also, you can be the Person you want to be, if you want to steadily enough. Whatever your age, you can be what you want to be. Opportunity keeps right on knocking, day in and day out.

SOME PEOPLE I ADMIRE

I first met Ann Astaire in the 1930's when her two famous children, Fred and Adele Astaire, were starring in *The Bandwagon*. A friend took me to the Astaires' New York apartment to tea. The conversation turned to health and youthfulness, whether it was possible to remain healthy and young by will power.

I said, "Not by will power. Those are the middle-aged men in bright neckties, the women who turn girlish in their fifties and go in for bright red shoes and hats. These people are trying to look young by force, as it were. I think being youthful is a matter of *wanting* to be youthful, steadily, all day, every day."

Mrs. Astaire smiled at me. "I am supposed to need glasses," she said. "I have a prescription for them. Do you think that I can avoid wearing glasses by wanting to, steadily enough?"

I told her that there were excellent eye exercises; that if she wanted to avoid glasses enough to exercise her eyes steadily—

"I'll do it," she said, with the note of quiet confidence that I like so much to hear.

I am introducing Ann Astaire to you for several reasons. One reason is that she is my very good friend. Another reason is that, although she is definitely one of my People, she is neither a celebrity, a career woman, nor a society leader. She is an unassuming, typically American woman, at home wherever she finds herself.

Born and raised in Omaha, Nebraska, she taught school for a time before her marriage. She was early left a widow with two small children who were soon to become a famous dancing team. Her children were the center of her life; wherever they were booked to perform, she went with them and made a home. She accomplished effortlessly the transition from Omaha to sophisticated New York. When her daughter Adele left the cast of *The Bandwagon* to marry the English nobleman, Lord Charles Cavendish, Ann Astaire made the transition from New York society to London society with equal ease and grace.

Her gentle, natural dignity amounts almost to nobility; she is internationally adored; the members of the British royal family are her friends. As her friend, I, myself, was welcomed into London's most brilliant and influential circles when I went there in the late 1930's to lecture on nutrition. In that way I was able to introduce to England the Hauser way of eating, which proved to be so helpful during the bitter, deprived war years that were to follow.

During the war, Ann Astaire took over the entire management of Lismore, Lord Cavendish's huge estate in Ireland, in order to free Lady Charles Cavendish for Red Cross work. Lismore Castle, already famous for its hospitality, now became equally famous for its cuisine; short-cooked vegetables and big bowls of crisp, tossed salads were a novelty, a seven-days' wonder. When food became very scarce in Ireland, fresh vegetables were still plentiful at Lismore Castle. Mrs. Astaire saw to the raising of them herself.

Now in her eighties, she has the same quality that she had in her fifties when I first met her—a quality not of youth but of youthfulness, of warm young dignity.

Her complexion is soft and unlined; she has healthy, shiny white hair highlighted with a bit of blue; her tall, slender figure is the envy of women in their twenties. She dresses simply, in quiet elegance, walks a great deal, gardens, enjoys her grandchildren.

She is an active churchwoman, a believer in service to humanity and in the power of the mind to accomplish, little by little, the good it sets out to do.

She uses a lorgnette for theater programs and the telephone book, but she still does not need to wear glasses; she never had that prescription filled. That first day I met her, she began making a part of her life not only the eye exercises I recommended, but the entire Hauser regime. With her characteristic quiet thoroughness, she has followed it ever since.

She eats intelligently; she has formed the habit of liking what is good for her, not because she must but because she wants to. She always undereats—again, not because she must but because she wants to. And she is always relaxed, for true relaxation comes from knowledge that you have yourself and your body under your own control, not because you must but because you want to have it that way.

Meet Albert Schweitzer

I have met only two people in my life whose inner serenity is so great that in their presence I have felt at the same time humble yet inspired, relaxed yet exhilarated. One was Ghandi. The other is Dr. Albert Schweitzer.

The life and work of Albert Schweitzer, who gave up his career as a world-famous musician and theologian to found and run a hospital for the most primitive people in the heart of Africa, has long been one of my most helpful sources of spiritual refreshment. And I had long wanted to meet him, partly because I was born in the Black Forest, only an hour from his native village of Günzbach in Alsace.

One day when I was in Paris I learned that he had returned to Günzbach. The next day Marion Preminger and I were on our way to see him. In Strasbourg, no one had ever heard of Günzbach, so we went on to Colmar. At Colmar they said, "Günzbach? Oh, you mean Dr. Schweitzer's village."

When we arrived we heard the sounds of organ music from the little whitewashed church. We entered and found Dr. Schweitzer, seated at the console of an organ built to his own design, playing Bach.

He finished the chorale, and then turned and greeted us with the warmth, kindness, and simplicity of an old friend.

"You enjoy music?" he asked. There was no need for us to reply. So he nodded and said, "Sit in the back of the church; you will hear better there."

He played the chorale "When We Are in Deepest Need." I have never been so moved and transported in my life as the glorious music filled that little church under Albert Schwcitzer's divine touch.

And when we walked out of the church, too full of emotion to speak, I was thankful to find that the moment had been captured for the whole world. For outside, incongruous in that ancient village, stood two great recording trucks which had come all the way from America to Günzbach. Albert Schweitzer was making a new record; and once again the money would go to his hospital in Africa.

"You will join us for lunch?" he asked.

The meal, as I had expected, was perfectly simple and simply perfect. A green salad with tomatoes in a white porcelain bowl. Cold meats, with Swiss and cottage cheese. A basket of Alsace grapes, and a bottle of dry Rhine wine. There was one cooked vegetable, a dish of soybeans.

I asked Dr. Schweitzer whether he was a vegetarian. He answered: "No, unfortunately I am not. I realize that we need meat and fish. The higher life must live on the lower. But we must kill only as much as necessary, and never wantonly."

I told him that the only "life" I had around me was my Sealyham, Deucy, and I confessed a great love for dogs.

"I hope you talk with them," he said at once. "They understand. Animals, of course, do not use our language, but they understand it.

"At my hospital in Lambarene wild animals often come, and I talk to them. A wild pig called one day and I spoke to him. So he came again. Now he is a regular visitor. He often sleeps there, though he has grown rather big and awkward. I cover him up with a rug at nights; and if he rolls out of it, I have to wake him up and put him back to bed."

We were now sitting in the living room. I mentioned a large picture of his hospital hanging on the wall.

"That bird in the foreground," said Dr. Schweitzer, "is the famous Monsieur Pelican. He came into the hospital one evening and apparently liked it. So he appointed himself night-watchman.

"Every evening he came to the hospital at the same time and took up his post in front of the building. If anyone approached, he would make a peculiar noise and flap his wings. And before he went off duty in the morning, he would 'report' to one of my African helpers. It was amusing to watch them have their daily chat."

The Africans flock to Dr. Schweitzer. He has won their love, and they know he is there to heal them.

Throughout the afternoon this great man talked of his hospital and his hopes for humanity, and I think perhaps the primitive buildings at Lambarene are a symbol of those hopes. For there he has established not only a white-walled center of healing, but a small kingdom where he rules by love.

He told me how he controls his helpers with a minimum of discipline. If an African boy steals a chicken or commits some other offense that gets him in jail, the Great Doctor, as the Africans call him, goes to see the boy. If the boy promises not to do it again, Dr. Schweitzer immediately releases him. He knows that if he trusts his helpers, they will not betray that trust.

In that simple home, surrounded by books and pictures, by the quiet atmosphere of humane culture, I experienced a most remarkable afternoon—one which changed my life permanently for the better.

Meet Lillian Martin

For a magnificent example of life lived to the full for almost a hundred years, read books by and about Dr. Lillian J. Martin of California. In her youth, Dr. Martin taught high school chemistry. In her thirties, she went to Germany to study psychology (then a new science), took a professorship at Leland Stanford University, made ten fresh contributions to psychological research, and then was retired, in the natural order of things, at the age of sixty-five.

Did Dr. Martin "retire"? Assuredly not. She then *began* her great work. Believing that the secret of youthfulness lay in breaking with the old and tackling the new, she launched into child-guidance work and opened the first mental hygiene clinic for preschool children in San Francisco. Working with children, she became interested in their grandparents also. Then she opened an Old Age Clinic in San Francisco, now world-famous, with branches in Los Angeles and New York City.

Dr. Martin learned to type at 65. She learned to drive a car in her seventies. At 75 she went alone to Russia. At 81 she toured Mexico alone in her car. At 88 she made a tour of South America, including a journey up the Amazon. At 89 she managed a 64-acre farm (at a profit) with four 60-year-old helpers.

If you are interested in art or architecture, read about Anna Mary Robertson Moses of Eagle Bridge, New York; and Frank Lloyd Wright of Spring Green, Wisconsin. Grandma Moses took up painting seriously at the age of 76. She had more than 35 exhibitions; some of her canvases have sold for $3,000. At the age of 88, she was awarded the Women's National Press Club award "for outstanding contribution to contemporary thought and achievement." Grandma Moses said (and artist friends of mine have corroborated this), "Anyone can paint who wants to. All you have to do is get the brush and paint and start in."

Frank Lloyd Wright was little known as an architect in his youth and middle life. But in his later years he became world-famous. He was in his eighties when he received the highest professional honors from the American Institute of Architects. His comment on age was, "A creative life is a young one. What makes everybody think that 80 is old?"

Geraldine Farrar, the famous opera star, is now over eighty. She recently said, "So much is pressing in on humans today that no one has time to stand still long enough to evaluate it. They gulp life and taste nothing. They eat life and have no savor." Still in good health, she spends most of her time in her ranch-type home in Ridgefield, Connecticut. She also drives her own car into town on periodic shopping trips.

Mrs. Edgar Ferry is a tiny great-grandmother from St. Paul, Minnesota. Recently she celebrated her hundredth birthday by flying to New York. When asked about her secret for living such a long and happy life, she said, "I eat carefully, and have a strong personal faith." Mrs. Ferry prefers fresh food, avoids all white flour and white sugar; honey is her favorite sweetener, and yogurt is one of her favorite foods. She gives credit to two of her favorite heroes, Gayelord Hauser and the late Bernarr MacFadden.

A gold medal for distinguished service to humanity was awarded to Dr. Lillian M. Gilbreth—engineer, psychologist, and author—by the National Institute of Social Sciences when she was in her seventies. She is not only an engineer, psychologist, and professor, but also mother of twelve children, author of ten books, recipient of nine academic degrees, and an industrial consultant now presiding over her own corporation.

Billie Burke, who in her twenties was called "America's favorite redhead," is still being called that, fifty years later. Gay, youthful, perennial, she became an author as well as a movie star, and declares that she still stands on her head and turns somersaults every morning before breakfast. This seems natural enough, since she is my friend and one of my favorite People, and a few years ago wrote glowingly of my diets which, she said, "have given pleasure and comfort to so many."

Clara Barton, founder of the American Red Cross, lived actively until the age of 91.

Sophocles wrote *Oedipus Rex* at 90.

Oliver Wendell Holmes wrote *Over the Teacups* at 85.

Titian painted his greatest masterpiece at 85, and lived to be 99.

The immortal Ninon de Lenclos has been called one of the most significant, as well as one of the most beautiful, women of the seventeenth century. A contemporary of her later years wrote of her: "Until she was over 60, she had lovers who loved her greatly and the most virtuous people of France for her friends. Until she was 90 she was sought by the best society of her time."

There is no limit to the proof that, as life goes on, energy can and does *increase*. Examples are limitless of men and women who, in the second half of their lives, have found their energy heightened, their creative powers intensified, their ability to learn doubled and redoubled. Wherever we look we find examples not just of continuing productivity, but of the new flowering of gifts, talents, and abilities at 40, 60, and beyond.

What is the secret? Let me repeat it:

Good health.

A strong, vibrant body.

A positive attitude of mind.

Meet Lady Mendl

Throughout this book I have spoken frequently of Elsie de Wolfe Mendl, a good friend and faithful student of nutrition, of whom I am very proud. In the first half of her life, Elsie de Wolfe was an actress. Born in a house which stood on the present site of Macy's department store (she liked to say she was born in Macy's basement), she was educated abroad, presented at Queen Victoria's court, and moved in the inner circle of the glittering society of the Edwardian Era in the United States and Europe. However, with the death of her father it became necessary to find some means of support for her mother and herself.

Elsie de Wolfe had always loved amateur theatricals, and she turned now to the professional stage for her living. David Belasco coached her. Charles Frohman was her producer. Later, she was star and manager of her own company. She starred with Sir Johnston Forbes-Robertson, John Drew, the Barrymores, Maude Adams, and many others. She was known as "the best-dressed woman on the American stage."

With her friend Elizabeth Marbury, with whom she shared houses in New York and in Versailles, just outside of Paris, Elsie de Wolfe became an internationally famous hostess as well. Her parties were breathtaking; her friends were kings and queens, princesses, diplomats, poets, painters, musicians, writers, admirals, generals, and stars of opera, stage, and screen.

One day she walked from the stage, through the wings, into her dressing room and sat down before the mirror to remove her makeup. Suddenly she heard, clearly and distinctly, the voice of her inner self saying, "Those are the last words you will ever speak in the theatre." She had always listened to her inner voice, sometimes even talked back to it. Now she said to herself, aloud, "All right. What are you afraid of?" And began to plan another career.

From earliest childhood, Elsie de Wolfe had hated ugliness. It was associated in her mind with the drawing room of her parents' house which was indeed ugly, "done" in the height of mid-Victorian elegance—tassels, lambrequins, depressing tan wallpapers with splotchy red-and-gray designs. She had made her life a quest for beauty. In the world of society and the theatre, she had learned to create beauty for herself, learned the arts of dress and make-up, studied her own good and bad points, and learned what to play up and what to play down.

Ugliness in her surroundings had always depressed her. Always conscious of rooms, she knew instinctively what was right or wrong about them. Closing her eyes in an ugly room (and in those days, the more lavish the room, the uglier it was), she would mentally re-create it and make it beautiful.

When Elsie de Wolfe decided to leave the theatre and become an interior decorator for the second half of her life, she was, therefore, turning back to a childhood dream. With no special training, no capital, nothing but many friends and an indomitable pioneering spirit, she became America's first woman interior decorator. Her first big assignment was the decoration of New York's celebrated Colony Club.

Stanford White, designer of the building, said, "Give the job of decorating to Elsie, and *let the girl alone.*" That assignment was uphill work; American women were accustomed to living in Victorian ugliness. But gradually Elsie de Wolfe won her crusade for beauty—warm, glowing colors on walls, bright chintzes in drawing rooms, indoor "garden rooms," furniture that was beautiful, useful, and comfortable, and mirrors, mirrors everywhere.

I have not space to tell you the whole story of Elsie de Wolfe, of her two careers, her marriage to Sir Charles Mendl, her parties, friends, houses, innovations, activities, her social, personal, and professional triumphs. That needs a book of its own and she herself wrote it, her delightful autobiography *After All.*

I recall as one of the most interesting occasions of my life the day in 1936 when I met this fabulous woman. Two of my friends took me to one of the famous "Sunday afternoons" at Lady Mendl's villa in Versailles. In the center of a group in which everybody was "somebody," I was received by a tiny lady, soignée, with shining dark eyes and platinum-white hair. She showed me her copy of my book, *Eat and Grow Beautiful.* It was well marked and underscored. Across the front she had written, "I *like* that man!"

Most of her life she had been interested in nutrition. As a child, she had wanted good teeth and a beautiful complexion; instinctively, she had avoided candy and other sweets. As the "best-dressed woman on the American stage," she had needed a perfect figure and had achieved it by teaching herself to like only fresh, vital foods, *under*eating always and cultivating the great art of relaxation. So important did she consider nutrition that for years her specially trained chef traveled with her wherever she went. Monsieur Fraise (Mr. Strawberry—a good name for a good chef) learned to prepare exactly the foods I recommended.

"What is the secret of being an internationally famous hostess?" I asked Lady Mendl. Her answer was, "Get a good chef; serve superb food." But we who knew Elsie know that it was her immense vitality, her love of life, which made her not only an internationally famous hostess, but one of the most adored women in the world.

Lady Mendl long ago adopted my Look Younger, Live Longer principles. "I have originated modern styles in clothes and decoration," she once told me. "You have originated the modern manner of eating." In 1937 she gave a large party in my honor at her Paris apartment. Her guests were some of her favorite people. They included a number of the world's most attractive women: the Duchess of Windsor, Lady Diana Manners, Lady Charles Cavendish, Mrs. Harrison Williams, Princess Karputhala. This was the first time these women had realized the limitless possibilities of good nutrition, for themselves and for the people of their countries. I gave them the first vegetable juice cocktail ever served in Paris and their enthusiasm was unbounded. The Duchess of Windsor, Lady Mendl, and my mother were the first three women in Europe to own the vegetable-juice extracting machine which was then my special innovation, and which I hope will someday be an indispensable part of household, restaurant, and hospital equipment everywhere.

Like all my People, Lady Mendl was ageless. She knew that keeping one's interests alive keeps old age from the door. Passionately devoted to France, she was active in that country's behalf during and after both World Wars. Lady Mendl was one of the few American women to have been awarded the Grand Croix de Guerre. Before her death, in addition to maintaining her Paris apartment and villa at Versailles, she became my neighbor in Beverly Hills, California. Wherever she was, her parties were wonderful; this fabulous Person was surrounded by the greatest talents, the greatest names, and the greatest minds of our time.

"The longer I live," she said, "the more I realize that it is never too late to learn. I have always been eager for the new and willing to discard the old in its favor. I never think of myself as being old —I never tell my age. I am deeply interested in all of the new movements which are taking shape around me. I am an optimist.

"I have lived and laughed and loved. I have waved over my life the magic wand of self-control. I love life. I have made it an adventure. I have thrived on opposition. I rejoice that I was born with the courage to live." And live she did, fully and beautifully, until she was 94.

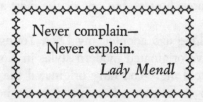

Never complain—
Never explain.

Lady Mendl

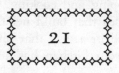

21

Helping Your Children

One day in Paris I was visiting the Louvre with a young American woman. As we strolled leisurely through the museum she told about her recent problems. Her children had been ill all winter with a series of colds and a sharp bout with pneumonia, and one child had required an operation for mastoiditis. Finally, she had become so exhausted from work and worry and sleepless nights that her husband insisted she should have a holiday in Paris.

At first glance she was fairly attractive, but close observation revealed that her face was furrowed with traces of dissatisfaction and unhappiness.

As we paused before Rodin's statue of "The Thinker," she remarked wistfully, "How I wish I might be an artist! It must be wonderful to be able to create such beauty. I spend my life cooking, shopping, and nursing the children. I'm nothing but a *Hausfrau*. It makes me feel so unimportant!"

She touched on one of my deepest convictions: that every mother can be an artist, a sculptor; she has it in her power to create and help develop live, vital beings.

"Don't you see that you can create beauty in building beautiful children?" I asked her. "Rodin worked with clay and bronze; you work with living flesh. Just as he molded his works of art, so are you molding the bodies and the spirits of your children. Just as he spent repeated hours in shaping and reshaping clay, you spend repeated hours in shopping and cooking. When the shopping is done with care and foods that build health are purchased, when those foods are prepared in a way that saves their vital elements to build beauty, then your kitchen has a dignity as great as the studio of any artist."

She considered this idea, and we went on to talk about the foods that must be chosen to create human works of art. She soon realized that this choice was as important as the choice Rodin made of which materials to work with. Gradually her dissatisfaction disappeared and her attitude toward housework and child care changed.

A few years later when I met her after a lecture I gave in Philadelphia, she proudly displayed for me her three wonderful children. She had created three works of art which were beautiful—beautiful in body, in mind, and in spirit.

If you are a mother, you should think of yourself as a sculptor. You can be a poor artist—and create sickly, underdeveloped children, or a great artist—and mold beautiful, happy lives. Keep this always in mind; it reflects the importance of your daily tasks.

YOUR INFANT

At birth a baby is as nearly perfect as Nature can make him. If the mother's diet, during pregnancy, does not include all the substances required for baby's body, her own body tissues are robbed to supply baby's needs. If her diet is adequate in all respects, perfection can be attained. If baby's diet supplies all of his needs, this perfection can be continued.

The best food for him is mother's milk. Breast-fed babies have a much lower death rate and suffer less frequently from allergies, infections, and abnormalities than do bottle-fed babies. Dr. Paul Gyorgy, of the Philadelphia General Hospital, states that breast feeding increases the infant's resistance to intestinal disturbances and to respiratory infections. However, the supply and quality of breast milk is determined by the adequacy of the mother's diet, especially in vitamins, minerals, and proteins, during pregnancy.

Whether breast milk or formula is given baby, certain supplements are necessary to keep him healthy. The amount of either breast milk or cow's milk likely to be taken in a day by a new-born infant supplies only about 1000 units of vitamin A. Twice this quantity is needed daily to keep his skin free of rashes and his resistance to infections high. The best source of vitamin A is fish liver oil, which also furnishes vitamin D.

Perhaps the most important nutrient during infancy and child-hood is vitamin D, which helps to develop a beautiful child. If vitamin D is lacking or is not absorbed into the blood, his teeth and bones may remain underdeveloped or become enlarged. Such abnormalities continue throughout life: narrow face, crooked or buck teeth, receding chin, pigeon chest, knock knees or bowed legs.

Liquid cod liver oil is probably superior to all other fish liver oils for baby because, in addition to vitamins, it contains useful unsaturated fat. However, because it is low in vitamin A, a table-spoonful (15 cc.) of plain halibut liver oil should be added to a pint of cod liver oil to increase its vitamin A content. Or, cod liver oil concentrate can be followed by a few drops of vegetable oil to provide the fat needed to stimulate bile flow; this also supplies unsaturated fatty acids. In any case, the cod liver oil should be given *after* morning and evening feedings, for only after feed-ing can baby's body properly absorb the vitamins in it.

If mother's diet includes adequate vitamin C, her breast milk will supply 100 milligrams of vitamin C in the amount of milk consumed in one day by a new-born baby. This amount is there-fore considered ideal for baby. However, cow's milk averages only 6 milligrams per quart. Baby would require almost seventeen quarts of cow's milk to get 100 milligrams of vitamin C from it. An ounce of orange juice has only 15 milligrams of vitamin C and an ounce of tomato juice only 5 or less. The best way to insure an adequate supply of vitamin C is to use 50-milligram ascorbic acid tablets. A tablet can be dissolved in one teaspoonful of water and added to baby's formula or drinking water. One tablet in the morning and another in the evening will supply the required 100 milligrams.

By the time baby is a week old, he should be given one table-spoonful of fresh, strained orange juice per day. This amount should be increased by one tablespoonful each week until eight ounces are being taken daily. As the amount of juice is increased, the amount of tablets is decreased.

The B vitamins are also important, for they help to maintain normal appetite, aid digestion and elimination, encourage sound sleep, and help prevent skin rashes and eczema. A teaspoonful of brewers' yeast, mixed with baby's formula, will supply B vitamins. Later, wheat germ, added to cereal or fruit, will provide more. Wheat germ can be softened in hot milk or quickly cooked, but never for more than five minutes.

Water in which short-cooked vegetables have been steamed will supply many valuable nutrients. A little iodized vegetable salt added to it will supply iodine, often neglected in baby's diet.

Sun baths should be given daily whenever possible. Start with three to five minutes and gradually increase the time up to a half hour. Be sure to coat baby lightly with a vegetable oil, such as avocado or peanut oil, before the sun bath. Then leave the oil on until it is completely absorbed.

Late in the fourth month, baby can be introduced to solid food. Start with no more than a half teaspoonful, and gradually increase the amount each time it is offered. Thus, if any food upsets him, the upset will not be severe. This method of introducing new foods also allows baby to grow gradually accustomed to new tastes and textures.

Whole-grain cereal, cooked in milk, can now be introduced. Wheat germ, added to cereals or fruit, should continue to be given daily. Baby can also have the yolk of a hard-cooked egg, mashed with a little milk or formula. (Soft-cooked egg and egg white are difficult for him to digest and sometimes cause an allergy.)

Dark green and yellow vegetables—such as carrots, broccoli, chard, and squash—as prepared for the family table, are now suitable for baby. Of course, they should be mashed or puréed; with a blender or liquefier, this can be done in just a few minutes.

By the fifth month, baby is ready for applesauce, very ripe mashed bananas, steamed and blended prunes and apples, or any fruit pulp. (Never, never add any white sugar.) He can also have cottage cheese and baked Irish or sweet potato.

Your Growing Child

When your child is five or six months old, new foods can be introduced rapidly. But there is no place in baby's diet for any refined foods; and such foods as crackers, melba toast, and zwieback should be completely avoided. Let him cut his teeth on such foods as raw carrot sticks, raw turnip sticks, and celery. He can now be given bite-size pieces of whole-grain bread and larger portions of salad, raw vegetables, and fruits.

At about the age of nine months, he should be ready to eat most of the foods prepared for the family—provided, of course, that the table holds no food which does not build health.

When the child is about a year and a half old, he should receive daily a tablespoonful of powdered food yeast, and this amount should continue to be given as he grows up. He should also have about six ounces of citrus juice daily, and two tablespoons of wheat germ. The fish liver oil should also be continued daily until the bones and teeth are completely developed. And vitamin D is also needed to keep his teeth and bones healthy.

Many mothers, anxious to provide all the nutrients they know their children need, try to overstuff them. A child will quickly learn that, by eating very little or not eating at all at regular mealtime, he gets extra attention—which he finds pleasant. If the mother is overanxious, this situation can snowball; so don't make an issue over his not eating, but proceed with the meal. What he fails to eat at one meal, he will make up at the next (unless he is ill or lacks vitamins). Lack of appetite can be caused by illness, excitement, emotional upset, or some other condition in which the child is better off not to eat very much. Continue to put small portions of proper food before him and, of course, permit between-meal snacks of natural foods. He will soon get over his eating problem.

If this method of feeding is continued as the child grows up, he should be able to reach maturity without illness of any kind and without digestive upsets, constipation, tooth decay, skin abnormalities, malformation of bones, nervousness, and dozens of other disturbances experienced by most children. He should have beauty and boundless energy. The mother-artist should take pride and pleasure in molding such a child.

Your Teen-Ager

Some people think teen-agers are terrible. I think they're terrific. But anyone that knows teen-agers will agree: They are terribly hungry. This is natural. During the teens the permanent foundations of bony structure, organic soundness, resistance to disease, nervous stability, and lifelong well (or ill) being are laid. For teen-agers good nutrition is, literally, the most important thing in life. Therefore, when I am asked what to *do* about them, my answer is, first of all, *feed 'em.*

Obviously, proteins, vitamins, and minerals are necessary for the growing body. But growing emotions and growing minds must also be fed.

Teen-agers may receive all the necessary proteins, carbohydrates, fats, minerals, and vitamins and still hunger for the most essential nutrient of all—vitamin X, better known as love. Vitamin X can have a two-way action. Enough of it means sturdy emotional and mental growth; but too much can create emotional and mental overdependence. Therefore, the full answer to what we are to do about our teen-agers is: *Feed 'em. Love 'em. And leave 'em alone.*

In spite of the fact that our nation's standard of living is at an all-time high, nearly half our teen-agers are gravely undernourished. An investigation at Pennsylvania State College showed that about three-fourths of them are not getting enough energy foods, such as whole-grain flours and cereals and natural sugar from fresh fruits and vegetables, to run the body efficiently. About half fail to get enough protein foods (meat, fish, cheese, eggs, milk) for building and repairing body tissues.

They do not get enough essential minerals—calcium and phosphorus (from milk, liver, eggs, fruits, vegetables, molasses) for good red blood. Their diets are lacking in B vitamins (from milk, whole-grain flours and cereals) required for proper growth and nervous stability; in vitamin C (citrus fruits and vegetable juices), important to health of gums and healing of injuries; in vitamin A (fish-liver oils, butter, cream, milk) essential to proper growth, clear skin, good vision.

These are shocking facts. But, you tell yourself, *your* teen-ager is well fed. This is not necessarily so. A well-fed youngster is not necessarily well-nourished. There is a 50-50 chance that your teen-ager is undernourished. He may have irregular and unbalanced meals at home; he may do haphazard between-meals snacking both at the local drive-in and at home. And he may be harassed by the poor example set by his parents!

What can we do about this?

Let me introduce you to my good friends, the Nobles. Tom Noble is a successful businessman. His wife Kathy is a radio and television actress. They have four teen-age children. Tom, Jr., 17, who had always been a brilliant student, was failing in his senior-high-school courses and had lost interest in college. Kathy, Jr., 16, had lost interest in boys; she had become a self-righteous bookworm, smug, superior, getting straight A's—and getting no fun out of life. Andy, 14, potentially handsome, had become fat, awkward, and antisocial, content with just television and comic books. Ruth, at 13, was disobedient, unruly, rebellious.

Tom and Kathy asked my advice. First, I suggested *feed 'em.* "Let's figure out an Eating-for-Fun program for each member of the family. Then let's get *every* member to agree to follow his or her program faithfully for one month."

There were three reasons for this. First, teen-agers are independent. No use making rules. No use coaxing, "Eat it—it's good for you." To get the four young Nobles to eat well, we had to get them interested in good eating.

Second, if teen-agers can discover the relation between the food they eat and the way they look and feel, their own natural desire to be as attractive as possible will do the rest.

Third, Tom and Kathy Noble set a poor example for their teenagers. Kathy zigzagged from one diet to another, with little regard for proper nutrition. Tom scorned her dietary rovings—and just plain overate.

The six Nobles agreed to follow the eating programs I drew up for them. These programs were based on the Nobles' nutritional needs, with variations according to age and sex. The results were gratifying to all six of them, long before the month was up—better health, glossier hair, clearer eyes, better complexions, and increased energy.

Tom, Jr.'s marks improved, and he showed increased ability and purpose. Kathy, Jr., discovered she could have fun on dates and still keep up her scholastic record. Andy lost weight and became interested in sports. And Ruth, with her improved complexion and added vitality, gained important self-confidence.

My second suggestion was: "Love 'em." Naturally, Kathy and Tom loved their children, and they were understandably indignant when I suggested that their children's emotional diet was deficient in vitamin X.

"Of course you love them," I agreed. "But do *they* know it?"

Like so many other worried parents of teen-agers, Tom and Kathy had been overconcerned about their children's "shortcomings." They had forgotten their own teen years—how pleasing and provoking, how beautiful and baffling, they were. They had forgotten that to develop confidence, good judgment, and emotional strength, teen-agers need, not just love, but a specialized kind of love—vitamin X *plus*, which is love-plus-approval. In short, less "You're terrible" and more "You're terrific!"

And, finally, "Leave 'em alone." Later, Kathy Noble told me: "Do you know why your Noble Experiment succeeded? Because you put it up to each one of us. We Nobles, like most Americans, are all-fired independent. We want to do the right thing, but we don't want to be pushed into it. I was startled when I first heard you say that the way to handle teen-agers was to 'Feed 'em, love 'em, and leave 'em alone.' It sounded too simple, even risky—especially the part about leaving 'em alone. But now I know you're right."

If we give our teen-agers the well-balanced meals and the well-balanced love they need for physical and emotional growth, we have equipped them for freedom. Give them the independence they crave—they'll thrive on it. Give them your confidence—they'll respect it.

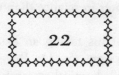

22

Helping Your Man

Although many thousands of men have learned to eat intelligently, there are many more thousands of women who tell me that their husbands refuse to consider the subject of nutrition and health. Therefore, this chapter is written for the woman who wants to help her man.

I know this is a most personal question, but: Is your husband in love with you?

If you have a man to love who also loves you, I hope you take good care of him. When I urge you to take care of your man, I do it as a reminder, because frequently people who have lived together for a while begin to take each other for granted. Still later, when the children have grown up and married, they confront each other almost like strangers. And I wonder if you know that there is a peak in divorces among people who have been married twenty years. I sincerely hope this does not happen to you. Take a good look at your man, and listen to him; let him do the talking for a change. What do you see and hear?

You may see thinning hair and a thickening waist. Can he still get into the suit in which he was married? You may hear minor complaints, aches and pains, the creaking of a body that is no longer joyfully active—a sure way to grow old young! You may hear and see signs of poor digestion, possibly of ulcers. Take note of them. Nothing is clearer in science than the connection between food and the emotions.

You may worry about his taking an extra drink somewhat too often. Take note of this sign, too. Dr. Roger J. Williams, who has done brilliant work in biochemical research, tells us that alcoholics are hungry, malnourished people. He says that in our American diet of highly saturated fats and over-refined starches and sugars, the hypothalamus—that center in the brain that guides the appetite —is starved for the relatively large quantities of minerals, vitamins, and amino acids that it requires. He believes that much alcoholism could be prevented, as well as cured, by sound nutrition which, interestingly enough, includes a tablespoon of golden vegetable oil, plus a vitamin concentrate especially high in the B vitamins. Should you be so unfortunate as to have an alcoholic problem in the family, I strongly suggest you read Dr. Williams' book, *Nutrition and Alcoholism.*

You may see your man constantly tired, sleepless, anxious, irritable. All the signs of psychiatry today point to the connection between healthy body chemistry and health of the mind, emotions, and behavior.

You may be troubled (perhaps he is, too) about a seeming loss of his masculine powers; this, to a man, is a profound anxiety. Yet this too is most often a result of tension, lack of energy, deficient nutrition—and deficient love.

Finally, you may be worried about his heart. What wife today is free of this worry?

It is not surprising that bachelors have a shorter life expectancy than married men. Certainly a man without a woman to love and care for him is not the best candidate for a happy, long life. Yet, from the thousands of questions married men ask me, it is evident that they face many problems. No doubt the strains and tensions of our competitive way of life are to blame, and to change all that is a large order for one lone woman!

Use Your Woman-Power

I believe that any intelligent woman has the power to change this hectic pace for her man. It is not as difficult as you may think. Its secrets are right in your own home, in your kitchen, your living room, and the bedroom you share with him.

In my many travels I have found that women—despite all the jokes about their unrealistic thinking—are the realistic, practical members of the human race. Men are the adventurers, the gamblers, often the self-deluders. Women are the ones who recognize a fact when they see it—they seem to have an extra sense!

What, then, are the facts behind that big phrase, our hectic "way of life"?

Our country enjoys the highest living standard in the world. Yet in seventeen other countries, men live longer past the age of forty-five than they do in the United States.

Of Americans who live past the age of forty, 50 percent die of cardio-vascular disease—disease of the heart or arteries. And of these, 77 percent die of arterial disease.

In our American high-standard diet, 44 percent of the daily food intake consists of fats, mostly the hard saturated variety.

Compare this with another set of facts:

In Japan, only 10 percent of men past the age of forty die of heart and artery disease. Only 10 percent of the Japanese food intake is fat, primarily the liquid fats.

What do these amazing figures tell you? Apparently a man's chances of dying of cardio-vascular disease are almost exactly as great as the percentage of hard fats in his diet.

Compare this with another finding, revealed during a recent conference at the New York Academy of Sciences on "Culture, Society, and Health." The increase in heart disease deaths among young American men—the "epidemic," as the medical world is beginning to call it—can be traced directly to changes in living habits in the past thirty years.

"Lack of exercise, coupled with rich snacks in front of television screens, may be a major factor," reported Dr. David M. Spain, pathologist of Beth-El Hospital and Columbia University College of Physicians and Surgeons.

There you have the man-killing American "way of life," pinned down to a few facts as simple as your own grocery list!

New Deal for Harassed Husbands

A leading women's magazine has been telling us for years, "Never underestimate the power of a woman." I never have, and neither do most men. In my observation, it is the women them-selves who fail to understand and use their power.

Once it was said that there was a woman behind every successful man—presumably, it was she who gently, subtly, directed him. That was in the days when women were slaves to housekeeping and child-rearing.

Today women are emancipated. They go out into the world, the equals of men. And now, it seems, there is a woman in *front* of every man, shaking a finger before his face and telling him what to do.

That is the picture I see, rising from the mountain of letters I have received through the years. "Dear Gayelord Hauser, How can I get my husband to take care of himself . . . to diet . . . to relax . . . to exercise . . . I keep telling him . . . etc. etc."

What has happened to the ancient feminine art of "getting around" a man?

I have a secret to share with you. Do you know the one complaint that men most often make about their wives? They say, "If she would only stop nagging!"

When a man says that to me, I see again that mountain of letters that show the other side of the picture, the letters from wives that say, "I *keep telling* my husband . . ."

Every woman knows that when she "keeps telling," she is nag-ging. Every woman knows in her heart, too, that nagging—or if you prefer, telling over and over again—does no good. Why does a woman continue to do this when she knows it accomplishes nothing? Does she do it, perhaps, to relieve her own tensions and irritations?

I am afraid she does. And I ask you, all you wives who love your husbands and want to take care of them, wouldn't you do better to find some other way of dealing with your tensions, instead of working them off on your long-suffering men?

Remember, constant dripping wears away stone! Constant nag-ging wears away the most patient man. Sooner or later he will flare up in answering irritation, and there will be a needless quarrel. Many husbands simply protect themselves by retiring behind the newspaper and turning a deaf ear. A wife may "keep telling" her husband, but he is no longer listening.

No, telling him does no good. You should know that a man does not like to be *told*. He does not *need* to be told. He knows all too well about his waistline, his flabby muscles, and the menace of a heart attack.

A man needs to take for granted in himself his manly strength and vigor. When you tell him that he has to watch his diet, watch his weight, watch his health, you undermine that belief in his manliness. You make him feel soft, unmanly—womanish! That is why he bristles with irritation or turns a deaf ear. He has to protect his ego.

If you are a womanly woman, you cherish the manliness of your man. You want to build up that ego, not break it down. You will quickly realize that what he needs from you is not talking about his health, but doing something about it.

If you have been trying to change his ways with words, give it up. Slip into a new gear. Change to the gentle, artful persuasion that only a woman knows how to do. Change his ways without even letting him know it.

You have the power to do this. You are still the mistress of the home. Above all, you are the queen of the kitchen, where so many of the sins of our modern way of life are committed.

You alone have the power to cook lean meals for him, without making announcements that will challenge him to resist. You alone can bring him serenity in his leisure hours. You can even get him to exercise, if you are wise in the way you go about it.

Remember, you are his new wife, who never nags. Give up "telling him" to take care of his health. Let him forget about his health while you take care of it for him.

THREE GIFTS EVERY MAN WANTS

In the fairy tales that we loved as children, there were always three magic gifts by which the prince made his way through perilous adventures and returned to his princess, to live happily ever after. Here are the three magic gifts you can give to your man:

Give him a new heart, one that will enable him to work and reach his life's goal.

Give him a new waistline, his youthful looks and vigor restored.

Last, but most important, *give him a new wife,* yourself transformed within and without.

By giving him these three great gifts, you will give yourself the greatest gift of all, a new husband, a better companion and a better lover, one whose pride and pleasure in you will keep you young and beautiful. If you have come with me this far, you are already creating the third magic gift. And this new wife, who now knows the power of good nutrition, also knows the power of her womanly wisdom to create for her man the other two gifts.

A STRONGER HEART

Here is good news: You can do, not merely something, but very nearly everything, about this way of life that threatens your man.

What I am about to tell you is vouched for by serious, conservative scientists. It is a hypothesis so far, but a strong and positive one.

Arteriosclerosis, the arterial disease that is the unrivaled, number-one killer today, can be foreseen, can be prevented, and sometimes can be cured. Dr. Harold Thomas Hyman greets this hope as "lighting a hitherto cheerless chamber with the first rays of hopeful prognosis."

Arteriosclerosis is a sort of porridge that forms in the arteries. It leads to a thickening and stiffening of the arterial walls that cuts off circulation to the heart. It does not have a single cause, but a combination of them. Inherited factors, and certain metabolic diseases, such as diabetes, make some men more susceptible than others, as is true with most diseases. But the crucial combination of factors are these: sedentary occupation, overweight, possibly with low thyroid function, and the stress and strain of modern living.

Dr. Hyman points to the "lush American diet" compared to the frugal diet of Chinese, Japanese, Italians, among whom heart attacks are relatively rare. As the immediate causes of arteriosclerosis he lists: "Sustained and prolonged hyperalimentation (overeating); excessive salting of foods; and undue dietary dependence on concentrated carbohydrate foods and on saturated fats which, in the process of refinement, have lost certain essential amino acids, minerals, fatty acids, and vitamins."

Most doctors now test for cholesterol level in the blood, and if the level is above normal, they prescribe a diet low in cholesterol-producing foods, mainly the saturated fats. (See also pages 191–192.) If you are at all worried about your husband's heart, I strongly urge you to discuss this test with his doctor. As Dr. Hyman says in his textbook for physicians, it is especially valuable to the doctor in general practice because it gives him a way of detecting, *in advance,* those "overtly healthy individuals" who are *prone* to arteriosclerosis.

A SMALLER WAISTLINE

You have known for a long time that overweight is a menace to your looks. Now you know also that it is a menace to your man's health and peace of mind. Not only motion picture Don Juans are reducing their waistlines today; all serious men are learning to eat intelligently.

The Senate restaurant offers a special reducing menu; all dishes contain the minimum amount of fat. The official physician to Congress, Dr. George W. Calver, urged leaner diets on representatives and senators as early as 1928. He worries especially about the freshmen legislators, men between thirty-five and fifty years old. So much of their work is sedentary—and so much of it involves not only sitting, but eating too, at the political banquet tables—that they have a constant struggle against excess pounds. Dr. Calver enlists their wives and even their secretaries in keeping track of what his charges are eating.

Vice President Lyndon B. Johnson believes that his heart attack saved his life. After he recovered, he wondered whether it could have been prevented. His doctors told him that the same regime he had to follow to prevent a recurrence might well forestall a heart attack in the first place. He had been working at a breathless pace, without pause for relaxation or exercise. His breakfast was coffee and cigarettes, his lunch a hurried hamburger, his dinner a heavy meal of fried meat and potatoes. One of his new rules is to keep down weight. The tall Texan (he is six feet three) reduced from 202 to a lean 174 pounds. A second rule is that he must have no more than 50 grams of fat each day. Mrs. Johnson promptly equipped her kitchen for leaner cooking.

IF YOUR MAN IS SEDENTARY

The second step, both to trim looks and good health, is exercise.

Men were hunters before they were farmers, and farmers before they were businessmen and desk-sitters. The human body, Dr. Laurence E. Morehouse tells us, was built for the rigors of the hunt. This professor of physical education at the University of California reminds us of what I have already mentioned in urging you to exercise for your own sake:

"Movement of the skeletal muscles in man not only performed his external work in primitive days, but also acted as supplemental heart muscles in moving fluids through the body. The modern sitting man relies on his heart muscle alone to pump fluids which support the internal environment of the body. The heart cannot do the job of circulation without the aid of other muscle pumps and sitting man soon begins to suffer."

Sitting man soon begins to suffer. Mighty important words, these, and the shouting will become louder and louder, because movement or exercise is important not only for your man's heart, but for every part of his body—even his hair!

From many years of experience, however, I have learned that you cannot force a tired, flabby body to exercise. How many mechanical exercisers, stretchers, bicycles, and rowing machines are gathering dust in American attics and basements! Many homes have one or two in the storeroom. All these appliances cost money, and they were bought with the most earnest resolutions.

But resolutions are not enough. Your husband, first of all, needs new energy. You must build up your man's body to the point where it will demand exercise, so much so that exercise will become a pleasure.

Begin your magic, right in your shining, push-button American kitchen. Right there is where you can create your man's new waistline and his new heart.

MILLION DOLLAR KITCHEN SECRETS

You are going to give your man, not a diet, but a new way of eating. You are going to put before him tasty, delicious meals, rich in proteins, vitamins, minerals, fatty acids; low in sugars and starches and especially lean in saturated fats. You are going to replace the refined sugars with natural sugars, full of their own good minerals and vitamins, and the refined starches you will replace with the whole, natural variety. You are going to replace the killing, hard fats with golden vegetable oils that contain the lifesaving, essential fatty acids. You are going to stop oversalting, oversugaring, overcooking; and flavor his food instead with delightful spices, herbs, and flavors.

With even a single change in his menu, the change from hard fats to vegetable oils, you can protect the health of your man's arteries and at the same time relieve him of those extra inches around his waistline. And with the change of the whole spectrum from empty foods to sound nutrition, you will give him new vigor and zest for living. You will boost his morale along with his metabolism.

So throw away the hardened hydrogenated fats that you have been using as shortening, even if they are vegetable fats. Look at the label on your margarine; make sure it is not the hydrogenated kind. Have your butcher trim the fat off the meat you buy, or sharpen your best knife and trim it off yourself.

Soya oil, which the Japanese housewife uses; sunflower oil, which the Soviet Ministry of Nutrition is devoting thousands of extra acres to produce; peanut, sesame, avocado, and wheat-germ oils are all insurance for your man's heart and general health. (See also pages 31–32.)

Something exciting has been recently discovered about wheat-germ oil and wheat germ. Experiments with athletes show a direct connection between this little heart of the wheat and the stamina of the human heart. At the Physical Fitness Laboratory of the University of Illinois, fitness scores were higher with wheat germ or its oil added to the diet than with exercise alone. Just one teaspoon of wheat-germ oil taken daily increased athletes' physical capacity and endurance by as much as 51.5 percent.

Now wheat germ is rich in vitamin E, and there is one school of thought that considers vitamin E a specific vitamin for the health of the heart. Whether it is this vitamin in the wheat germ or some other factor, it is clear that this food element provides something that gives men added endurance under physical stress.

Yet this very precious substance is refined out of American bread and cereals. But you, performing your magic in the kitchen, can easily learn how to restore it to your man's food. You simply add some golden wheat germ oil to your salad dressing. Sprinkle wheat germ kernels over salads and cereals. You can even make a delicious wheat germ pie crust. (See page 516.)

Another valuable nutrition supplement is lecithin. Dr. Lester M. Morrison, in his fine book, *The Low Fat Way to Health and Longer Life*, describes lecithin as one of the most important nutritional supplements developed in the last fifty years. I have known about lecithin since I was a schoolboy in Germany. Our family doctor insisted that we children, and especially my sisters, must have it in its natural form of beaten egg yolk, in fruit juice or sherry wine; it was the only form in which we knew it then. In Germany at that time it was considered a very good food for the nerves.

Lecithin is better known now. We know today that it can be a lifesaver because it is a natural emulsifier of fat, and fat is the enemy of the heart, whether it is part of the added burden of overweight or a direct cause of high cholesterol in the arteries.

I have mentioned that the Chinese and Japanese suffer very little heart disease. It is also a curious fact that in their diet—so poor by our standards—the soybean has been the keystone. They call it their holy bean, their meat without a bone. It has been their flesh, fowl, milk, cheese, and oil for thousands of years. And here is the most surprising fact of all: The soybean is one of the richest natural sources of lecithin. I beg you to use soybean oil; also try some of the soybean dishes. (See page 468.)

More About Lecithin

Mr. Edward R. Hewitt, the New Yorker who wrote that charming book *The Years Between 75 and 90*, learned about the tremendous benefits of lecithin while studying in Germany. Here is what he has to say: "Lecithin is well known to have a very great emulsifying action on fats. It is reasonable to suppose that it would have the same emulsifying action in the body. . . . With older people the fats remain high in the blood for from 5 to 7 hours, and in some cases as long as 20 hours, thus giving the fats more time to become located in the tissues. If lecithin is given to older people before a fatty meal it has been found that the fats in the blood return to normal in a short time, in the same way they do in younger people. . . . I myself also have observed that my memory is better than it was before I took lecithin regularly. My nervous reactions are still perfectly normal at 88. My hands are much steadier than those of any doctor who tested me."

THE OUTER MAN

Next to loss of sexual potency, a man worries most about losing his hair. Most men do not admit it, but it is one of the questions I am most often asked at my lectures before men's clubs, and today there is a booming business in toupees. Medical science, as a whole, pays little attention to this problem. Yet I think it is important, otherwise men would not spend millions of dollars on useless hair tonics.

The whole question of baldness is confusing. There are many theories. Some researchers claim that men lose their hair more often than women because an excess of male sex hormones affects the quantity or quality of the oil produced in the sebaceous glands of the skin and scalp. The laboratory evidence for this claim is that when the oil was rubbed on the bodies of mice and rabbits, all the rabbits and many of the mice lost their hair in ten days.

When female hormones were injected into bald-headed men, the men stopped losing their hair; but they also began developing breasts, so obviously that was not the solution. A good endocrinologist can determine whether an excess of male hormones is in fact the cause of your man's falling hair, and can give him a prescription for an oil lotion containing the recommended female hormones in the proper dosage. An estrogenic hair lotion, offered by a New York endocrinologist to be applied directly to the scalp, is reported to be helping some men keep their hair.

Some American doctors believe that a lack of proteins can cause extensive loss of hair, and some Scandinavian doctors believe that too much salt in the diet can cause baldness. According to them, cutting down on salt significantly reduced hair loss. This is right in line with Dr. Eugene Foldes, of New York, who has been able to arrest hair loss by reducing the salt content of the body. Dr. Franz Halla in Vienna claims that pork fat has extremely bad effects on hair growth and blood circulation.

Dr. Irwin I. Lubowe, the distinguished New York dermatologist, pays a great deal of attention to nutrition in his excellent book, *New Hope for Your Hair,* and in his discussions on the importance of vitamins he points out that nicotinic acid or niacin causes marked vasodilation of the scalp. This means dilation of the capillaries bringing increased circulation and thus increased nutrition to the hair follicles.

A method closer to home holds out promise that your man's chance for hanging onto his hair is good as long as he keeps the muscles under his scalp in good tone. Dr. M. Wharton Young of Howard University in Washington, D.C., in order to test his theory that good scalp muscles prevent baldness, applied electrodes to hairy and hairless parts on the scalp of balding people. Then the subjects were asked to move the scalp and wiggle the ears. The muscle contractions registered on the machine as electrical impulses, but only in areas with hair; the bald spots showed no movement or muscular activity whatsoever. This proved to the experimenters that it is the muscles under the scalp, with their rich supply of blood vessels, which bring nourishment to the hair follicles in a healthy loose scalp.

According to Dr. Young's theory, massage fails to stop baldness because it does not strengthen the muscles under the scalp. Only exercise can strengthen muscles, in the scalp as everywhere else. According to Dr. Young, this can be accomplished by wrinkling the forehead as hard as possible. At first it seems difficult, but with a little practice it becomes easier.

If your man is losing his hair, tell him about this most important exercise. Here is what he should do:

Pull the forehead up as much as possible without the use of the hands. Then pull it down as hard as possible. He will find as he does this scalp lifting exercise that the ears also move, and that is as it should be. Encourage him to do this exercise regularly, moving his forehead and ears up and down ten times or more, at night, in the morning, and whenever he thinks of it. After a while he will notice that he can move his scalp and wiggle his ears quite easily.

This takes only a few moments of his time and is well worth doing if he wants to stop his receding hairline.

A more drastic, but seemingly successful, treatment for baldness has recently come into the spotlight. Dr. Norman Orenthreich, Assistant Clinical Professor of Dermatology at New York University, has been able to transplant healthy hair from the sides of the head to the bald spots. The treatment is given in the office, under local anesthetic. Only six or seven hairs at a time are taken from

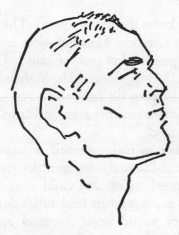

Modern hair transplants are 90% successful

the base of the neck, where the hair is thickest, and transplanted into the bald spots. While this is a drastic and expensive way of adding hair to a bald pate, it is most welcome to actors and other people whose jobs depend on their looks. Dr. Orenthreich has done more than 500 of these transplantations, and 90 percent have been successful. But never forget that all hair, transplanted or otherwise, gets its proper nourishment via the blood stream.

You Can Be the New Wife

I began this chapter by saying that love is the greatest beauty-giver a woman may be fortunate enough to enjoy. Let me say now that it is also the greatest source of contentment and well-being, yes, and morale, that a woman can give to her husband.

I am not a marriage counsellor. But a vast number of women

have written to me, asking for advice in their anxiety, and it is sadly apparent that many American women who truly love their husbands do not know how to show their love. They simply do not understand the psychosexual nature of the male.

European women on the whole have had a better education in this respect. There is a gem of Continental wisdom that mothers have passed on to their daughters for generations: *A wife should be a chef in the kitchen, a lady in the drawing room, and a mistress in the bedroom.*

A man needs to know that he is wanted. The most masculine of men—to quote Dr. Gregorio Marañon—does not aggressively woo women once he is past the hot years of youth. The most masculine man is a faithful, loving, dependable husband and father, who devotes himself to keeping his family safe and cared for. He is not likely to force his attentions, not even on his wife. He needs to be invited and encouraged.

Do you remember to make yourself attractive for him? I am sure you are never deliberately negligent in your appearance. But in the press of housekeeping and child care, perhaps also work outside the home, many women tend to let down their standards at home when they would never dream of appearing before an outsider in pin curls and cold cream.

The fact is that many women who do let down in this way are the first to complain that their husbands are no longer ardent lovers!

Habit and routine are deadly to love. Why do so many men approaching middle years fall prey to temptation outside the home?

Many a man's eyes stray because his love is not courted, but merely taken for granted at home. But another reason for infidelity is that a man is worried about his dwindling potency and is seeking reassurance wherever he can find it. This is such a sensitive subject with a man that he may never mention it to his wife. He may not even admit it consciously to himself.

There is still a widespread belief that a man's sexual prowess ends with a change of life like the end of child-bearing in a woman. Somehow you should convey to your man that this is simply not so.

Here is what the recently published, medically endorsed book, *Sexual Pleasure in Marriage*, by Jerome and Julia Rainer, says on this troubling subject:

"The theory that there is a male climacteric with symptoms similar to those of the female has long been obsolete. If he suffers somatic ailments or states of depression . . . the causes are not to be sought in a nonexistent climacteric. Neither is a sudden slackening of sexual desire and potency, in a man otherwise physically well, a result of physiological decline. These phenomena have a psychic origin."

In other words, it is all in the mind! A man may lose confidence in his manhood when his wife does not seem to invite his attentions, when she does not bother to make herself attractive, even seductive, just for him. And it is a sad fact, which no wife should forget for an instant, that there are some 25,000,000 women without men in the United States, widowed, divorced, or unmarried, many of whom would give anything to have a man of their own.

No wife can afford to be careless about her man's health, or his happiness, or his love.

FOOD AND LOVE

Can you strengthen your man's sexual powers with food?

Some years back I wrote an article for *Esquire* on the care and feeding of executives. It won a tremendous response and brought me many invitations to lecture to men's clubs. I remember especially a luncheon at the Athletic Club in Philadelphia. As usual I answered all kinds of questions on diet and health, on how to relax, how to get rid of tiredness.

Then there was a lull, in which I could plainly hear some snickering from a table at the end of the room. Finally a small, slight man stood up and blurted, "Is there any connection between food and sex, and what should a man eat when his love life is on the blink?"

The whole room shook with laughter, but I admired that courageous little man. He looked tired and worried, but he was the only one who had dared to ask the question that haunts most men past the age of forty, and even some who have not reached that fortieth birthday. I answered him in all seriousness. I told him that, of course, there is a relationship between a man's diet and his sex drive. I said, "I only wish I could give you one potent recipe, food, or formula to make you a romantic, carefree lover, but unfortunately, it is not that simple."

I went on to tell him what I now want to tell you. The search for a more satisfying sex life has been going on ever since Adam found the first gray hair in his beard. The ancient Greeks and Romans had books full of strange formulas for waning sex powers. Some of them contained dangerous poisons—the Roman poet, Lucretius, died of one of these "love philters."

And some were frankly based on magic. For instance, the early Greeks swore by onions and garlic because both of these root vegetables have the shape of male testes. Another favorite was wine made from the mandrake root, simply because this two-legged root looked rather like a miniature man.

But strangely enough, many of those ancient love potions contained such highly nutritious foods as eggs, snails, fish, all of which are full of vitamins and minerals; liver, the richest source of iron and the B vitamins; wild game, which we know today ranks higher than domestic meats in many vitamins and is also much leaner. Among the vegetables they recommended were cabbage, a fine source of B vitamins and C, and peas, which are high in vegetable protein. High on the ancient lists of love foods was honey, one of nature's finest sugars.

Listen, now, to a 2000-year-old tip on foods for sexual prowess: wild honey, ginger, vinegar, wild garlic, shallots, cinnamon, nutmeg, wild seeds, pepper, and all heat-producing spices.

Today we laugh at such concoctions. But do you recognize in this list some health-giving foods? Of course you do. As for the spices, we know today that they stimulate the stomach to produce gastric juice and thus promote good appetite.

Actually, we do not need to go back to antiquity to find love potions. In my boyhood days in the Black Forest, the country folk staunchly believed in their "potent potage for lovers," and to this day in some parts of Europe, women prepare this soup when they feel neglected by their husbands. Its chief contents are glandular meats such as liver, heart, tripe, cock's comb and testes, cut up fine and simmered in a powerful broth of onions, leek, garlic, celery root, parsley, and every other available garden green. It is a very thick soup and must on no account be strained, for, say the peasants, to derive the "strength" from this potent potage a man has to eat every bit, its meats and vegetables as well as its broth.

Pumpkin Seeds, a Man's Best Friend

During my lectures at the Titania Palast in Berlin, it was my pleasure to meet an unusual man, Dr. Devrient. He is a medical doctor who specializes in nutrition. Dr. Devrient complimented me on my work; but, he said, "Hauser, you neglect telling your students about one of nature's most potent foods, the seeds. Seeds have been used since Biblical times, and they are an excellent food. They contain protein, vitamins, minerals, and some of them contain hormones." Then the Berlin physician gave me a copy of an article he published in the German journal of health *Androgen;* "Hormonal Curative Influence of a Neglected Plant." In this article he said:

"Only the plain people knew the open secret of pumpkin seeds, a secret which was handed down from father to son for countless generations. No matter if it was the Hungarian gypsy, the mountain-dwelling Bulgarian, the Anatolian Turk, the Ukranian, or the Transylvanian German, they all knew that pumpkin seeds preserve the prostate gland and thereby, also, male potency. In these countries people eat pumpkin seeds the way they devour sunflower seeds in Russia, as an inexhaustible source of vigor offered by nature."

My Paris office informs me that pumpkin seed oil is highly valued in France and it is used to fortify other vegetable oils. Here is another proof of what Hippocrates knew 500 years before Christ: "And your food shall be your medicine."

In France even today, their beloved bouillabaisse is considered a dish for lovers; and as you know, it contains every conceivable fish and shellfish, every nutrition-rich gift of their Mediterranean Sea.

Today we know that there are no mysterious love potions for tired lovers. But we also know that many of those fantastic formulas did really perform miracles—not through magic, but through good nutrition! The good proteins and the high vitamin and mineral content of those love dishes invigorated men in those days as they do today.

And this is the truth about the ancient love potions, which science confirms today. Good nutrition is not only the basis for health and beauty, but also for a healthy and happy sex life.

As a loving and understanding wife, you can perform this same miracle for your man. You can sustain his manhood, strengthen his morale, and satisfy his deepest hunger. You need no magic recipes, formulas, or tricks—nothing else but good nourishing food, potent with nature's own potency. That is what science knows about food and sex today.

CARE AND FEEDING OF HUSBANDS

All hard-working husbands should be treated and fed as VIPs. Good meals are doubly enjoyed and give double value when eaten in a relaxed atmosphere. Feeding a husband in the modern manner means *cutting down* on hard fats, starches, and sugars, and *increasing* the protein foods. (Remember, he needs half a gram of protein for each pound of his ideal body weight—not his overweight. If your man weighs 160 pounds, he needs 80 grams of protein every day.) Also, include as many fresh fruits and vegetables as possible. You may have difficulty at first changing your man's eating habits, so use your womanpower—do it gently and gradually. By all means begin by serving good protein breakfasts because this greatly determines whether the day ahead will be hectic or whether things are taken calmly.

BREAKFAST

Unlimited choice of fresh or frozen fruit juices, tomato juice, or fresh fruits in season. (You can make an irritable husband amiable by handing him his fruit juice while he is dressing; this ups the blood sugar level by the time he comes to breakfast.)

Choice of proteins: 2 eggs: poached, boiled, scrambled, or fried in golden oil. Or: omelet, ½ cup cottage cheese, lean broiled meat patty, liver, fish, or ham. When bacon is served, make sure it is lean and crisp.

Cereals: Serve only whole-grain varieties. If he insists on cold cereal, serve it à la mode, fortified with 2 tablespoons of fresh wheat germ and half a cup Hi-Vi lean milk.

Breads: Muffins, biscuits—only the whole-grain variety. Also introduce high-protein wheat germ and soya muffins. Breads are better eaten untoasted. If he insists on toast, make it light brown; only one piece should be eaten and this can be buttered lightly. If a more generous spread is desired, serve homemade lean cream cheese or cottage cheese.

Coffee: Freshly made, preferably Swiss coffee made with fresh milk, or tea with milk.

HI-VI RITUAL:

So that there is no possible chance of missing any important nutrients, see to it that he takes the prescribed vitamin-mineral concentrates before leaving the breakfast table. It is a wise plan to keep the concentrates on a special tray.

LUNCHEON

Choice: Vegetable espresso, tomato juice, or hot bouillon, if desired.

Choice of proteins: Lean meat, cheese, fish, eggs, cottage cheese. Serve with a portion of green salad or, better still, mix the proteins into a bowl of crisp salad greens and marinate with golden oil dressing.

Add: One slice of good bread or a muffin, lightly buttered.

Beverage: Choice of coffee, milk, tea, or yogurt.

MIDAFTERNOON

To prevent any let-down, choice of a glass of vegetable espresso—carrot, celery, or apple—or a glass of milk, yogurt, or tomato juice, fortified with a teaspoon of food yeast

DINNERTIME

Give your husband a chance to unwind. Serve a cool vegetable espresso with a handful of pumpkin seeds.

Choice of: Lean meat, fish, or fowl—broiled, baked, or stewed
                   Mixed green salad with golden oil dressing
                   One or two short-cooked green vegetables (twice a week, a Light-Hearted Baked Potato)

Dessert: Fresh fruit, compote, honey custard; occasionally, open-face fruit pie or lean cheese with an apple or pear

Beverage: Demitasse, milk, or yogurt

BEFORE RETIRING

A glass of lean milk, cottage cheese with cracker, yogurt, or hot Swiss broth

How to Cook a Husband

One day while being interviewed on television by that knowing and attractive Pamela Mason in Hollywood, we discussed everything from how to feed babies to how to handle husbands. I mentioned that husbands, especially in America, sometimes have tough going. I also spoke of the three things most husbands want more than anything—a smaller waistline, a younger heart, and a new wife.

Pamela agreed with me on the first two points, especially when I said that a good wife certainly can help to give the smaller waistline and a healthier heart by spending a little more time in the kitchen, doing some tender loving cooking with less hard fat and fewer carbohydrates. I also insisted that any woman who really wants to, regardless of birthdays, can make herself slimmer and more attractive, and stop nagging (the No. 1 complaint of millions of husbands) and become that new wife.

Then I read a note that appeared in the New York *World-Telegram*. This is what Mrs. Walter Ferguson wrote: "We hear that scientists are working to see if they can find out what is killing off so many men in the prime of life. That's a real easy one. *It's the women*. We aren't doing it on purpose, of course; we love our men and are worried about their shortened life span. But we also love having mink coats, air-conditioned cars, large houses with lovely gardens, stylish clothes, and all the latest gadgets for the kitchen. It's killing the men to supply them. The pressure of getting 'things' for their women, and gratifying their own material wants, puts them in a rat race."

Well, that did it. My telephone never stopped ringing that afternoon. Women were furious with me for putting all the blame on them; but the men thanked me. One of them said, "It's even worse in my house. All the wife wants is more money. No matter how much I turn over, there are days and weeks when she will have nothing to do with me." Several others said that their wives keep them constantly in hot water.

Only a few days after that, a very nice letter arrived from a woman doctor living in the San Fernando Valley. She thanked me and Pamela Mason for the frank discussion. She also reminded me that I said there are many ways of cooking a husband and that most women do it the wrong way. Enclosed in the letter was a recipe which a friend of her mother's had made many years ago.

It is so true to life, and full of common sense, and expressed so charmingly, that I would like to have cards printed of it for every wife to place on her mirror as a daily reminder of the real million dollar secret of handling her man. It is reprinted on the next page.

HOW TO COOK A HUSBAND

A good many husbands are utterly spoiled by mismanagement in cooking and so are not tender and good. Some women keep them constantly in hot water; others let them freeze by their carelessness and indifference. Some keep them in a stew with irritating ways and words. Some wives keep them pickled, while others waste them shamefully. It cannot be supposed that any husband will be tender and good when so managed, but they are really delicious when prepared properly.

In selecting a husband, you should not be guided by the silvery appearance as in buying a mackerel; nor by the golden tint as if you wanted salmon. Do not go to the market for him as the best ones are always brought to the door. Be sure to select him yourself as tastes differ. It is far better to have none unless you will patiently learn how to cook him.

Of course, a preserving kettle of the finest porcelain is best, but if you have nothing better than an earthenware pipkin, it will do—with care. Like crabs and lobsters, husbands are cooked alive. They sometimes fly out of the kettle and so become burned and crusty on the edges, so it is wise to secure him in the kettle with a strong silken cord called Comfort, as the one called Duty is apt to be weak. Make a clear, steady flame of love, warmth and cheerfulness. Set him as near this as seems to agree with him.

If he sputters, do not be anxious, for some husbands do this until they are quite done. Add a little sugar in the form of what confectioners call kisses, but use no pepper or vinegar on any account. Season to taste with spices, good humor and gaiety preferred, but seasoning must always be used with great discretion and caution. Avoid sharpness in testing him for tenderness. Stir him gently, lest he lie too flat and close to the kettle and become useless. You cannot fail to know when he is done. If so treated, you will find him very digestible, agreeing with you perfectly; and he will keep as long as you choose unless you become careless and allow the home fires to grow cold. Thus prepared, he will serve a lifetime of happiness.

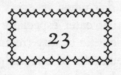

23

Look Younger, Live Longer Goals

What are our Look Younger, Live Longer goals? Here are some of them. As you read, sit back and be comfortable, relax your body, and let your imagination strike off sparks of its own, kindle its own enthusiasm. Let your wisdom, your own knowledge and experience, show you your own particular goal.

LOOK YOUNGER BEAUTY SHOPS

Some years ago, when I wrote my book *Eat and Grow Beautiful,* I expressed the hope that in time my inside-and-outside plan would be incorporated by some of our smart New York and Beverly Hills beauty salons. I had not long to wait. Dorothy Gray engaged one of my assistants and opened a beauty bar in New York. Helena Rubenstein opened a "food for beauty" restaurant, and Ann Delafield set up her famous and profitable Success School at Richard Hudnut's.

So far, so good. But that was only the beginning. Americans are beauty-conscious. American women are by nature the most beautiful women in the world; the mixture of our nationalities, diets, and clothes all help. American women in the second half of life already are learning to give more, rather than less, attention to grooming and appearance.

I look forward to the day when in every city there will be Look Younger beauty shops that cater especially to the mature woman. Such shops will give scientific beauty treatments in the Yoga Slant position to improve circulation in our scalps and faces. They will serve fortified milk drinks and fresh vegetable juice cocktails—enrichment for the blood stream, bringing beauty from within.

Such shops will be run by mature beauty operators who understand the special needs of adult American women and have special interest in teaching them the art and science of agelessness. Here will develop new fashions in smart and conservative hair-dos, in dignified and natural make-up.

Already, such organizations as Beautymasters (of Detroit, Michigan) are instructing their women representatives according to a coordinated beauty plan. After thorough training in diet, exercise, reducing, hair care, eye care, make-up, and the art of relaxation, these representatives are taught to present this plan in the privacy of the client's home.

Here is a business with a future. Teaching others the art of youthfulness is a good way to keep youthful oneself. And beauty is a profession which knows no depression.

MEDICAL CENTERS

Here is the job for the wise older general practitioners, the specialists in chronic and degenerative diseases, eye and ear specialists, research scientists—to establish "human machine shops" for geriatrics and prevention of the disabilities of older people in every city of our country. The Mayo brothers, Johns Hopkins Hospital, and others have proved that this can be done very successfully. A group of doctors, members of the Class of 1900 of the College of Physicians and Surgeons at New York's Columbia University, organized themselves into a Committee on Longevity to study their own old-age health problems and those of patients in their own age group. The findings of this group can be made the basis of a strong, nationwide movement. My great hope is that these doctors will give nutrition the attention it deserves. Specialized work by these and other distinguished physicians will be of immense value to all Americans in the second half of life.

HEALTH PROTECTION CENTERS

Much time, thought, and money are given to planning for the health of our pedigreed animals. Is it not high time that we stop using haphazard methods for humans, and mobilize our American efficiency for long-range health planning for ourselves, our children, and their children? I am much impressed with the health-protection experiment conducted by two English physicians who set up, in the London district of Peckham, a health center with all the equipment of a modern clinic plus a modern swimming pool and gymnastic facilities for exercise and play. The reports of increased health and disease prevention are amazing. Another health-protection center is in Dornach, Switzerland, where, under the leadership of Dr. Rudolph Steiner, a group of physicians built a magnificent place called the Goetheanum, where health protection starts with the correction of the soil.

I envision such health centers as focal points of community life, social gathering places for all age groups, where each family can be examined as a biological unit, where hidden disorders can be detected and corrected before they have a chance to become chronic. I envision these centers also as opportunities for health re-education, for teaching people how to relax, how to exercise, and, above all, how to eat. Such health centers will also offer golden opportunities for the teaching of simple, basic rules of mental hygiene; and surely psychosomatic medicine has convinced us that for true health protection, we need not only sound bodies but sound minds, not only a physical but also a "mental" diet.

This is a big job for doctors, psychiatrists, psychiatric social workers, and also for nutritionists, dietitians, former champion athletes, physical education and recreation directors.

SENIOR COUNSELING

Dr. Lillian J. Martin of California and Dr. George Lawton of New York have demonstrated the way in which universally tested principles of clinical psychology can be applied to the needs of men and women in the second half of life. I look forward to the day when every city will have its senior counseling bureau, staffed by psychologists, vocational guidance experts, aptitude testers, rehabilitation workers who already have spent a "lifetime" of work in these fields; who know the eternal resilience of the human spirit; and who passionately believe, as Dr. Lawton has so well said, that "to lose interest in setting up personal goals, some distant, some near, and to give up the struggle for their achievement—this [and only this] is growing old."

New York University's Testing and Advisement Center is another example of what can and should be done. Men and women who are not happy in whatever work they happened into, or who want to develop other talents for the second half of life, are given scrupulously careful, objective analyses of their aptitudes and personalities. At the end of the testing, they are given practical advice on the field in which they would be happiest and most useful.

LEGISLATIVE PLANNING

Here is the job for older statesmen, legislators, lawyers, politicians, sociologists, economists, members of professional groups and unions. These are men and women who have had many years of experience in "getting things done." Theirs is the responsibility to work for broader Social Security programs, retirement planning, old-age benefits that are realistic and not "crackpot," and dynamic, not makeshift. So far as I know, only two countries, Sweden and New Zealand, have well-organized systems for social protection. This is because citizens of both countries have unusual longevity and have, in addition, an unusually high general cultural level.

INDUSTRIAL PLANNING

There is great need for industry to "come of age," to curtail automatic retirement of workers at a fixed birthday regardless of whether or not the power and desire for work has lessened. Here is a job for older industrial executives who not only have the interests of their contemporaries at heart, but also know from experience that the older worker is just as effective a producer as the younger man. In a recent survey of 1,000 business firms, more than three-quarters of the firms reported that older men are as productive and efficient as younger men, and there is less absenteeism.

Jobs can be shifted, working hours shortened, wages and pension benefits altered as workers grow older. To keep older workers productive is today's challenge to industry. Ford and General Motors have pioneered in this; other industries are following suit. *Time* Magazine cites an interesting example, the Ithaca Gun Company, in which "A man is not considered experienced until he is past eighty."

ADULT EDUCATION

Here is a wide-open field for retired educators—to adapt and revitalize educational methods to meet the growing demand of those who believe that it is never too late to learn. Older people want to go back to school, to learn new subjects and to learn more about themselves. Dr. George Lawton's course, "Aging Successfully," which was given at Cooper Union in New York City, was attended by several hundred students, half over 60, some over 80. Some husbands and wives attended together.

JOB PLACEMENT BUREAUS

I like to think that one day there will be in every city an employment bureau with a sign on its door: No One Under Fifty Need Apply. That office would be staffed entirely by people of well-seasoned maturity, "retired" personnel experts and job analysts, whose aim is to secure for older applicants their share in the world's work. Such employment services already are part of many philanthropic organizations and nonprofit public welfare societies.

"Forty Plus" organizations, notably the one in New York City, are dedicated to placing *only* men over forty in desirable positions. They analyze each job-seeker, prepare job-getting resumés, and give pointers on the techniques of getting the right position.

It is my belief that in the coming years such bureaus can be operated on a sound business basis, making it their special function to develop a new repertory of ways to utilize the judgment and experience of older people.

SMALL BUSINESS OPPORTUNITIES

Have you always wanted a business of your own? Go to your public library for books on business opportunities. They are written for younger people, but what of that? Dr. George Lawton recommends one such book, *A Business of My Own, Possibilities in Small Community Occupations and Industries,* published by Community Service, Inc., Yellow Springs, Ohio. There are many others. Also, there are in your community many other such seasoned businessmen and -women as yourself, eager and able to launch a new venture. Find them. Put an ad in the newspaper, if necessary. Remember that at 89, Dr. Lillian J. Martin, a retired schoolteacher, ran a profitable farm with four 60-year-old assistants.

TRAINING SCHOOLS AND WORKSHOPS

We need training schools in every city where older people can know the joy of rediscovering their creative selves. Edward T. Hall, founder and director of the Universal School of Handicrafts in New York, calls this rediscovery "vitamin V" in human behavior. His students refuse to grow old; the oldest ones look younger, shed symptoms of advancing age and fears of the future, and set themselves up in new business ventures. Another model enterprise is the Opportunity School in Denver, Colorado, which for many years has trained women in their sixties for new careers.

VOLUNTEER BUREAUS

War years have proved the inestimable value of volunteer workers; they are often called "our greatest unused national resource." We need training courses for older volunteer workers, especially to work with and in behalf of the handicapped. It is not enough to give money and shed tears; active work must be done if we are to have, for example, compulsory hearing tests in schools to prevent deafness, and compulsory eye drills to prevent poor vision in later life. These and many similar reforms are projects of special interest to older volunteer workers. Also, older people are the logical choice to work in behalf of other older people. The Council of Social Agencies in Chicago offers training courses for volunteers who visit the aged, listen to their problems, help in countless ways. In many communities the Red Cross Chapter includes services for the aged as part of the voluntary service program.

RECREATION CENTERS AND CLUBS

Here and there around the country, isolated "straws" show which way the wind of the future is blowing: Forty-plus clubs; the Walkers' Club of New York, all of whose members are between 60 and 80; Benjamin Rose Institute in Chicago, which has pioneered in promoting a model recreational program for older people. Philadelphia is outstanding, with forty-three clubs for older people, drawing their membership from all cultural and economic levels. I am also told of a Grandmothers' Club—a large group of amazingly young and good-looking grandmothers—who have regular get-togethers, give dances, put on shows. (Yes, they have their annual "Grandmothers' Follies.")

There will be increasing opportunities for older people to meet and make friends with others of like tastes and interests. Not just "Lonely Hearts" clubs, but active, lively groups of people gathered together to do what they most enjoy. Dancing, choral singing, discussion groups, travel clubs, vacation camps—the possibilities are boundless. Being a nutritionist, I am most interested in seeing groups form for the congenial purpose of eating together—Eaters Anonymous Clubs of reformed overeaters, who help one another to follow the Look Younger, Live Longer dietary program. Why not start such a club in your city? It takes only one capable man or woman to do it. Already there are enthusiastic Eaters Anonymous Clubs in Detroit, Milwaukee, and Los Angeles; their numbers are increasing rapidly.

HOUSING

Growing awareness of the housing problems presented by our increasingly older population is indicated in projects developing in different parts of the country, especially in mild climates. It is my belief that coming generations of men and women in the second half of life will prefer to live with their contemporaries rather than with married children, and that the ideal arrangement will be self-managed, co-operative housing developments, apartments, and residence clubs.

Let us forever banish the old concept of Homes for the Aged, dreary places to wither away, and think constructively, from now on, in terms of homes for the aged where longer living can be a pleasure. Such projects would include resident doctors and nurses, recreational facilities, workshops; they would have co-operative dining rooms where, instead of dreary Old-Ladies'-Home dishes, vital, living, delicious foods will be served, organically grown vegetables straight from their own gardens, fresh or short-cooked.

St. Petersburg, Florida, is noted for its "planned living" for older people; some 60,000 have made it their home. Moosehaven, in Orange Park, Florida, has co-operative residence clubs and apartments especially adapted to the needs of oldsters. Another interesting project is the Colony Club for Older People in Roosevelt Park, Millville, New Jersey, which offers residents individual cottages at low rentals. There are others in California and elsewhere.

Here is a job to quicken the imagination of every architect, city planner, decorator, furniture designer, gadgeteer, dietitian, and home-economics expert in the second half of life—to visualize and create the living quarters they themselves want, in terms of millions of their contemporaries. The proposal of Dr. Martin Gumpert that small villages be built in Southern states, planned for the social, physical, and educational requirements of older people (why not financed by insurance companies?), is a forward step in the right direction.

I am happy to report that in Yucca Valley, near Palm Springs, 20,000 acres have been acquired to set up a new community dedicated to happy living. This tract of land includes Pioneer City (California), for many years a location for Western movies.

This fertile land has a stimulating combination of sun, soil, air, and water. It has an ideal year-around climate, and the soil is excellent for organic gardening. There are hot springs nearby.

Home sites are of various sizes; they can be large enough to provide space for ten children or small enough for a retired couple to manage without help. The ranch-type houses are spaced to allow plenty of fresh air and sunshine—and they are available as low as ten thousand dollars.

Many sports are planned—swimming, riding, walking, golf—and

gardens will provide not only recreation, but also a chance to grow beauty-full foods. Of course there will be shops, as well as a country club.

This beautiful spot is only 25 minutes from Palm Springs and less than 3 hours from America's largest city, Los Angeles. It promises to be a community devoted to fun and healthy living. It is *not* a retirement village; indeed, young people are welcome because they help to keep older people young. It is *not* a place to dry up, but a place to enjoy all your long life.

PUBLIC RELATIONS

At the present time, America has gone "youth crazy." We hear of young presidents, young executives, young actors, young singers. Why do we not hear more about the tried and true mature people?

We need to work vigorously to restore the prestige of age and to break down existing social and economic prejudices against older people, in the American way, by means of planned, intelligent, long-range public relations. There is work to be done, changing existing ideas of what constitutes the useful span of life; there is work to be done to convince newspaper editors, advertising directors, and entertainment entrepreneurs that people who have lived many decades are neither marvels nor freaks, but mature human beings with talent, dignity, importance, and buying power.

Here is a job for writers, artists, publicity experts, lecturers, fashion designers, entertainers in the second half of life: to re-create America's mental concept of age. It is also the individual job of every man and woman over the age of fifty to demonstrate by example that the second half of life can be the best half. Dr. George Lawton has said, "We are as young as society says we are." It is up to *you* to re-educate society.

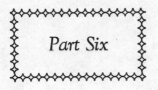

Part Six

INTELLIGENT DIETING

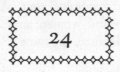

24

Reduce and Rejuvenate

HOW TO MAKE REDUCING A PLEASURE

Once I wrote an entire book on reducing: *New Guide to Intelligent Reducing*. I did many years of research on that book. In it I explained why so many people overeat and described their physical and emotional problems. I gave recipes galore, diets and low-calorie menus, all worked out to perfection. I received hundreds of letters, in many languages, telling me that somehow, when excess pounds disappeared, feelings of depression and inferiority also disappeared; and all who wrote me agreed that they felt and looked much younger. Naturally, I was delighted that through this book I could help so many people. If you have a reducing problem and want to solve it for a lifetime, I suggest you read it. It is published by Farrar, Straus & Co., New York.

But looking back over the years, and talking to thousands of people here and abroad, I discovered that there is something wrong with all reducing diets and books in the past—including mine. Men and women the world over have developed a deep hatred for all prescribed diets and the pains associated with reducing. The chores of following a severely restricted diet are the greatest obstacles to slimness. Why, you ask? Let me remind you of what that wise man Sigmund Freud said: "The most powerful urge is to seek pleasure and avoid pain." This is the pleasure-pain principle, a biological and psychological truth. Dieters and doctors, nutritionists and dietitians, all must remember that pleasure-pain is the most basic motivation of men and women; and unless we can turn the pains of reducing into pleasure, the most scientifically planned diets are of no avail.

Let me tell you of an interesting lesson I learned in Paris. Lady Mendl arranged a lecture for me in her Avenue D'Iena salon and invited ten of her closest friends. Before me sat the Duchess of Windsor, Lady Duff Cooper, Princess Aspasia of Greece, Princess Karputhala of India, Lady Cavendish (Adele Astaire), Lady Carnarvon (Tilly Losch), the beautiful French Ambassadress Madame de Saint Hardouin, Madame Ruth Dubonnet, Madame Arturo Lopez, and the famous beauty Mona Williams, now the Countess Bismarck. I had addressed audiences of thousands, but they were mostly Mrs. Smiths and Mrs. Browns. Here were women with position, looks, worldly goods—what could I tell them? It was one of the most difficult lectures I ever gave. Lady Mendl had warned me not to talk too long, so I discussed my Eat and Grow Beautiful plan— with special emphasis on *staying* slim, since not one of those glamorous ladies was overweight. I stressed the fact that they could remain slim without boring dieting; that wise Mother Nature has given us unlimited varieties of food for our enjoyment; food should be prepared attractively, since sophisticated people also "eat" with their eyes; but above all we should get pleasure from our meals and eat them slowly, gratefully, in a pleasant and relaxed atmosphere. That was 24 years ago and not *one* of those women has become overweight. Some still make the yearly "best-dressed" list. And most of them tell me: We don't diet, we have learned to like lean meats, we eat big salads, our cooks undercook vegetables and spike them with herbs, we don't like starchy dishes and gooey sweets, we prefer fresh fruits or fruit compotes for dessert. In other words, they have learned to eat intelligently.

Why Most Diets Fail

Let us be absolutely realistic. Every month, hard-working beauty editors beat the bushes for a new diet or exercise regime to take off pounds and inches. How many of them have you tried? How many have been successful for you? And how long has it taken you to get back to your old weight and measurements?

Quick-reducing schemes are all deceptive. They often show sensational results. But they do not change your eating habits. And so the quick miracle is a mirage. It cannot last; the pounds come back.

Lose It the Same Way You Gained It

No healthy person gains weight overnight. It is the day-by-day overeating of starches and sweets, plus the extra cocktail or cream in the coffee, that puts on perhaps ten, perhaps fifteen pounds in a year or two or three. Sometimes one begins eating a little more; sometimes one eats the same as ever but spends more time sitting at work or riding in cars or watching television.

It probably has taken you two or three years to gain those ten or fifteen pounds; but you are not going to work for two or three years—or even one year—to lose them, and I can't blame you. Yet neither can you expect to lose them, and lose them permanently, in a few days.

Every time you try one of those quick methods and fail, you lose, not your excess weight, but your courage and confidence. All that work wasted! All those daily self-denials, those sacrifices of good spirits and good temper! If the overweight is much more than ten pounds, if it is perhaps twenty-five or fifty, the disappointment in quick-reducing diets, in gimmicks and gadgets and drugs, is a real morale-destroyer.

The Simple Arithmetic of Weight-Losing

Once and forever, let us look squarely at the mathematical facts of gaining and losing. The food that you take into your body each day is fuel. Your body uses up as much as it needs for the day's activities. What it does not use, it stores.

The body has three levels of storage. A certain amount it keeps in circulation as glucose—blood sugar—for immediate use. The next level of storage is in the form of body starch, called glycogen, and it is stored in the liver.

The third, the long-term fuel storage form, is body fat. This is the most compact form of stored energy. Any food that you eat in excess of your body's needs, especially the over-refined starches and sugars, eventually ends up as stored energy in the form of body fat.

These are the mathematical facts. There are no other explanations, no alibis. And don't blame your glands!

Women especially have a tendency to retain fluid in the body tissues, and this adds both weight and inches. These pounds and inches are the first to come off when you begin a reducing regime, and that is why the results of a quick-reducing program seem so gratifying. But the moment the program ends, and you return to your normal eating and activity, the fluid seeps back into the tissues; and there you are, right back where you started.

In most of these quick-reducing schemes you do not make a dent in your body's fat. All you do is lose water. Test it and see: Weigh yourself, drink two glasses of water, and weigh yourself again. You will find you have gained about a pound!

The biggest handicap is that you try to lose weight without ever knowing *how* you gained it. You feel guilty, dissatisfied with yourself, obsessed with the question of just what to eat. But you have no real guide to how you can achieve your best contours *permanently*, until you know how you gained weight in the first place.

Let us check up a little. Compare your weight today with your best weight since your twenties. What did you weigh on your wedding day? What was the size of the dress or suit you wore at your wedding?

Now consider: What has changed in your way of life since then? Are you eating more? Or are you using your body less?

Perhaps you have changed dwellings during these years. Have you, like so many, moved from a two-story into a ranch-type house with no stairs, or into an apartment?

One woman tells me that she has been able to trace her gradual gain in weight from the time her children started to school. Another, from the time she went back to a job, at which she sits all day. Still another, from the time she moved six blocks nearer to the bus stop.

And many people, searching for the cause with real honesty, tell me that they began to gain weight when the family acquired its first television set, or its second car! Or from the time when their circle of friends expanded and they began "cocktailing" every weekend!

And then there are people who eat more out of loneliness, boredom, anxiety. Diet alone will not overcome this kind of eating. You need to find new interests and goals. Some very overweight people need psychiatric help or hypnosis under a competent doctor's care.

The most worthwhile new goal is making yourself over into the person you were meant to be. I can promise you a happier you, not so lonely, or so bored, or so anxious. You must break the vicious circle somewhere. Why not break it with a program for your new slim body? And remember the cause of your own particular weight gain; you can lose the same way you gained, safely, easily, and permanently. You can lose one pound per week. In ten weeks you can lose ten pounds. In a year you can lose fifty pounds—or even more, if you apply the million dollar secret which was discovered by an Englishman who had tried all sorts of low calorie diets and became desperate.

For the Hard to Reduce

One hundred years ago, an Englishman named Banning made a marvelous discovery. He was short—five feet, five inches—and he was vain; his bulkiness made his life miserable. When he became so fat (202 pounds) that he could no longer see his feet, Banning became frantic. He visited one doctor after another. They all told him he was eating too much and put him on very low calorie diets. These made him feel even more miserable; his whole life seemed a hopeless battle against his excess layers of fat. Then a new misery descended on Banning. He started to lose his hearing. Friends sent him to a fine ear surgeon, who obviously was a wise man. Instead of ordering surgery, this doctor put Banning on a diet different from any other he had ever followed. This time he did not follow a 1000-calorie restricted diet; he ate the foods he liked best. In less than a year the hard-to-reduce Banning lost 50 pounds and 12 inches around the middle. But what made Banning happiest was that his hearing came back. So elated was Banning that he put his experience in a booklet called "Letter on Corpulence." In it he reported just what he ate and drank. Here was his daily fare:

BREAKFAST: 4 oz. beef, mutton, kidney, liver, fish,
                                  bacon, or cold meat (no pork)
                          one slice of toast
                          cup of tea without sugar

LUNCHEON: 5 oz. fish or meat (no pork), or any kind
                                  of poultry, especially game
                          choice of any vegetable (no potato)
                          one slice of toast
                          fruit for dessert
                          one glass of claret, sherry, or Madeira
                                  wine (no beer or champagne)

TEA TIME: 2 or 3 oz. fresh fruit
                          one slice of toast
                          tea without sugar

DINNER: Same as luncheon

BEFORE RETIRING: If wanted, a glass of grog or a glass of
                          sherry

As you can see, the Banning regime was very high in calories. Thus, it could *not* have been low caloric intake that did the reducing; it was the low, low amount of carbohydrates, as Banning himself wrote in his book—and which every modern nutritionist, dietitian, and doctor should write in *his* book: "I can now confidently say that quantity of diet may be safely left to the natural appetite and it is the quality only which is essential to abate and cure corpulence." Banning stuck to his diet. He omitted concentrated starches and sugars and kept his weight down to normal. He lived a comfortable and long life.

More Scientific Proof

In 1950, another distinguished Englishman, Sir Charles Dodds, before the Royal Society of Medicine in London, threw a monkey wrench into the well-established low-calorie diet theory. He tested both men and women who had kept their normal weight for years. He now had them eat two or three times as much food as they were accustomed to. All of them stuffed themselves, yet none of them gained weight. It was discovered that with these normal-weight people, the body metabolism automatically was increased; or, in simple language, the body fires burned brighter and did away with the excess food.

Then Sir Charles picked another group of men and women. This time he selected those who had weight problems and whose weight constantly fluctuated. These people were also asked to eat much more than usual. Of this second group, all gained weight and inches. Obviously, their metabolism did not rise; the extra foods were not burned and were turned into fat.

Here, then, was scientific proof of what happens to people when, sitting at the same table, eating the same meals, one gains weight and the other stays slim. People blamed glands, nerves, disposition, digestion—but now, with the help of isotopes, scientists have been able to tag many food and chemical substances; and we no longer need to guess. The action of the isotopes can be watched and followed throughout the body. The metabolism of the foods we eat—the proteins, carbohydrates, the fats—is no longer a mystery. *What Banning found out the hard way, scientists can vouch for today: It is the large group of carbohydrates, especialy the denatured, over-refined ones, that are the real troublemakers; they are the real enemies of the millions of men and women who gain weight easily and who are hard to reduce.*

If you are that type, you should remember that your body obviously is not equipped to handle carbohydrates—the starches and sweets. For that reason, shun the empty flours, sugars, and cereals, and use even the whole, natural carbohydrates in modest amounts. Here is how William Banning expressed it:

"For the sake of argument and illustration, I will presume that certain articles of ordinary diet, however beneficial to youth, are prejudicial in advanced life. . . . The items from which I was advised to abstain as much as possible were: bread, butter, sugar, beer and potatoes. These, said my excellent advisor, contain starch, and saccharine matter, tending to create fat, and should be avoided altogether."

Turning Point

As is so frequently the case, this new idea was not easily accepted. The doctors in England did not like to give up their established ideas that overweight is caused by overeating and that the way to correct it is to count calories and eat less. No one wanted to admit that Banning was right, until the Doctors Kekwik and Pawan published their scientific tests of Banning's diet carried out in London's Middlesex Hospital. They announced: "The composition of the diet can alter the expenditure of calories in obese persons, increasing it when fat and proteins are given, and decreasing it when carbohydrates are given."

When the results of this testing appeared in the United States, Pennington went one step further. In 1951, he wrote an important report based on his research with fat and high-protein diets: "The Use of Fat in a Weight-Reducing Diet." In it he had the courage to say: "Contrary to the claims of the low-calorie school of thought, low-calorie diets have failed." Dr. Pennington also insisted that "the ability of tissues to oxidize fat in contrast to carbohydrates is unlimited."

He also discovered that some people can burn only small amounts of carbohydrates—and any excess is turned into fat. At long last there was scientific proof of what Banning already knew and applied a hundred years ago: *Carbohydrates are the fat person's poison!*

Easy Does It

And now, instead of giving you a neatly worked-out 1000- or 1500-calorie diet, with dry toast, half squares of butter, vegetables without salt, and a carefully measured piece of fish or liver, let me pass on to you another important and almost forgotten biologic secret (especially if you are sick and tired of calorie charts and regimented eating): There is an easier, relaxed, and sure way to get back into shape. For my students in America, France, Germany, and England, it has proved to be the best and shortest short-cut to most reducing problems. You need only to remember these four major points:

Eat slowly, in a relaxed atmosphere.
Enjoy first-class proteins with each and every meal.
Cut carbohydrates (starches and sugars) to minimum.
Chew your food twice as long; you will have twice the pleasure, it will help your blood sugar to rise, and you will feel nourished and satisfied with less food.

It sounds too simple to be true. Yet it is the simplest possible rule to follow. And it works—for reasons which are not quite so simple. If you would follow your natural appetite, and if your foods came to you directly from the fields instead of the supermarkets, it would be very simple: You would eat only what your body needs, and you would never weigh one extra ounce. *I am really more concerned with what you eat, rather than how much. If your foods were truly full of their natural nourishment, you probably would never overeat.* And you would not have to count your calories, for calories *alone* don't count.

Get More Pleasure from Your Food

We do not eat only to appease hunger. We also eat for satisfaction and pleasure. But most of the time we miss the pleasure. We gobble our food absent-mindedly, not knowing what we are eating. This gulping of food is an ugly habit, not only because lumps of food are harder to digest, but also because so much more food must be eaten before hunger is appeased. Long before I talked about this, Burton, in his book *Anatomy of Melancholy,* stressed the importance of *slow, conscious eating and careful chewing. In that way the appetite is thoroughly appeased with only half the usual amount of food.*

Perhaps some of my older students remember Dr. Horace Fletcher who, fifty years ago, taught his followers to "Fletcherize" everything they took into their mouths. At the "Nut and Berry Club," as we used to call their eating place in New York, they sat chewing like cows; they even chewed water! Often a good and wise idea is made ridiculous when carried to extremes. But believe me, basically "Fletcherizing" is sound. At any rate, all of Dr. Fletcher's followers were slim!

Our teeth, our jaws, our facial muscles, all were made for chewing. But what benefits most of all from chewing is the mind. When you chew twice as long, you also taste your food twice as long, and it gives you twice the pleasure.

Last, but not least, masticating your food slowly gives the blood sugar level a chance to rise so that it can send signals to the appetite control center (in the hypothalamus) that your hunger has been really satisfied. You automatically lose the urge to overeat. You will no longer need to diet. You can throw away all reducing books, including mine, because your psychological appetite, as well as your physical appetite, will be satisfied. That, I believe, is the real million dollar secret to most reducing problems.

When my friend Martha Deane, in New York, interviewed Carl Sandburg, the earthy and outspoken American poet said: "People eat too fast; they don't take time to appreciate their food."

I only wish that my American readers (who are the champion gobblers and gulpers) would have the pleasure of dining with a French family. In France they still take time to eat *slowly* and get the maximum amount of pleasure from their food; and they have only half as many overweighters as we have in the United States.

Stop Stretching Your Stomach

A woman of average size has a stomach that can hold a quart of food. Yes, just one quart. A large person, a six-foot-three man like myself, has a stomach capacity of one and one-half quarts. Those are normal capacities. But a habitual overeater, a real *fresser* as they say in German, or a *gourmand* as they say in French, can stretch his stomach to hold as much as six quarts! And once he has stretched it to that size, it will clamor for that quantity of food—until he disciplines it and trains it back to normal.

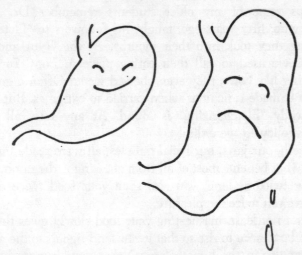

An overloaded stomach groans, prolapses, and eventually goes on strike

You do not have a six-quart stomach—far from it. But you can easily stretch your stomach by eating until it groans. You do not need all that food; you cannot possibly use it all up. But your thrifty body will not waste it. Your digestive system will process it, your liver will convert it, and your body will store it away—as body fat.

Seven Secrets to Smart Eating

1. *Chew*, slowly, pleasantly. The longer you chew, the less you will eat, as thousands of my students have proved.

2. *Enjoy* and appreciate every bit consciously. No more absent-minded eating which stretches the stomach.

3. *See* what you eat. We eat with our eyes, too (no TV dinners in the dark).

4. *Taste* what you eat. Satisfy your need for pleasure in eating.

5. *Refuse* to eat anything that does not satisfy your body's needs. No more empty, foodless carbohydrates.

6. *Take time* to eat. Satisfy your psychological need for un-hurried pleasure in food, and give your blood sugar a chance to rise.

7. *Eat only for eating's sake.* Find other remedies for boredom, tenseness, and emotions. Thousands have done it.

If you satisfy your physical appetite with truly wholesome, nu-tritious foods and your psychological appetite with the fullest pleasure in eating, you will lose your extra weight and you will never again have a weight problem.

Your Ideal Weight

Most people are at their best weight between the ages of twenty-five and twenty-eight. After thirty, with a general lessening of movement and exercise, weight seems to pile on gradually.

The following weights for both women and men have been painstakingly tabulated by the Society of Actuaries, an organiza-tion of experts, after studying five million policy holders. The Metropolitan Life Insurance Company has prepared these charts. Compare your weight with these new figures, according to your height and the size of your body frame. If you have difficulty as-certaining whether you are small-, medium-, or large-boned, let your doctor help you.

Remember that your ideal weight should be figured out according to these new findings, regardless of your age.

CHART

IDEAL WEIGHT FOR WOMEN				IDEAL WEIGHT FOR MEN		
Small Bones	Medium Bones	Large Bones		Small Bones	Medium Bones	Large Bones
4'10" 92-98	96-107	104-119	5'2"	112-120	118-129	126-141
5'0" 96-104	101-113	109-125	5'4"	118-126	124-136	132-148
5'2" 102-110	107-119	115-131	5'6"	124-133	130-143	138-156
5'4" 108-116	113-126	121-138	5'8"	132-141	138-152	147-166
5'6" 114-123	120-135	129-146	5'10"	140-150	146-160	155-174
5'8" 122-131	128-143	137-154	6'0"	148-158	154-170	164-184
5'10" 130-140	136-151	145-163	6'2"	156-167	162-180	173-194
6'0" 138-148	144-159	153-173	6'4"	164-175	172-190	182-204

NONREGIMENTED REDUCING REGIME

(High-Protein, Medium-Fat, Low-Carbohydrate)

Have a Good Breakfast

I cannot repeat this often enough: Breakfast is the most important meal of the day. Start with a glass of fruit juice, preferably fresh (but canned and frozen juices are permissible, provided they are unsweetened). If you are tired and irritable in the morning, drink your juice as soon as you get up. As your blood-sugar level rises, your spirits will also rise, and the world will look brighter. For your all-important protein, you can choose from the following: Fresh eggs, preferably boiled, scrambled, or poached, with bacon; French omelet; cheese omelet; chipped beef; or a quarter- to a half-pound of your favorite lean meat: ground beef, liver, chops, steak, mixed grill; or ⅔ cup of cottage cheese. With any one of these you can enjoy *one* slice of bread, whole-wheat, gluten, or rye, toasted if you like, buttered lightly, or still better, spread generously with sun-butter (see page 33). Large cup of fresh or instant Swiss coffee (see page 524). While reducing, it is best to forego ready-to-eat cereals. If you like, you may have a cooked whole-grain cereal, but it should be cooked in skim milk and sprinkled with a tablespoon of toasted wheat germ.

Let your conscience and your waistline be your guides. Eat lots of protein, some fat (golden oils or sunbutter), and be a miser with carbohydrates (starches and sugars).

So that there is no possible chance of missing any important nutrient, take your vitamin-mineral concentrate at breakfast and be fortified for the day ahead.

Luncheon Time Should Be Salad Time

Heap a generous portion of your favorite protein food on a bed of green salad leaves (other vegetables such as tomatoes, cucumbers, radishes, and green peppers are permitted, but green leaves are more important). Take your choice of: hard-cooked eggs, lean meat, lean fish, Swiss cheese, soybeans, cottage cheese, or yogurt-cheese. Salads should be mixed with a tablespoon of French mayonnaise or golden oil dressing. For office workers, a pint of milk, yogurt, or buttermilk, or two hard-cooked eggs, with an apple or orange, makes a nutritious and satisfying lunch.

Midafternoon, If Hungry

Your choice of large glass yogurt, buttermilk, or egg tonic (see page 473). For office workers, a handful of unsalted almonds or pumpkin seeds.

Dinnertime Is Relaxing Time

A half hour before dinner, enjoy a tall cool Vitality Drink— your choice of fresh vegetable espresso (see page 505) or a glass of Hi-Vi tomato juice (see page 78). Take your time, relax and unwind, and give your blood sugar level a chance to rise. Then, enjoy a large portion (at least half a pound) of lean meat, fish, fowl, or cheese; a large green salad mixed with a tablespoon of golden vegetable oil or mayonnaise; one short-cooked green vegetable with a teaspoon of sunbutter, vegetable oil, or margarine. Once a week, a Light-Hearted Baked Potato (page 501). Dessert should be fresh fruit, although nuts or lean cheese may be substituted.

One piece of toast, spread generously with sunbutter, may be eaten at each meal (but only if wanted). Milk drinks or Swiss coffee are the best mealtime beverages, taken at the end of meals. Under no circumstances should water be drunk while eating—only between meals.

These suggestions offer you a diet that gives you a wide choice of foods and a chance to eat freely of the foods you like best. Anyone can plan tasty, balanced meals following the above outline. There is no more excuse for anyone carrying around excess weight when such unregimented eating will slowly but surely help to burn up ugly fat deposits. I cannot with good conscience recommend an all-meat-and-fat diet or any other unbalanced regime. Such diets may work with ditchdiggers, farmers, day laborers, or Eskimos, but not with most men and women in the jet and pushbutton age. I believe now, as I always have, that in balance there is strength and health. With a high-protein, medium-fat, and low-carbohydrate diet, you should not only lose fat but gain in health and vitality.

"Any nobleness," says Thoreau, "begins at once to refine a man's features." This is especially true of overweighters who take the great step forward to reclaim their normal body.

SAMPLE MENUS FOR REDUCING

Here are some menus to get you started. You can follow these or make up your own. But remember, lots of protein and fresh foods; and use at least 2 tablespoons of golden vegetable oil each day; and go easy on carbohydrates.

First Day

BREAKFAST: Half grapefruit
2 poached eggs
1 slice whole-wheat toast, with sunbutter or margarine
Swiss coffee
Best time to take your vitamins

LUNCHEON: Salad bowl with half-cup cooked shrimp, golden oil dressing
1 slice gluten bread or toast
1 glass buttermilk

DINNER: Green salad with golden oil dressing
Large lean beefburger, broiled
Short-cooked green vegetable
Fresh fruit in season
Demitasse

Second Day

BREAKFAST: Sliced orange
2 scrambled eggs with fresh sliced mushrooms
1 slice gluten toast, with sunbutter or margarine
Swiss coffee
Best time to take your vitamins

LUNCHEON: Salad bowl with half-cup cottage cheese, golden oil dressing
1 slice rye bread or toast
1 cup yogurt

DINNER: Fresh vegetable espresso
Half broiled chicken
Short-cooked green peas
Fresh fruit in season
Demitasse

Third Day

BREAKFAST: Grapefruit juice
Chipped beef simmered in milk
1 slice rye bread or toast, with sunbutter or margarine
Swiss coffee
Best time to take your vitamins

LUNCHEON: Salad bowl with half-cup lean ham and Swiss
                     cheese, golden oil dressing
                     1 slice whole-wheat bread or toast
                     1 glass buttermilk

DINNER: Green salad, with golden oil dressing
                     Broiled lean steak
                     Short-cooked string beans
                     Fruit gelatin
                     Mint coffee

Fourth Day

BREAKFAST: Fortified tomato juice
                     Broiled lean fish
                     1 slice gluten bread or toast, with sunbutter
                     or margarine
                     Swiss coffee
                     Best time to take your vitamins

LUNCHEON: Half-cup cooked lean chicken or meat,
(*Hot liquid lunch*)   blended smooth in 1½ cups chicken broth,
                     with stalk of celery and slice of onion. Heat
                     in double boiler.

DINNER: Green salad, with golden oil dressing
                     Broiled lean ham steak
                     Light-Hearted Baked Potato (page 501)
                     Short-cooked green vegetable
                     Wine jelly
                     Mint coffee

Fifth Day

BREAKFAST: Half grapefruit
                     Broiled lean ham slice
                     1 whole-wheat muffin, with sunbutter or
                     margarine
                     Swiss coffee
                     Best time to take your vitamins

LUNCHEON: Half-cup cottage cheese blended smooth in
(*Cold liquid lunch*) electric blender with 1½ cups tomato juice
                     and 1 tablespoon parsley

DINNER: Green salad, golden oil dressing
                   Large portion broiled lean fish
                   Stewed tomatoes
                   Fresh fruit in season
                   Demitasse

GOOD NEWS: Russian doctors discovered that the constantly hungry and overweight man or woman should not despair on a reducing diet. With every pound of fat that is lost, the appetite will also decrease; the more you lose, the faster you will lose the desire to overeat.

Sixth Day

BREAKFAST: Melon or fresh fruit in season
                   French omelet (page 473)
                   1 slice gluten bread or toast, with sunbutter
                     or margarine
                   Swiss coffee
                   Best time to take your vitamins

LUNCHEON: Salad bowl, with cream cheese and pineapple
                   1 slice rye bread or toast
                   1 cup yogurt

DINNER: Fresh carrot espresso (page 506)
                   Large portion baked soybeans with lean bacon (page 470)
                   Short-cooked spinach
                   Baked apple
                   Mint coffee

Seventh Day

BREAKFAST: Fresh fruit in season
                   Whole-wheat waffle with tablespoon honey
                   2 slices lean bacon, broiled crisp
                   Swiss coffee
                   Best time to take your vitamins

LUNCHEON: Salad bowl, with two hard-cooked eggs
             1 slice whole-wheat bread or toast
             Glass of buttermilk

DINNER: Green salad, golden oil dressing
             Lean cold cuts
             Homemade potato chips (page 502)
             Fruit sherbet
             Demitasse

Eighth Day

BREAKFAST: Fortified tomato juice
             Broiled lean beefburger
             1 slice rye bread or toast, with sunbutter or
                margarine
             Swiss coffee
             Best time to take your vitamins

LUNCHEON: Salad bowl, with half-cup tuna fish
             1 slice whole-wheat bread or toast
             1 cup of yogurt

DINNER: Fresh vegetable espresso
             2 lean lamb chops, broiled
             Short-cooked green vegetable
             Open-face apple pie
             Demitasse

Ninth Day

BREAKFAST: Orange juice
             2 soft-boiled eggs
             1 slice whole-wheat toast, with sunbutter or
                margarine
             Swiss coffee
             Best time to take your vitamins

LUNCHEON: Salad bowl: Waldorf salad, with half-cup of
                walnuts, yogurt dressing
             1 slice rye bread or toast
             1 glass of buttermilk

DINNER: Fresh vegetable espresso
                 Walnut loaf (page 465)
                 Short-cooked vegetable
                 Custard
                 Demitasse

Tenth Day

BREAKFAST: Fresh fruit in season
                 Whole-wheat cereal, sprinkled with 2 table-
                     spoons of wheat germ, Hi-Vi milk (page
                     528)
                 Swiss coffee
                 Best time to take your vitamins

LUNCHEON: Salad bowl with half-cup of diced cooked
                     chicken, golden oil dressing
                 1 slice gluten bread or toast
                 1 cup yogurt

DINNER: Fresh vegetable espresso
                 Large portion broiled liver
                 1 medium parsley potato
                 Applesauce
                 Demitasse

You will not be hungry if you eat slowly and chew your food
well; the longer you chew, the less food your appestat demands.
You can always eat celery, carrot sticks, radishes, green and red
ripe peppers to your heart's content; these are wonderful appetite
trainers, and they keep an overdemanding stomach filled.

Should you be hungry between meals, have a glass of yogurt,
buttermilk, or Hi-Vi milk. These help to feed the friendly "flora"
in the intestines. Do not tolerate constipation; if necessary, use
natural laxative herbs (page 202)—never mineral oil or synthetic
laxatives. Office workers can satisfy any between-meal hunger
with one or two apples. Before retiring, check up on your protein
intake; it should be at least 70 grams for ladies and 80 grams for
gentlemen. Make up any deficiency with a glass of Hi-Vi milk, hot
or cold.

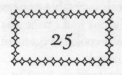

Reducing Plans from All Over the World

How the French Reduce without Tears

Some of the most elegant people in the world come to our **Life and Beauty Center** at 4, Rue Faubourg Saint Honoré in Paris, where, under the direction of chic Colette Lefort, thousands of men and women have been shown how to eat intelligently.

The French are special people. They do not fall for fads and trick reducing schemes. For one thing, good food and pleasurable eating are probably more important to the French than to any other people in the world. Any diet that takes away the pleasure in eating is doomed from the start.

The 900-calorie liquid diet that fooled millions of Americans had no success in France whatsoever. Neither did the "Safflower Capsules and Fried Food" diet have any success there, because no Frenchman would live on such a one-sided, rich, oily, fried-food diet. Every Frenchman knows that rich fried foods are bound to play havoc, especially with the liver (the French are the most liver-conscious people in the world). French homemakers would never give up serving their butter, the sweetest in all the world; nor would they deny themselves their delicious fruits and fruit juices.

The thousands of French ladies and gentlemen who come to or write to the Life and Beauty Center in Paris are told to forget their reducing problem for a while, to throw away their calorie charts and scales, and, instead, to concentrate on one thing only: to build up health and vitality. This means *stepping up* the basal metabolism—making the body fires burn more brightly—with the foods that do it best: the first-class proteins. For about a month, or until the ideal weight is reached, they are invited to eat freely of lean fish and sea food of all kinds; fowl, preferably wild; lean meat, especially liver of all kinds; kidney and other organ meats, including tripe, which is a great favorite in France. These meats are never fried, but broiled, baked, or stewed (with any excess fat removed).

Green Salads Are Most Important

The French love their salad greens, the greener the better. Fortunately, they never heard of iceberg lettuce, the palest and least nourishing of all. Instead, escarole, endive, Bibb lettuce, romaine, and watercress are piled high in Les Halles and all the other farmers' markets, and every homemaker takes pride in making a tossed salad that looks like shiny green gold. Such a salad, the bigger the better, is eaten with a good helping of meat or fish for lunch and for dinner. This protein and green salad combination helps immeasurably to pep up lazy metabolism, and the green leaves help to balance the high acid content of the meats.

Golden Oils Burn Brightly

Fresh raw or cold-pressed vegetable oils are more easily metabolized than animal or hydrogenated fats. France offers a good example of that. In Provence, where they cook predominately with fresh oils, they have fewer metabolic disturbances and overweight than in Normandy, with their rich cream cookery, or in Alsace-Lorraine, bordering on Germany, where the majority still cook with lard and goose grease.

A crude example of the burning qualities of animal versus vegetable fats is known to every cook. If you put animal fat in one pan and vegetable oil in another, you can see with your own eyes that the vegetable oil cooks cleaner and smokes less. But, in order to get all the benefits of vegetable oils, they should be fresh and cold-pressed. Use them not only for cooking but also for salad dressing and mayonnaise. Most French women still make their own mayonnaise, which is utterly delicious and has no fillers or artificial preservatives. At least two tablespoons of fresh vegetable oil should be used each day. The favorite French salad and cooking oils are: olive oil, peanut oil, poppyseed oil, walnut oil, sesame oil, sunflower oil, and pumpkin seed oil.

Remember: Meat and fish proteins, eaten with a green salad tossed with a rich oil dressing, are ideal for pepping up basal metabolism and getting rid of unwanted weight without going hungry.

To prevent monotony, the following protein foods may also be eaten: Eggs, not more than two a day (try a delicious omelet made fluffy in 40 seconds with the French dry thermo pan cover). French yogurt, the best in all the world, made with lean milk, can be eaten two or three times a day, plain or with unsweetened fruit; this custardy milk food plays an important part in reducing and is easily made at home with an inexpensive automatic yogurt maker. Short-cooked vegetables, especially the green leafy kind, can be added to meals if the large green salad is not enough. Fresh fruits make the best desserts. Lean milk or decaffeinated coffee and milk is the ideal mealtime drink while building up vitality and losing weight.

Foods That Dampen Body Metabolism

These trouble-makers should *not* be used if you want to get your body back to normal: All cereals, with the exception of wheat germ. White sugar and white flour in all forms. White bread (one slice of 100-percent whole-wheat or gluten bread is allowed each meal). Cola drinks and all other pops (luckily, the French never accepted cola drinks). All hard and hydrogenated fats, with the exception of a tablespoon of sweet butter or nonhydrogenated margarine to be used on bread or toast.

Remember: Starches, sweets, especially the over-refined ones, white flour and white sugar, colas and all other sweet drinks, plus the hydrogenated fats, put a damper on body fires. Many people cannot metabolize them completely, so they are responsible for excess weight that destroys health and good looks.

Vive la Différence!

The difference between the dynamic French diet and the many starvation diets is immense. First of all, you can eat generous portions of first-class proteins, plus green salads with at least one tablespoon of fresh vegetable oil dressing. This mixture satisfies even an overdemanding appetite more than any other combination because it stays with your stomach longer than any so-called reducing food which "guarantees" that you lose a pound each day (but which you will gain back as soon as you start eating normally). These high-protein and salad meals will step up your basal metabolism and thus increase your energy. Men and women on both sides of the Atlantic report that this way of eating eliminates "that tired feeling" and re-creates a natural urge to exercise. The loss of weight is gradual—and permanent. Best of all, eating these natural, wholesome foods retrains the appetite so that the craving for foodless starches and sweets is gone forever. This is as it should be. When first-class proteins keep the blood sugar level at an all-time high, false cravings stop automatically and you have solved your reducing problem for a lifetime.

Here is a bird's-eye view of the French reducing regime:

Most Popular French Reducing Secret

Superlevure, a high-protein, high-vitamin, good-tasting brewers' yeast, has become a tremendous success. It can now be purchased, in powder form or in compressed tablets, all over France. Even their supermarkets carry it. They take this Superlevure regularly, much as Americans take their vitamins. When on a reducing diet, the Superlevure is taken ten to fifteen minutes *before* each meal. Two teaspoons of the powdered yeast is taken in a bit of fruit juice or tomato juice; or four compressed yeast tablets can be swallowed with a bit of water. Thousands of French men and women who have reduced successfully insist that regular use of their good-tasting yeast has helped them from being hungry and helped them to normalize their hungerstats. Since brewers' yeast is rich in both protein and B vitamins, it also helps to prevent tiredness while reducing.

More French Reducing Tips

Use absolutely no white sugar or saccharin; brown sugar or honey should be used instead—and only in small amounts.

One slice of wholesome bread is permitted with each meal. High-protein bread made with gluten flour, skim milk, and soy flour is very popular.

A large cup of coffee with foamy, hot, lean milk, half and half, can be taken with each meal.

French yogurt or lean French cream cheese, made from yogurt (see page 540), makes excellent high-protein desserts, eaten plain or with fresh fruit.

The big secret of this, as well as any other, successful reducing regime is eating a big portion of protein with each meal. These include lean meats, fish, and especially eggs. (The fabulous new French thermo-pan cover tenderizes the toughest meats and preserves all nutrients.)

Here is one week's menus, which the French call *une semaine de menus manneguins*:

French Reducing Menus

MONDAY

BREAKFAST: 10 minutes before eating: Superlevure
Fruit juice, unsweetened
French omelet (see page 473)
One slice high-protein bread, buttered lightly
Café au lait or tea

LUNCH: 10 minutes before eating: Superlevure
Small lean steak
Large fresh salad with oil dressing
One slice high-protein bread, buttered lightly
Café au lait or yogurt

DINNER: 10 minutes before eating: Superlevure
Fresh vegetable juice cocktail
Broiled fish with tomatoes
One slice of high-protein bread or one parsleyed
   potato
Fruit compote, sweetened with honey

TUESDAY

BREAKFAST: 10 minutes before eating: Superlevure
Sliced orange with three heaping tablespoons
   fresh cottage cheese
One slice high-protein toast, lightly buttered
Café au lait or tea

LUNCH: 10 minutes before eating: Superlevure
Breast of chicken, broiled
Mixed green salad with vegetable oil dressing
One slice high-protein toast, buttered lightly
Café au lait or yogurt

DINNER: 10 minutes before eating: Superlevure
Vegetable soup
Boiled beef with carrots and leeks, French
mustard
Fresh fruit salad with yogurt
Café au lait or demitasse with honey

WEDNESDAY

BREAKFAST: 10 minutes before eating: Superlevure
Half grapefruit
One or two boiled eggs
One slice high-protein toast, buttered lightly
Café au lait or tea

LUNCH: 10 minutes before eating: Superlevure
Large tomato salad, French dressing
Two lean lamb chops
One slice high-protein bread, buttered lightly
Yogurt with fresh fruit
Café au lait or tea

DINNER: 10 minutes before eating: Superlevure
Mixed green salad, vegetable oil dressing
Broiled fish with tomatoes
Parsleyed potato
Melon
Café au lait or demitasse

THURSDAY

BREAKFAST: 10 minutes before eating: Superlevure
Pineapple juice, unsweetened
Yogurt with honey
One slice high-protein bread, buttered lightly
Café au lait or tea

LUNCH: 10 minutes before eating: Superlevure
          Large endive salad with vegetable oil dressing
          Large veal chop, broiled
          One slice high-protein bread, buttered lightly
          Fraise de bois (strawberries) sprinkled with
              honey, or melon in season
          Café au lait or tea

DINNER: 10 minutes before eating: Superlevure
          Large green salad, olive oil dressing
          Slice of lean broiled ham
          Braised celery
          One slice high-protein bread, buttered lightly
          Fresh fruit
          Café au lait or demitasse

FRIDAY

BREAKFAST: 10 minutes before eating: Superlevure
            Orange juice
            Two tablespoons fresh cream cheese with a bit of
                honey
            One slice high-protein bread, buttered lightly
            Café au lait or tea

LUNCH: 10 minutes before eating: Superlevure
          Broiled lean fish with tomatoes
          Watercress salad, vegetable oil dressing
          One slice high-protein bread, buttered lightly
          Café au lait or tea

DINNER: 10 minutes before eating: Superlevure
          Fresh vegetable juice cocktail
          French omelet with cheese
          One slice high-protein toast, buttered lightly
          Café au lait or demitasse

SATURDAY

BREAKFAST: 10 minutes before eating: Superlevure
            Apple juice
            Large slice of lean ham
            One slice high-protein toast, buttered lightly
            Café au lait or tea

LUNCH: 10 minutes before eating: Superlevure
              Fresh vegetable juice cocktail
              Two slices calves' liver, broiled
              Two small parsleyed potatoes
              Café au lait or yogurt

DINNER: 10 minutes before eating: Superlevure
              Cucumber salad, olive oil dressing
              Cheese omelet
              Spinach
              Sliced pineapple
              Café au lait or demitasse

SUNDAY

BREAKFAST: 10 minutes before eating: Superlevure
              Fresh prune juice
              Two eggs, any way but fried
              One slice high-protein toast with butter and
              honey
              Café au lait or tea

LUNCH: 10 minutes before eating: Superlevure
              Tomato salad with fine herbs and oil dressing
              Lean beefsteak, broiled
              Green beans
              Fresh fruit
              Café au lait or tea

DINNER: 10 minutes before eating: Superlevure
              Vegetable broth
              Roast chicken
              Braised endive
              One slice of high-protein toast, if wanted
              Melon or fresh berries
              Café au lait or demitasse

If Hungry between Meals:
              French people prefer these snacks:
              Lean yogurt
              Protein cookie
              Cream cheese made from yogurt
              Hard-cooked eggs

How the Russians Fight Bulging Waistlines

While in Moscow, I could see for myself that the Russians also have a serious overweight problem. After watching them eat, it became clear that one reason for their overweight is their shortage of good proteins. The average Russian diet is made up chiefly of grains, potatoes, cabbage, and cottage cheese. Meat is expensive and so are eggs.

Their best and cheapest sources of protein are cottage cheese, milk, and yogurt. Russian doctors emphasize exercise more than diet. After two conferences with Dr. Menshikov in his nutrition clinic, I learned how the Russians fight bulging waistlines.

To say that food alone is the main cause of overweight is like saying walking causes the feet to be sore. As an example, they say, take a secretary who sits all day doing boring routine work, getting fatter and fatter; then all of a sudden when she gets a promotion and is doing interesting work, she gets slim.

Dr. K. M. Bykov, one of the most respected researchers, has an interesting theory. He claims that basal metabolism is controlled by the brain. The idea of overweight being caused by being starved for love or security is ridiculed. Millions who lack love and security are skinny, and millions of overweighters are happy with their mates and their jobs. According to Bykov and Pavlov, *the most important thing in reducing weight is the effect our muscles have on the brain and the whole body. Muscular activity, they say, rules metabolism.*

In reducing menus they stress raw vegetables, fresh fruits, lean milk, meat, yogurt, and kumiss; they permit one slice of dark rye bread with each meal.

Russian nutritionists agree with American nutritionists that you should not feel hungry while reducing, and suggest that you eat raw vegetables and fruits for bulk and satisfaction. They ask you to go easy on vitamin B_1 because it stimulates the appetite, and, above all, avoid the slightest case of constipation. To Russian doctors, this is a major necessity in every reducing program because an active bowel helps to get rid of cholestrin. They also stress having a big meal for breakfast, a midmorning snack, the main meal in the afternoon, and a light supper at night. The before-going-to-bed snack should be milk or an apple. Weight should be lost slowly—about one to one-and-a-half pounds a week.

Russian Unloading Day

After reaching the proper weight, Russian nutritionists recommend an Unloading Day each week to prevent excess weight from creeping back. On an Unloading Day you can choose from different kinds of foods, but it is best to stick to one or two basic foods.

Milk Day: This is a popular one-day diet. On it, you may drink a quart and a half of fresh milk. If you are more than ten pounds overweight, use skim milk. If you are suffering from constipation, use yogurt in place of milk.

Apple Day: This is probably the most popular Unloading Day. It is made up of apples and apple juice. You can eat about three pounds of apples a day. The juicier the apples, the better.

Salad Day: On this day you can eat great big bowls of salad all day long. The more green leafy vegetables you use, the better. Always serve salad with simple vinegar-oil dressing, spiked with dill or your favorite herbs.

Fruit and Meat Day: On such an Unloading Day, you are permitted to eat two pounds of your favorite fresh fruit, and, for your noonday meal, you are permitted half a pound of lean meat, any way but fried. A cup of tea or coffee (nothing added) is permitted with meals.

On Unloading Days it is suggested that you space your meals two or three hours apart, such as eight o'clock, eleven, two, four, seven, and nine. Remember, these are just one-day-a-week diets.

Exercise Breaks, not Coffee Breaks

The Russians believe that exercise, done willingly and with pleasure, such as walking, swimming, bicycling, and dancing, brings joy to the body and stimulation to the brain and nervous system and peps up metabolism. The real control of body weight, according to Russian scientists, is physical exercise—or, as they call it, "Muscular Joy."

Each and every day of the week there are morning and afternoon "Exercise Breaks," with the radio blasting full force. Millions stop their work and twist and bend and stretch. How I wish President

Kennedy would engage Bonnie Prudden to give a daily exercise break on the radio. Millions could be made happier with such cheerful exercise breaks, instead of bad coffee breaks and those foodless rolls!

They say that a man or woman climbing a mildly sloping hill can burn up to six ounces of excess weight; climbing 300 yards on a fairly steep hill can burn up ten ounces of fat; climbing a hill for just two miles can burn up twelve ounces of fat. The favorite muscular joy is bicycling (few Russians can afford cars); going to and from work they can burn up four ounces of fat. I know that these figures seem greatly exaggerated to us in America. But in any case, muscular joy, or good sensible exercise in the fresh air, is of tremendous value in keeping the body fires burning brightly (increased metabolism). I only wish that more Americans would go in for more muscular joy.

Muscular Joy Gymnastics

That is what the tough Russians call their exercises when done with gusto and in fresh air. Before explaining what Russian researchers taught me about muscular joy exercise, let me quote Dr. Jean Mayer of Harvard, who says: "Combatting overweight by diet alone is like fighting with one hand behind your back. Exercise is the other fist that enables us to deal the knockout punch."

Here is how Dr. K. M. Bykov, Russia's most advanced researcher, explains that knockout punch. He says that *exercise not only helps to burn up food; it also stimulates the brain to such an extent that it sends joyous signals to all parts of the body.* He insists that metabolism is controlled by the brain, and that the impulses from the cortex and centers of the brain control the adding and taking off excess fat; therefore, muscular exercise is the important key to controlling weight.

Swiss Apple Diet

A short time ago the Swiss Fruit Association, in cooperation with Dr. Edouard Jenny, introduced an apple diet to the thrifty Swiss people. It proved eminently successful. Nothing was actually forbidden to the participants; only the over-all daily intake was restricted. The Swiss nutritionists emphasized a point that is important to every dieter the world over: that the dieters could eat the foods they were accustomed to eating. But to overcome the feeling of hunger between meals, they recommended eating apples.

Apples are low in calories, as everyone knows; but what most people do not know is that apples quickly satisfy the appetite, which obviously makes them an ideal food for a reducing regime. The Apple Diet was more popular and more successful than any other diet the Swiss people have ever followed. More than 30,000 men and women who followed the diet wrote glowing reports to the Swiss Fruit Association. (Of the 30,000 participants, 78 percent were women and 22 percent were men.) The diet became so popular that many hospitals and more than six hundred Swiss doctors recommended it. As a whole, the men had greater success than the women—and those who followed their doctor's advice had the greatest success of all.

Swiss doctors were delighted to discover that an extra bonus resulted from the Apple Diet: *People with high blood pressure, after a few weeks on the Apple Diet, reduced their blood pressure to normal, without any additional medication.*

Dr. Ancel Keys' research in the United States proved that it is the rich content of pectin in apples that is responsible for the lowering of blood pressure. In these experiments, 15 grams of pectin were given, which equals the amount of pectin in about two apples. (The peeling of the apple contains the greatest amount; therefore, apples should not be peeled, only thoroughly washed.)

My American students who eat apples when hungry between meals discovered the following: Apples seem to satisfy more than any other fruit. Apples are cheaper and taste better than those between-meal preparations that come in cans. Three apples a day seem to give extra-soft bulkage, which improves bowel elimination. No rigid menu planning is necessary; the usual foods are eaten. And apples between meals seem to prevent overeating at the next meal, especially if the apples are chewed well.

The weight loss is gradual—no hectic seven- or ten-day diet—but a pleasant way of eating and retraining a spoiled, overdemanding stomach with a vitamin-, mineral-, and pectin-rich fruit that is obtainable at every grocery store. Slow and pleasant weight reduction avoids the tiredness, loose skin, and wrinkling so characteristic of "crash" diets. Homemakers do not have to prepare different diets for each member of the family. The diet remains a pleasant one, with sufficient proteins, vitamins, minerals, unsaturated fats, and carbohydrates of the wholesome kind—no empty starches or sugars!

One medium apple contains:

vitamin A	120	I.U.
thiamine	.05	milligrams
riboflavin	.03	milligrams
niacin	.2	milligrams
vitamin C	6.	milligrams

Plus minerals, especially calcium, phosphorus, and iron

Eating apples when you are hungry between meals will also help to train your appetite away from sweets such as candies and colas. Most people do not realize that one candy bar has sugar value equal to that of about twelve apples. Our normal appetite control (appestat) automatically prevents us from overeating on apples; but it doesn't know how to deal with the highly concentrated sweets, because they confuse a normal appetite. Cutting out sweets and other harmful snacks, and substituting apples whenever hungry between meals, can within a few weeks help to normalize the craving for concentrated sweets.

Apple Diet as Served in Switzerland

BREAKFAST:	Large cup Swiss coffee (see page 524)
	One slice rye bread, buttered lightly
MIDMORNING:	One large juicy apple
LUNCHEON:	(The Swiss take their main meal at noon.)
	Large cup clear broth
	One veal chop
	Large helping red cabbage, cooked with apple
	One potato boiled in jacket
	Green salad with golden oil dressing
MIDAFTERNOON:	One large juicy apple

EVENING MEAL: Two hard-cooked eggs or Bircher Apple
                 Muesli (see page 411)
                 One slice rye bread, buttered lightly
                 Clear tea or Swiss coffee

BEFORE RETIRING: One large juicy apple, or glass of apple
                   milk (see page 411)

Apple Diet a l'Americain

Not too many Americans will follow such frugal fare, so here
is a bird's-eye view of the Swiss Apple Diet adapted to American
tastes:

BREAKFAST: Your favorite fruit or fresh apple juice
              (see page 411)
              Your choice of eggs, cheese, fish, or meat
              (Once a week have the Bircher Apple
              Muesli [see page 411] sprinkled with
              fresh wheat germ.)
              One slice whole-wheat, rye, soya, or
              gluten bread, buttered lightly
              (toasted, if you like)
              Large cup Swiss coffee

MIDMORNING: Good-sized juicy apple, peeling and all,
              and eat it s-l-o-w-l-y

LUNCHEON: Salad bowl (Be sure it contains a good
              helping of fish, lean meat, cheese,
              chicken, or egg, with golden oil
              dressing.)
              One slice of good bread, buttered lightly
              Clear tea or Swiss coffee

MIDAFTERNOON: One juicy apple, peeling and all, and eat
                it s-l-o-w-l-y

DINNER: Apple juice, fresh vegetable espresso,
              tomato juice spiked with lemon and
              herbs, fruit cup, or salad with golden
              oil dressing
              Good helping of lean meat, liver, fish, or
              eggs

One or two short-cooked green vege-
tables; twice a week, a Light-Hearted
Baked Potato (see page 501)
Fresh fruit or five-minute apple sauce
Demitasse or tea

BEFORE RETIRING: Another juicy apple, glass of apple milk,
or apple juice

This is how one day's menu would look:

BREAKFAST: Sliced orange or glass apple juice
Soft-cooked eggs, spiked with herbs
One slice rye, whole-wheat, or gluten
toast
Swiss coffee

MIDMORNING: One juicy apple—be sure to eat it
s-l-o-w-l-y

LUNCHEON: Large cottage cheese and apple salad,
golden oil dressing and parsley
One slice rye bread, lightly buttered
Tea or Swiss coffee

MIDAFTERNOON: One juicy apple—be sure to eat it
s-l-o-w-l-y

DINNER: Waldorf salad, golden oil dressing
Broiled lean meat, liver, or fish
Short-cooked spinach
Light-Hearted Baked Potato
Fresh berries or melon
Demitasse or tea

BEFORE RETIRING: One juicy apple, apple milk, or apple
juice

Use Different Kinds of Apples

For variety's sake, try different kinds of apples. It would be ideal
if you could get the fresh, home-grown variety, but not many of us
are so lucky. The best-tasting apples, and richest in vitamin C,
are: Pippin, Northern Spy, Yellow Newton, Baldwin, Golden De-

licious, and Winesap. These can be stored in a cool, dry place without refrigeration. (The Swiss keep them all winter long in their attics.) Ease of storage is a special advantage for those who spend their days in an office.

Swiss Apple Milk

Cut one medium-sized apple into one cup of skim milk. Add one teaspoon of honey, and mix in blender until smooth.

Bircher Apple Muesli

For thirty years this simple apple dish has been the mainstay at the Bircher-Benner Sanatorium in Zurich, Switzerland. They serve it for breakfast and dinner. When prepared correctly, the Muesli is creamy and delicious. Simply soak overnight one level table-spoon of whole cereal (at the sanatorium they use oatmeal) in two tablespoons of water. Next morning, add the juice of half a lemon, one tablespoon of condensed milk, and mix. Quickly shred one large unpeeled apple into the mixture, and stir in a table-spoon each of honey and fresh wheat germ. Serve at once. To in-crease the protein content you may also add a tablespoon of chopped walnuts, almonds, or sunflower seeds. Thousands of thrifty Swiss are thriving on this simple and nutritious dish.

Fresh Apple Juice

Many people have never tasted this delightful nectar made from fresh ripe apples. Now that Dr. Ancel Keys has reported his amaz-ing results with pectin in apples (normalizing high blood pressure), no doubt many people will eat and drink more juicy ripe apples. When eaten slowly, apples give bulk and fill up an overdemanding stomach. Fresh apple juice, with its vitamins, minerals, and pectin, gives a natural lift when taken between meals, and curbs an unruly appetite when taken twenty minutes *before* meals, due to its natu-ral sugar content. Since most of the pectin is in the peeling of the apple, when making juice you simply cut the fruit into quarters—peeling, seeds, and all—and put through your rustproof vegetable juice espressor. Drink this foamy white juice immediately; or add a few drops of lemon juice to prevent apple juice from turning dark, refrigerate, and serve chilled.

Tip to the apple growers of America: Millions prefer the milder acid of apple juice to citrus juices. Why not serve it in every bar and corner drugstore? The benefits would be tremendous.

Fresh Raw Apple Sauce

Shred unpeeled juicy red or yellow apples on medium shredder. To prevent turning dark, sprinkle with lemon juice. Sweeten with honey, if you wish. Serve at once in sherbet glasses.

Five-Minute Apple Dessert

Shred apples as above; sprinkle with lemon juice. Heat half butter and half golden oil in heavy skillet, to prevent burning. Mix apple shreds with butter and oil and heat. When thoroughly hot, flavor with honey and a tablespoon of toasted sesame seed. Serve hot. A good substitute for apple pie.

THE JAPANESE WAY TO HEALTH AND LONGEVITY

In Japan, where food is scarce, the people usually eat only two meals a day. Compared with American standards, their meals are frugal. Fish and soybean products are their main sources of protein, for milk, eggs, and meat are expensive. There are many fresh vegetables; these are always undercooked, in vegetable oil, and they are used to stretch their small amounts of meat, as in their beloved sukiyaki.

More than any other people, the Japanese cultivate sea farming—not only for all kinds of fish, but also for sea vegetables and sea greens of all kinds. In a Japanese market you may find a dozen varieties of sea kelp, sea lettuce, sea bulbs, and sea herbs. These are eaten daily, fresh or dried. A typical Japanese breakfast consists of a bowl of brown rice, a piece of *tofu* (a cheese made from soybeans and dried sea greens), and a cup of tea.

It is well known that all food coming from the oceans is rich in minerals, especially iodine, plus the many trace elements. But Japanese scientists claim that certain seaweeds are the best source of vitamin K, the vitamin discovered by the Danish chemist Dam.

Dr. Shichiro Goto, M.D., Professor at Kyushu University, has written a booklet explaining the virtues of seaweeds, stressing their high content of vitamin K. Dr. Goto, after reading my book *Look Younger, Live Longer*, sent me his book, *A Way to Health and Longevity*. He quotes many Japanese scientists who stress the importance of undereating, rather than overeating, as a means of staying slim and young. In the Mishi Health Program, which is so very popular in Japan today, the scientist Kondo, at the University of Tohoku, insists that the diet of long-lived individuals consists of large quantities of seaweeds and vegetables that are rich in vitamin K. According to these investigators, vitamin K has many functions in human nutrition. Goto claims that vitamin K regulates the functions of the liver, adrenals, and reticuloendothelial system, and has potent detoxifying and antihistamin action. They even claim that a lack of vitamin K is one of the underlying causes of heart and kidney disorders. Goto also points out that the rich supply of fish and seaweeds eaten by the fishermen and -women who cultivate the sea farms and dive for their living, is responsible for their superior strength and long life.

I hope that scientists of the Western world will investigate and verify some of the claims Japanese scientists are making for foods coming from the oceans. Is it the iodine or is it vitamin K that makes the Japanese so active and slim? These and many other questions need to be answered by our biologists. From the many case reports Dr. Goto so kindly sent me, let me give you just one.

A man of forty years—overweight, high blood pressure, and almost white hair—as a last resort studied various dietary programs and came to the conclusion that he should add seaweeds to his diet. For over twenty years he has taken seaweeds daily with his meals. Today, according to Dr. Goto, his weight and blood pressure are ideal. He does not have a single white hair, and he looks ten years younger than his age. For my American and European students who may be interested, here are the nine vital points in Dr. Goto's Japanese-type rejuvenation and road to long life:

1. Have regular habits, avoiding mental and physical overwork.
2. Stop drinking and smoking.
3. Avoid physical and mental work under direct sunlight or in high temperature. (Overheating is definitely aging.)
4. Ventilate your living and work areas, and cool them as much as possible without discomfort. Clothes and bedclothes should be light.

5. Do not take over-hot baths. It is better to take baths of low temperature, even cold, especially in summer. If possible, take a rubdown with a *cold* wet towel every morning.

6. Do not eat to excess. (Taking meals only twice a day is of significance.) Follow a diet rich in vitamin K, especially seaweeds and green leafy vegetables. If sufficient fish is eaten, eggs and milk are not especially needed. It is better to take meats in small quantities, and *no* animal fat. When large quantities of meat are eaten, large quantities of leafy vegetables should be taken at the same time in order to neutralize the acidity caused by meats.

7. Drink fresh water on an empty stomach, especially in the morning, instead of boiled water (as in coffee or tea).

8. Regulate bowel movements.

9. Vitamin K, taken daily in small doses by mouth, is recommended to prevent disorder to cardiac function due to physiological decrease of vitamin K in older people.

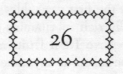

26

My Seven-Day Elimination Diet

I created this, which is probably my best-known diet, in 1922, when I started my first food clinic in Chicago. This was one of the most interesting periods in my long career. People came to me from all over the country—rich and poor, fat and thin, young and old. They were sick. They had "been everywhere, tried everything." Now they came to me as a last resort. Many were skeptical about trying "food science," as I then called it. I had to work fast to convince them, do something basic to help all these overfed and undernourished people—overfed with foodless starches and sugars, undernourished in proteins, vitamins, and minerals.

Like all overfed and undernourished people, they were burdened with excess fat, while the tissues and fluids of their bodies, in varying degrees, were starved of vitamins and minerals.

My Seven-Day Elimination Diet is a seven-day housecleaning, a putting of one's house in order. It restores to the tissues and fluids of the body much-needed vitamins and minerals, and affords an opportunity for the body to eliminate accumulated waste products.

What it does is to give the "inner man" a much-needed rest from past dietetic mistakes, and give Nature a perfect opportunity to exert her marvelous capacity to reinforce the body.

You can go on this Seven-Day Elimination Diet (actually it is a feast) whenever you feel the need for a thorough cleansing.

Springtime is ideal, for the first vegetables and fruits coming from the garden are especially rich in vitamins and minerals. But here in America, where we have fresh fruits and vegetables the year around, the diet can be taken at any time of the year. I, myself, and thousands of my students, go on the Seven-Day Elimination Diet twice a year: before Easter and again in the fall. I am convinced that such periodic cleansings and removal of body wastes can prevent much suffering and premature aging.

Here, then, are the foods which you can eat to your heart's content for seven days and at the same time give your body a Seven-Day Housecleaning:

Bird's-Eye View of the Seven-Day Elimination Diet

BREAKFAST: Upon arising, after cleansing your mouth, drink a large glass of fruit juice, preferably fresh orange, grapefruit, pineapple, or apple juice. In addition to the fruit juice, you have one or two cups of fragrant herb tea such as peppermint, strawberry, or papaya. These can be flavored with a bit of honey and a slice of lemon. It is best to do without coffee. However, if you simply cannot get along without it, have one cup of fresh coffee and drink it clear. Should the fruit juice and a hot beverage not satisfy you, you might add some fresh or stewed fruit sweetened with a little honey.

MIDMORNING: If you want something more substantial, have a cup of yogurt, plain or flavored. You could also have a finger salad consisting of celery sticks, carrot sticks, slices of green pepper, or bits of cauliflower spiked with vegetable salt. If chewing is a problem, have a glass of vegetable espresso (see page 505).

LUNCHEON: One cup of Hauser Broth (see page 425), a fresh fruit or vegetable salad, a dish of yogurt, hot tea with lemon.

MIDAFTERNOON: A glass of your favorite fruit or vegetable juice, fresh if possible. If something hot is wanted, one cup of peppermint tea with lemon and honey.

DINNER: A cup of broth, one short-cooked vegetable, a fresh green salad, a cup of herb tea or demitasse.

BEDTIME: Take a 20-minute warm relaxing bath. If bowels have not been moving freely, take some mild herbal laxative. If hungry, have some fresh fruit, fruit juice, or fat-free yogurt.

You can make up your own menus from the lists of fruits and vegetables that follow, or you can follow the day-by-day plan given further on. *The pint of yogurt which I have added to the daily menu is of great help, but do not use more than a pint if you are overweight, and be sure to use skim milk.*

Here Are the Fruits to Choose from

1st Choice: Oranges, grapefruit, pineapple (whole or in juice form), lemon and lime juices in water.

2nd Choice: Apples, peaches, grapes, pears, apricots, and all berries.

3rd Choice: All melons, also papayas, pomegranates, and persimmons. (No bananas during this week.)

Here Are the Vegetables to Choose from

1st Choice: Celery, carrots, spinach, parsley, beet tops, watercress, and okra.

2nd Choice: Celery roots, cucumbers, asparagus, green and red peppers, bean sprouts, and eggplant.

3rd Choice: Red and white cabbage, sauerkraut, cauliflower, beets, zucchini, and young peas.

Cooked vegetables can be spiked with herbs or soy sauce, not butter.

Don't let yourself get hungry. If you are working, take some fresh fruit, or some celery and carrots, to the office so that you will have something to eat during the morning and afternoon.

And Here Are Your Menus

First Day

BREAKFAST: Large glass orange juice or grapefruit juice
Hot beverage: your choice of: peppermint, papaya, or strawberry tea with a bit of honey. Clear coffee, if you must.
If still hungry, you may add some fruit

such as melon, berries, peaches, or apples; pears, fresh or baked.

MIDMORNING: Your choice of any *one* of the following:

Fresh fruit in season or fruit juice (no bananas)

Raw vegetables in season or vegetable juice

Tomato and sauerkraut juice (equal amounts mixed—an excellent reducing cocktail)

Yogurt (not more than a pint a day)

If you prefer something hot, your choice of: hot Hauser Broth, hot tomato juice, hot herb tea (peppermint, papaya, strawberry), weak tea with lemon—sweetened only with a bit of honey or brown sugar. Clear coffee, if you must.

LUNCHTIME: Hot Hauser Broth or tomato juice

Yogurt—one cup

Salad: cucumber, lettuce, green pepper (or your own combination), with yogurt dressing

Choice of hot beverage as above

MIDAFTERNOON: Same as midmorning

DINNERTIME: Hot Hauser Broth

Spinach, or other greens, steamed with thin slices of onion

Yogurt

Baked apple

Choice of hot beverage as above

BEDTIME: Same as midmorning

Check up on your elimination. Take a simple herbal laxative when needed.

Second Day

BREAKFAST: Large glass orange or grapefruit juice

Hot beverage: your choice of: pepper-

mint, papaya, or strawberry tea with a
bit of honey. Clear coffee, if you must.

If still hungry, you may add some fruit
such as melon, berries, peaches, or apples; pears, fresh or baked.

MIDMORNING:
Your choice of any *one* of the following:

Fresh fruit in season (no bananas) or fruit
juice

Raw vegetables in season or vegetable
espresso

Tomato and sauerkraut juice (equal
amounts mixed—an excellent reducing
cocktail)

Yogurt (not more than a pint a day)

If you prefer something hot, your choice
of: one or two cups hot Hauser Broth,
hot tomato juice, hot herb tea (peppermint, papaya, strawberry), weak tea
with lemon—sweetened only with a bit
of honey or brown sugar. Clear coffee,
if you must.

LUNCHTIME:
Hot Hauser Broth or tomato juice
Yogurt—one cup
Salad: pineapple, carrot, and raisins
Choice of hot beverage as above

MIDAFTERNOON: Same as midmorning

DINNERTIME:
Hot Hauser Broth
Steamed cauliflower
Salad: celery hearts and strips of green
peppers
Yogurt
Fresh or broiled grapefruit
Choice of hot beverage as above

BEDTIME: Same as midmorning.

Check up on your elimination. Take a simple herbal laxative when
needed.

Third Day

BREAKFAST: Large glass orange or grapefruit juice

Hot beverage: your choice of: peppermint, papaya, or strawberry tea with a bit of honey. Clear coffee, if you must.

If still hungry, you may add some fruit, such as melon, berries, peaches, or apples; pears, fresh or baked.

MIDMORNING: Your choice of any *one* of the following:

Fresh fruit in season (no bananas) or fruit juice

Raw vegetables in season or vegetable espresso

Tomato and sauerkraut juice (equal amounts mixed—an excellent reducing cocktail)

Yogurt (not more than a pint a day)

If you prefer something hot, your choice of: one or two cups hot Hauser Broth, hot tomato juice, hot herb tea (peppermint, papaya, strawberry), weak tea with lemon—sweetened only with a bit of honey or brown sugar. Clear coffee, if you must.

LUNCHTIME: Hot Hauser Broth or tomato juice

Salad: cabbage and pineapple with yogurt dressing

Yogurt

Choice of hot beverage as above

MIDAFTERNOON: Same as midmorning

DINNERTIME: Hot Hauser Broth

Broiled eggplant (inch-thick slices) or summer squash

Salad: sliced cucumbers

Yogurt

Fresh or stewed fruit

Choice of hot beverage as above

BEDTIME: Same as midmorning

Check up on your elimination. Take a simple herbal laxative when
needed.

Fourth Day

BREAKFAST: Large glass orange or grapefruit juice
                        Hot beverage: your choice of: pepper-
                            mint, papaya, or strawberry tea with a
                            bit of honey. Clear coffee, if you must.
                        If still hungry, you may add some fruit
                            such as melon, berries, peaches, or ap-
                            ples; pears, fresh or baked

MIDMORNING: Your choice of any *one* of the following:
                        Fresh fruit in season (no bananas) or
                            fruit juice
                        Raw vegetables in season or vegetable
                            espresso
                        Tomato and sauerkraut juice (equal
                            amounts mixed—an excellent reducing
                            cocktail)
                        Yogurt (not more than a pint a day)
                        If you prefer something hot, your choice
                            of: one or two cups of hot Hauser Broth,
                            hot tomato juice, hot herb tea (pepper-
                            mint, papaya, strawberry), weak tea
                            with lemon—sweetened only with a bit
                            of honey or brown sugar. Clear coffee,
                            if you must.

LUNCHTIME: Hot Hauser Broth or tomato juice
                        Salad: apple, celery, and orange, diced
                        Yogurt
                        Choice of hot beverage as above

MIDAFTERNOON: Same as midmorning

DINNERTIME: Hot Hauser Broth
                        Stewed tomatoes

Finger salad: celery and carrot sticks and
green onions
Yogurt
Berries or fruit in season
Choice of hot beverage as above

BEDTIME: Same as midmorning

Check up on your elimination. Take a simple herbal laxative when
needed.

Fifth Day

BREAKFAST: Large glass orange or grapefruit juice
Hot beverage: your choice of: pepper-
mint, papaya, or strawberry tea, with
a bit of honey. Clear coffee, if you must.
If still hungry, you may add some fresh
fruit such as melon, berries, peaches, or
apples; pears, fresh or baked.

MIDMORNING: Your choice of any *one* of the following:
Fresh fruit in season or fruit juice (no
bananas)
Raw vegetables in season or vegetable
espresso
Tomato and sauerkraut juice (equal
amounts mixed—an excellent reducing
cocktail)
Yogurt (not more than a pint a day)
If you prefer something hot, your choice
of: one or two cups hot Hauser Broth,
hot tomato juice, hot herb tea (peppermint, papaya, strawberry), weak tea
with lemon—sweetened only with a bit
of honey or brown sugar. Clear coffee,
if you must.

LUNCHTIME: Hot Hauser Broth or tomato juice
Yogurt
Fruit salad
Choice of hot beverage as above

MIDAFTERNOON: Same as midmorning

DINNERTIME: Hot Hauser Broth
                Vegetable Chop Suey (equal amounts of
                    diced celery, onions, and bean sprouts,
                    when available, spiked with soy sauce)
                Salad: sliced tomatoes
                Yogurt
                Peaches or fruit in season
                Choice of hot beverage as above

BEDTIME: Same as midmorning

Check up on your elimination. Take a simple herbal laxative when
needed.

Sixth Day

BREAKFAST: Large glass orange or grapefruit juice
                Hot beverage: your choice of: pepper-
                    mint, papaya, or strawberry tea with
                    a bit of honey. Clear coffee, if you must.
                If still hungry, you may add some fruit
                    such as melon, berries, peaches, or ap-
                    ples; pears, fresh or baked.

MIDMORNING: Your choice of any *one* of the following:
                Fresh fruit in season or fruit juice (no
                    bananas)
                Raw vegetables in season or vegetable
                    espresso
                Tomato and sauerkraut juice (equal
                    amounts mixed—an excellent reducing
                    cocktail)
                Yogurt (not more than a pint a day)
                If you prefer something hot, your choice
                    of: one or two cups hot Hauser Broth,
                    hot tomato juice, hot herb tea (pepper-
                    mint, papaya, strawberry), weak tea
                    with lemon—sweetened only with
                    honey or brown sugar. Clear coffee, if
                    you must.

LUNCHTIME: Hot Hauser Broth or tomato juice

Yogurt

Finger salad: cauliflower buds, green onions, carrot and celery sticks, and other
raw vegetables in season

Choice of hot beverage as above

MIDAFTERNOON: Same as midmorning

DINNERTIME: Hot Hauser Broth

Stew of tomatoes, onions, and green peppers—okra, if available

Salad: chopped pineapple, carrot, and
cabbage

Yogurt

Fresh pears or fruit in season

Choice of hot beverage as above

BEDTIME: Same as midmorning

Check up on your elimination. Take a simple herbal laxative when
needed.

Seventh Day

BREAKFAST: Large glass orange or grapefruit juice

Hot beverage: your choice of: peppermint, papaya, or strawberry tea with a
bit of honey. Clear coffee, if you must.

If still hungry, you may add some fresh
fruit such as melon, berries, peaches, or
apples; pears, fresh or baked.

MIDMORNING: Your choice of any *one* of the following:

Fresh fruit in season or fruit juice (no
bananas)

Raw vegetables in season or vegetable
espresso

Tomato and sauerkraut juice (equal
amounts mixed—an excellent reducing
cocktail)

Yogurt (not more than a pint a day)

> If you prefer something hot, your choice of: one or two cups hot Hauser Broth, hot tomato juice, hot herb tea (peppermint, papaya, strawberry), weak tea with lemon—sweetened only with honey or brown sugar. Clear coffee, if you must.

LUNCHTIME: Hot Hauser Broth or tomato juice
Yogurt
Salad: raw sauerkraut with lemon juice
Choice of hot beverage as above

MIDAFTERNOON: Same as midmorning

DINNERTIME: Hot Hauser Broth
Cooked young green peas
Salad: chopped celery hearts, watercress, and orange
Yogurt
Sliced pineapple or fruit in season
Choice of hot beverage as above

BEDTIME: Same as midmorning

Check up on your elimination. Take a simple herbal laxative when needed.

Hauser Broth

> 1 cup finely shredded celery, leaves and all
> 1 cup finely shredded carrots
> ½ cup shredded spinach
> 1 tablespoon shredded parsley
> 1 teaspoon vegetable salt
> 1 quart water
> 1 cup tomato juice
> Brown sugar or honey

Put all shredded vegetables into the quart of water, cover and cook slowly for about 25 minutes; then add tomato juice, a teaspoon vegetable salt, and a pinch of brown sugar or honey. Let cook for a few more minutes. Strain and serve.

Should you be hungry as a bear and *not* overweight, you may eat the broth unstrained. Added vegetable juices give variety and flavor to the broth. If you are unable to buy them and do not possess a juicer, you may add any of your favorite vegetables or herbs. Some days add a bit of onion (fresh or dried flakes), green peppers, beet tops, chives, etc. This broth has been a "comfort to thousands" as Billie Burke once wrote. It has been used by many beautyfarms. If you are unable to prepare this broth, you can use any prepared dry vegetable broth and heat it to simmering point in tomato juice. Or you can buy canned mixed vegetable juice, spike it with vegetable salt, and heat, but do not boil.

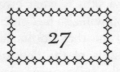

27

How to Gain Weight

If you are slightly underweight, thank your lucky stars and stay that way. But if you are *too* thin, do something about it. Obviously you are not eating the right kind of food. Perhaps, also, you are too tense and carry the burdens of the world on your shoulders.

It is important that the diet eaten by thin people be rich in all body-building elements, especially the vitamins of the B family and the easily digested fatty acids found in the golden vegetable oils. If you are painfully thin and have not been able to gain in the past, by all means learn to "let go"—to relax completely. Your diet may be deficient in calcium and vitamin D. If so, calcium foods and vitamin D, in the form of fortified milk drinks, yogurt, and cheese, should be increased in the daily diet. If you are very deficient in calcium, add calcium and vitamin D concentrate to your daily meals. Sun baths are especially helpful to thin people not only because of their soothing and relaxing effect upon the whole body, but also because direct sunshine delivers vitamin D to the body. (But do not overdo.)

While gaining weight and health, use only those foods that are easily digested and absorbed by the body. Do not stuff yourself with so-called fattening foods, but eat smaller meals and *more often*. The midmorning, midafternoon, and before-retiring refreshments are very helpful. After you have gained all the necessary pounds, you will find that you not only look much better (the thin padding of fat directly under the skin is what gives those pleasant curves to face and body) but you will also *feel* much better.

Most thin people tell me they do not like fats; but when I tell them to use extra amounts of the delicious and easily digestible golden oils, they usually follow my advice—and with excellent results.

A delicious weight-gaining salad dressing with peanut oil will help you to put on healthy pounds and curves. Mix two parts of peanut oil with one part of lemon juice or cider vinegar. Add a little honey, vegetable salt, garlic, or any herb of your choice. Pour this over salad greens. Sprinkle with a spoonful of wheat germ and mix.

To help underweight people get more benefit from their meals, hot broth (rather than a cold appetizer) is given at the *beginning* of the meal, and hot peppermint tea is given at the *end* of the meal. The heat seems to help relax nervous and sensitive stomachs and thus promotes digestion.

Then there are those wonderfully nutritious nut milks. All nuts, especially almonds, pecans, and walnuts, are good building foods. However, most people do not chew them sufficiently, so much of their food value is lost. Fortunately, a gadget has been invented that whips nuts into a milklike consistency. You simply put one glass of your favorite fruit juice (fresh or frozen) into the electric gadget. To this you add a handful of nut meats, a teaspoonful of honey, and mix. In exactly half a minute, you will have a delicious beverage, with the nuts finely Fletcherized and easily assimilated.

Last but not least, very ripe bananas are the best of all weight-builders for thin people. They should be used when the skin is almost black. Simply whip a very ripe banana and a teaspoonful of honey or molasses into a glass of hot or cold milk.

I highly recommend a glass of this banana milk to all the skinnies who really want to gain weight. Drink it right with your meals. It seems that the potent enzymes in very ripe bananas aid the digestion and help to get more good from all the other foods eaten at that meal.

And Here Are Some Weight-Gaining Menus to Guide You:

MONDAY

BREAKFAST:
Large glass of pineapple juice
One or 2 eggs, any way but fried
Two slices of 100% whole-wheat bread with butter and honey
One glass of vitamin D banana milk
If desired, *café au lait* with honey

MIDMORNING:
Your choice of: large glass of fortified milk, carrot juice, or yogurt mixed with teaspoon of brewers' yeast, molasses, and honey

LUNCH:
Cup of hot broth
Finely chopped carrot and raisin salad with lots of golden oil dressing
One whole-wheat or corn muffin with honey and butter
Cup of yogurt, flavored with honey or jam, if you like
Hot peppermint tea or New Orleans cup

MIDAFTERNOON:
Same as midmorning, or glass of banana milk, or Curvaceous cocktail

DINNER:
Finely chopped vegetable salad with yogurt dressing
Lamb roast
Green peas
Parsley potatoes
Sliced bananas with coconut and honey
Peppermint tea or demitasse

BEDTIME:
For deeper sleep and relaxation, your choice of: hot banana milk or glass of yogurt with teaspoon of brewers' yeast. This is also a good time to take your calcium–vitamin D concentrate and other vitamins.

TUESDAY

BREAKFAST: Large glass of orange juice
               Cooked whole-wheat cereal with honey, sprinkled with wheat germ
               Whole-wheat muffin with butter and honey
               One glass of vitamin D banana milk
               If desired, *café au lait* with honey

MIDMORNING: Your choice of: large glass of fortified milk, carrot juice, or yogurt mixed with teaspoon of brewers' yeast and honey

LUNCH: Cup of hot broth
               Tomatoes stuffed with cottage cheese
               Wheat-germ muffin with butter and honey
               Cup of yogurt, flavored with honey or jam, if you like
               Hot peppermint tea or New Orleans cup

MIDAFTERNOON: Same as midmorning, or glass of banana milk, nut milk, or Curvaceous cocktail

DINNER: Fruit cup or hot broth
               Broiled liver and bacon
               Potatoes boiled in jackets
               Creamed spinach
               Head lettuce with golden oil dressing
               Baked apple with cream
               Peppermint tea or demitasse

BEDTIME: For deeper sleep and relaxation, your choice of: hot banana milk or glass of yogurt with teaspoon of brewers' yeast. This is also a good time to take your calcium–vitamin D concentrate and other vitamins.

WEDNESDAY

BREAKFAST: Large glass of apple juice
               Four slices of crisp bacon, lean

Two slices 100% whole-wheat bread with butter and honey
Glass of vitamin D banana milk
If desired, *café au lait*

MIDMORNING: Your choice of: large glass of fortified milk, carrot juice, or yogurt mixed with teaspoon of brewers' yeast and honey

LUNCH: Cup of hot broth
Creamed chicken on whole-wheat toast
Fruit salad sprinkled with nuts
Cup of yogurt, flavored with honey or jam, if you like
Hot peppermint tea or New Orleans cup

MIDAFTERNOON: Same as midmorning, or glass of banana milk, nut milk, or Curvaceous cocktail

DINNER: Hot broth or chopped mixed green salad
Broiled tender steak
New potatoes with parsley
Cauliflower sprinkled with American cheese
Fresh fruit with honey
Peppermint tea or demitasse

BEDTIME: For deeper sleep and relaxation, your choice of: hot banana milk or glass of yogurt with teaspoon of brewers' yeast. This is also a good time to take your calcium–vitamin D concentrate and other vitamins.

THURSDAY

BREAKFAST: Large glass of orange juice
Oatmeal, Scotch style, with honey and milk
Whole-wheat muffin with butter and honey
Glass of vitamin D banana milk
If desired, *café au lait*

MIDMORNING: Your choice of: large glass of fortified milk, carrot juice, or yogurt mixed with teaspoon of brewers' yeast and honey

LUNCH: Cup of hot broth
                   Avocado and orange salad with golden oil dressing
                   Corn bread
                   Cup of yogurt, flavored with honey or jam, if you like
                   Hot peppermint tea or New Orleans cup

MIDAFTERNOON: Same as midmorning, or glass of banana milk, nut milk, or Curvaceous cocktail

DINNER: Hot broth or Waldorf salad with wheat germ
                   Beef stew with potatoes and carrots
                   Turnip tops or spinach
                   Apple pie with cheese
                   Peppermint tea or demitasse

BEDTIME: For deeper sleep and relaxation, your choice of: hot banana milk or glass of yogurt with teaspoon of brewers' yeast. This is also a good time to take your calcium–vitamin D concentrate and other vitamins.

FRIDAY

BREAKFAST: Large glass of tomato juice
                   One or 2 eggs, any way but fried
                   Two slices of whole-wheat toast with butter and honey
                   One glass of vitamin D banana milk
                   If desired, *café au lait*

MIDMORNING: Your choice of: large glass of fortified milk, carrot juice, or yogurt mixed with teaspoon of brewers' yeast and honey

LUNCH: Cup of hot broth
Shrimp and celery salad with golden oil dressing
Whole-wheat muffin
Cup of yogurt, flavored with a bit of honey or jam, if you like
Hot peppermint tea or New Orleans cup

MIDAFTERNOON: Same as midmorning, or glass of banana milk, nut milk, or Curvaceous cocktail

DINNER: Hot broth or mixed green salad
Broiled fish or lobster
Parsley potatoes
Hot applesauce with cream and honey
Peppermint tea or demitasse

BEDTIME: For deeper sleep and relaxation, your choice of: hot banana milk or glass of yogurt with teaspoon of brewers' yeast. This is also a good time to take your calcium–vitamin D concentrate and other vitamins.

SATURDAY

BREAKFAST: Large glass of orange juice
Whole-wheat pancakes or waffle with honey or real maple syrup
One glass of vitamin D banana milk
If desired, *café au lait*

MIDMORNING: Your choice of: large glass of fortified milk, carrot juice, or yogurt mixed with teaspoon of brewers' yeast and honey

LUNCH: Cup of hot broth
Large fruit salad with bananas
Two slices whole-wheat cinnamon toast
One cup of yogurt, flavored with a bit of honey or jam, if you like
Hot peppermint tea or New Orleans cup

MIDAFTERNOON: Same as midmorning, or glass of banana milk, nut milk, or Curvaceous cocktail

DINNER: Hot broth, or coleslaw with yogurt dressing
Large beefburger mixed with parsley and wheat germ
Hashed-brown potatoes
Short-cooked beets
Ice cream with fruit
Peppermint tea or demitasse

BEDTIME: For deeper sleep and relaxation, your choice of: hot banana milk or glass of yogurt with teaspoon of brewers' yeast. This is also a good time to take your calcium–vitamin D concentrate and other vitamins.

SUNDAY

BREAKFAST: Large glass of pineapple juice
Cooked, mixed cereal (whole-wheat, rye, barley, millet, etc.) with milk and molasses
Muffin with butter and honey
Glass of vitamin D milk mixed with tablespoon of wheat germ
If desired, café au lait

MIDMORNING: Your choice of: large glass of fortified milk, carrot juice, or yogurt mixed with teaspoon of brewers' yeast and honey

LUNCH: Cup of hot broth
Two scrambled eggs with fresh stewed tomatoes on whole-wheat toast
Cup of yogurt, flavored with honey or jam, if you like
Hot peppermint tea or New Orleans cup

MIDAFTERNOON: Same as midmorning, or glass of banana milk, nut milk, or Curvaceous cocktail

DINNER: Hot broth or finger salad
                            Roast chicken with dressing
                            Baked potato with butter
                            Broccoli
                            Sliced bananas with honey
                            Peppermint tea or demitasse

BEDTIME: For deeper sleep and relaxation, your
                            choice of: hot banana milk or glass of
                            yogurt with teaspoon of brewers' yeast.
                            This is also a good time to take your
                            calcium—vitamin D concentrate and
                            other vitamins.

French Doctor's Weight-Gaining Secret

Extremely thin people should learn to let go, r-e-l-a-x, and get rid of their inner tensions *before* they sit down to eat. Then *after* meals they should lie down and relax another fifteen minutes. This, according to the doctor, gives the body a chance to assimilate better and get more benefit from the foods eaten.

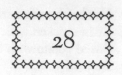

More Million Dollar Secrets

Diet and Health Secrets of the Famous

Queen Elizabeth II of England transformed herself into a glamour Queen by eating frugal, balanced meals predominating in proteins. The Queen is deeply in love with her Prince Charming, and the desire to be beautiful in his eyes made it easy to give up rich pastries.

Former President Eisenhower learned a lifetime lesson in intelligent eating from his wise physician, Dr. Paul Dudley White, who prescribed more lean proteins, less saturated fat (including his beloved bacon), and less salt. Mr. Eisenhower also increased his muscular activity, doing the exercise he likes best—playing a relaxed game of golf.

Garbo, the only one, a reformed vegetarian, now enjoys lean beef, even steak tartar, and lean lamb with dill sauce. She starts dinner with a huge salad and ends with fresh fruit. She is a champion walker (in space shoes) one hour each day, rain or shine.

Maurice Chevalier, raised on French cuisine, learned to eat lean while in Hollywood. He takes daily walks and likes to dance. While in Sicily, he enjoyed climbing the steep hills of Taormina.

Mrs. Kingman Douglass, the vivacious Adele Astaire, believes that your menus can make you or mar you. She trained her cook to prepare her favorite Southern dishes—but minus the hard fat and grease. Such delightful meals are kind not only to her waistline, but also to her guests'. Dancing has always been the favorite exercise of the Astaires; and Adele's elegant double twist, after meals, has become her favorite waistline whittler.

Cary Grant believes that seeing yourself slim in your mind's eye helps you to develop a dislike for all fattening foods. It seems to work for Cary!

Bob Hope keeps fit with a balanced protein diet prescribed by his doctor. He also does specific muscle-tensing exercises and takes sauna baths at the famous Terry Hunt gymnasium in Hollywood. When Bob is asked about his secret for staying young, he says: "I lie about my age."

Jessica Dragonette keeps her vest-pocket Venus figure by singing and dancing; and she drinks cool glasses of vegetable juices before meals and fresh orange juice with orange-blossom honey for quick energy before concerts and lectures.

Ann Delafield, the ageless beauty who directed Elizabeth Arden's beautyfarm, believes that a high-protein diet, plus two half-hour relaxing periods on the Yoga Slant board, keep the neck and face firm without surgery.

Ruth Dubonnet, internationally beloved hostess, helps to keep her guests' waistlines down by serving her famous Dubonnet-on-the-rocks before meals. Her famous Zen dinner parties are the talk of New York. Her cook spikes many dishes with a delightful mixture of vegetable salt and toasted sesame seeds.

Roger Dann, the handsome leading man of the London cast of *Sound of Music,* says that two tablets of sea greens, taken before his protein dinner, keep his waistline a firm twenty-eight inches.

Mary Garden, the unforgettable prima donna, now living in her beloved Scotland, believes that her lean Scottish meals, plus her nightcap of two drops of organic iodine in a glass of warm milk, is the secret of keeping her size-ten figure for decades.

Frances Carpenter's 18-inch waistline is the envy of the whole Du Pont dynasty. Whether in her home in Delaware or in Southampton, or on her yacht, you can be sure of superb protein meals. Caviar, wild game, and salads, lovingly tossed, are favorites. No gooey desserts are ever served in the Carpenter home, and all meals end with fresh fruit or honey compotes.

Lydia Lane, through her syndicated column, helps millions of women to achieve their heart's desire. She believes that beauty is an inside-outside job and writes with enthusiasm about beauty-full eating and scientific body care. In her forthcoming book she expresses what I so thoroughly believe: "A woman's beauty is not imprisoned by her skin; it permeates her entire home, creating warmth, love, and harmony . . ."

Julia Meade, one of our loveliest television personalities, is a protein-breakfast enthusiast. She always starts her day with a glass of unsweetened fruit juice, and she boosts her vitality during the day and before performances with protein snacks. She loves yogurt and Hi-Vi tomato juice.

Anita Loos, famous author of *Gentlemen Prefer Blondes,* still has her tiny 90-pound figure. Her favorite foods are broiled meats, especially calves' liver, plus huge salad bowls with golden olive oil dressings, spiked with fresh garden herbs.

Mae West, the endurable one, does not smoke or drink; she keeps her body beautifully fit. Her secret? Daily exercise. Says Sexy Mae, "My father was a muscle man, and I learned it from him."

Princess Grace of Monaco enjoyed her mother's delightful German cuisine until she came to Hollywood, where she learned to diet to keep her beautiful contours. Now, Her Grace eats a nourishing breakfast, a light luncheon, and a well-balanced dinner with lean meat. To banish between-meal hunger, there is always French yogurt in the palace refrigerator, as well as unlimited amounts of fresh raw vegetables and fruits.

Paulette Goddard is a high-protein enthusiast. She not only insists on lean broiled meats, but also has taught her cook in Porto Ronco to make protein bread and soy muffins. Her favorite sport, waterskiing on Lake Garda, also provides an outlet for her tremendous verve and vitality.

Princess Marusia Toumanoff has her favorite Russian dishes prepared in the modern manner. Kasha is simmered in lean chicken broth; borscht and beef Stroganoff are made creamy with fresh yogurt. Toumanoff parties are the talk of the town. Besides enjoying gourmet food beautifully served, you can also count on a feast for the eyes. You meet the loveliest stars, handsomely dressed and bejeweled in Marusia gowns (Princess Toumanoff's profession is creating exquisite gowns).

Cobina Wright, socialite and Hollywood columnist, while in Rome said: "I've never had a reducing problem. All my life I've been too active to let fat accumulate. I'm a great believer in action."

Adelle Davis, author of *Let's Cook It Right,* says: "Fats are more satisfying than any other foods. If you forego eating 100 calories of fat per meal, you usually become so hungry that you eat 500 calories of starches and sugars, simply because you cannot resist them."

Mahatma Gandhi, when asked how he remained so slim all his life, said: "I only eat innocent foods, goat's milk and fruit."

Albert Schweitzer eats frugally at all times, and only on special occasions does he permit himself a glass of his native Alsace wine. When asked about the secret of his long and exemplary life, he said: "Every human being, whatever his place, can find full achievement to the very end of his life. He must always do the best he can, take care of his health, live and eat simply, never stop working, and give the greatest part of his time to others."

What Famous Doctors Discovered About Improved Nutrition

Dr. F. K. Menshikov, Russia's No. 1 nutritionist to its more than 200 million people, agrees that no seriously restricted diet can give permanent results. He also definitely recommends vegetable oils in place of animal fats. Based on experiments carried on over four years, the following report was made: In the Baltic region, where people are used to eating chiefly animal fats (including butter when available), among 100,000 people, 3 percent were stricken with heart attacks; but in Stalinbad, a poorer district where only vegetable oils are used for eating and cooking, only 1 percent had heart attacks. Dr. Menshikov also says that physical exercise definitely helps the heart. The Russian people are told: "Every time you move your muscles, you help your heart."

Dr. L. M. Morrison, M.D., author of *The Low Fat Diet* discovered that soya-lecithin is very effective in reducing blood serum cholesterol. He also discovered that adding brewers' yeast and wheat germ to the daily diet was helpful in the prevention of heart trouble.

Dr. Fred R. Klenner, M.D., writing in the *Tri-State Medical Journal,* feels that susceptibility to polio is definitely increased when there is a decrease in vitamin C; and that rapid recovery from polio may be possible with an intake of 250 to 400 milligrams of vitamin C around the clock.

Dr. O. W. Portman, Harvard School of Public Health, investigated the relationship between cholesterol and diets high in refined sugar; he discovered that diets high in refined sugar definitely increase blood cholesterol levels!

Dr. Thomas Cureton of the University of Illinois says: "One of the greatest needs for the average American, in addition to food, is *exercise*. . . . By taking mild exercise (and 1½ teaspoons of wheat germ oil daily) middle-aged men may reverse their age characteristics from ten to fifteen years."

Dr. Charles Best, discoverer of insulin, says he never diets; he eats balanced meals, with a little less of everything.

Dr. O. K. Alieva, head of the USSR Institute of Nutrition, tested four different fats on a hundred patients who had atherosclerosis and who had suffered from heart attacks. Patients were divided into four groups according to the fat consumed in their daily diets. The fats tested included sunflower oil (most popular in Russia), cottonseed oil, corn oil, and butter. The men and women eating straight butter had the least favorable results. Some improvement was reported by those eating cottonseed oil; those eating sunflower oil had still better results; but the best results were reported by those using cold-pressed corn oil exclusively.

Dr. Charlotte West, M.D., in her book, *Ageless Youth*, says: "Constipation is probably so little heeded because it rarely gives rise to actual pain. It does give rise to a vast amount of health and beauty defects. Who can be attractive with an offensive breath, a muddy skin, dull eyes, a listless manner and dullness of mind?"

Dr. Paul Dudley White, famous heart specialist, says: "Physical activity is just as necessary to life as food, air and water. People live by activity. It helps to keep your muscles in tone . . . it aids respiration, digestion, blood circulation and the elimination of body wastes. It is a law of nature that your organs as well as muscles grow stronger with use, weaker with disuse."

Dr. Michael M. Miller, at St. Elizabeth Hospital in Washington, D.C., reduced the amount of salt in the diet of some of his patients. Within just one week, these patients were able to fall asleep within 15 minutes after retiring—and most were able to sleep all night without waking up.

Dr. Paul C. Aebersold of the Atomic Energy Commission, doing research with radioactive isotopes, presented the world with the happy news that the body renews itself constantly. Dr. Aebersold could prove that 98 percent of the cells of the body are replaced each year (not every seven years!) through the air, food, and liquids we take into our bodies.

Dr. M. K. Horwitt, associate professor at the University of Illinois College of Medicine, presented evidence at a conference in Switzerland that an increased amount of polyunsaturated fats calls for increased amounts of vitamin E.

Dr. Laurance W. Kinsell, Director of the Institute for Metabolic Research in Oakland, announced, "We feel the evidence is sufficiently strong to advise people to use a low-fat diet and take vegetable oils . . . oils like safflower, corn, and cottonseed tend to dissolve cholesterol spots and lower the cholesterol level in the blood." Dr. Kinsell believes the cholesterol count should be maintained below 180. He also predicts that soon we will be able to get the important linoleic acid in our breakfast eggs; when chickens are given safflower oil, the linoleic acid in their eggs is increased up to 30 percent.

Dr. W. J. McCormick, M.D., in the *Archives of Pediatrics,* says he has reason to believe that a lack of vitamin C is the basis for the change in the connective tissue underlying the skin and mucous membranes which predisposes to cancer. A number of other scientists support Dr. McCormick's theory.

Dr. A. S. Church, in the New York State *Journal of Medicine,* states that there were serious evidences of malnutrition in over 80 percent of the 750 boys tested in a correctional institution; they were living on the worst possible diet of canned and processed meats, white bread, white sugar, jam, and soft drinks. When the diet of these delinquents was changed to include fresh fruits, fresh vegetables, nuts, salads, fish, cheese, and honey instead of sugar, these youngsters quickly became less aggressive and less quarrelsome. Their bad habits gradually disappeared. The most significant part of the experiments was that the difference in their *behavior* was amazing.

Dr. G. Lehmann, of the Max Planck Institute in Dortmund, Germany, discovered a million dollar secret for those who tire easily. Instead of relaxing for half an hour at the end of the day, Dr. Lehmann suggests six short relaxation pauses of five minutes each. This prevents exhaustion at the end of the day.

Dr. Royal Lee, D.D.S., of Milwaukee, Wisconsin, says that chalky teeth, as a rule, can be converted into normal teeth by the use of calcium lactate and vitamin F.

Dr. Melvin E. Page, D.D.S., says it is well known in the medical and dental professions that sugar is not essential in the diet as an energy food. The general public suffers from this misconception due to misleading advertisements.

Dr. W. Coda Martin, M.D., reports: "It is now believed that the greater number of hepatitis cases is caused by DDT spraying of green vegetables."

Dr. Anton J. Carlson, a professor at the University of Chicago, used to say: "On the whole, we can trust nature further than the chemist and his synthetics."

REDUCING SECRETS FROM ALL OVER THE WORLD

A wise husband can greatly help his wife to reduce by buying her an expensive and beautiful dress in the size she was when he fell in love with her. Results are magic for two reasons: the beauty of the dress and the fact that he *cares!*

A craving for rich, sweet foods is no manifestation of body need. It is a bad habit. Habits can be broken. Within thirty days you can replace your fondness for fattening sweets with a preference for fresh fruits.

Protein foods, with their specific dynamic effect, are 35 percent less fattening than starches or fats.

Lean meats, fish, and hard-cooked eggs keep the diet varied and flavorful and prevent that feeling of hardship while reducing.

French yogurt remains in the stomach longer and prevents between-meal hunger pains.

Chilled raw vegetables (see finger salads, pages 98–99) help to retrain an overstretched, overdemanding stomach by keeping it filled longer.

Taking a balanced vitamin-mineral concentrate in the morning makes reducing easier.

Be especially generous with the B vitamins; the food richest in B vitamins is brewers' yeast. A tall glass of chilled tomato juice, spiked with two teaspoons of brewers' yeast, gives a sustained lift that lasts for hours.

Dr. Lewis R. Wolberg, M.D., deflates the caloric bubble. He says, "The establishment of the calorie as a respectable household unit led to many disappointments. As a yardstick for gross energy exchanges, it was academically accurate, but as a means of arriving at a proper balanced ration, it was positively worthless."

Dr. William Coda Martin, M.D., says: "With over 50 percent of our daily diet made up of over-refined carbohydrates—chiefly, white sugar, white flour, white rice, and most breakfast cereals—it is no wonder we are developing more and more obesity."

Dr. Hilda Bruch, M.D., says, "Within every fat person is buried the real person, signaling frantically to be let out."

Tiredness while reducing is often due to a lack of B vitamins and protein. Brewers' yeast is rich in both; the more you use, the better you feel and the more active you become.

According to a Hollywood psychiatrist, feelings of inferiority and even emotional conflicts seem to melt away with the rolls of fat.

If you have many pounds to lose, do not be discouraged. Promise yourself that you will lose just five pounds. That's easy! When you have accomplished that, promise yourself just five more. With this accomplished, you experience one of life's greatest thrills, the feeling of victory. Now nothing can stop you!!

Don't bore your friends with the intimate workings of your body while reducing. Keep those secrets between yourself and your doctor; he will listen patiently and advise you professionally.

Before starting to reduce, make up your mind not to feel sorry for yourself. You will still get plenty to eat. In fact, millions would consider your rations a banquet.

Loving wives, while cooking, should remember that all solid fats tend to settle not only on hips, but also in hubby's arteries.

Sugar and cream in your coffee is a passé habit. Waistline watchers thrive better on Swiss coffee (see page 524). The milk gives added protein and keeps the stomach contented longer.

Dr. Herbert Pollack, of New York University, says: "You can loose ten pounds a year by simply walking one mile each day."

Dr. D. T. Quigley, M.D., says: "We overeat on carbohydrates because they have no self-limiting action on our appetites."

Dr. Herman Friedel, M.D., English author of *Slenderness through Psychology,* says: "Get to understand the reason why you reach for a sweet . . . and you've taken the first and most important step toward slenderness."

Dr. W. J. McCormick, M.D., of Toronto, Canada, testing his patients for vitamin C deficiency, discovered that the inhaling of one cigarette destroys about 25 milligrams of vitamin C (contents of average orange). Dr. McCormick believes that the major cause of prevalent vitamin C deficiency, often found in reducers, is due to excessive smoking.

Dr. Daniel Colin Munro, M.D., famous diet specialist, in his book *Slenderizing for Beauty,* says: "When you start to deposit fat on your abdomen, you then start your decline in virility. You may be sure that when you deposit layers of fat on your abdomen, you are also depositing its buddy, cholesterol, in your sex glands, hardening them as it does the arteries, and producing a decline in their function. This is what brings about the so-called change-of-life in both men and women."

Dr. Richard MacKarness, M.D., London, author of *Eat Fat and Grow Slim,* says: "It is still unfortunately true that many doctors do not understand obesity for what it is: an error of metabolism, an internal defect, affecting some people and not others, quite apart from the actual amount of food consumed."

Dr. George H. Gehmann, director of the Du Pont Medical Department, says: "Overweight and high blood pressure are Siamese twins."

Dr. Alfred Pennington, M.D., asked his patients not to sleep more than eight hours at night, because you burn up more fat while up and about.

Drs. Wilins and Boyd, well-known English physicians, say that useless fat overworks the heart, tires the feet, and disturbs the conscience!

When German biologists fed mutton fat to test animals, the animals would invariably gain weight around the abdomen. When they fed vegetable oil instead, the same animals would reduce.

Dr. William Brady, M.D. and beloved newspaper columnist, urges his patients and readers to speed up their metabolism and lose their blankets of fat with a daily iodine ration. His favorite prescription is a tablet of dry sea vegetables that contains as much organic iodine as a large fish. Dr. Brady also points out a fact that is well known to dermatologists: Dry skin, and dryness, thinness, and poor growth of hair are often signs of iodine deficiency.

Dr. Margaret Mead, says that the present phase of American "dieting" and "slimming" by counting calories, has something of the same pathetic rigidity that accompanied early bottle feeding.

Eventually bottle feeding was modified according to the needs of self-demand or self-regulation.

PURELY PERSONAL

For the past forty-five years I have followed my own teaching —eating intelligently most of the time. Twice each year I have gone on a week's housecleaning diet. Thousands of my students and I can vouch for the great benefits from such a yearly housecleaning (see my Seven-Day Elimination Diet, page 415). About three years ago I learned about the many diet sanatoriums where people from every walk of life go to take tea, vegetable juice, and fruit fasts. I have always been one of my own guinea pigs, so I decided to take a 14-day trial. I wanted to see what happens when you stop eating solid food for two weeks.

I had the first surprise when I registered at one of Germany's most famous fasting sanatoriums. I was impressed with the elegance and cheerfulness of the place. There were 150 sunny rooms and every room was occupied. After an examination by the head physician, I was put on a fruit day. I could eat two pounds of fresh fruit—peaches, apples, and plums. This seemed meager fare after my vacation in Taormina.

The next day the head nurse brought me a pitcher with a pint of hot *Bitter-Wasser*, a terrible-tasting laxative drink—and that pretty nurse stayed right there to see that I drank every drop of it. When I thought I just could not take another swallow, she gave me a spoonful of sweet raspberry juice. Eventually I emptied the whole pitcher of *Bitter-Wasser*. (I knew, of course that this *Bitter-Wasser* was a terrific laxative, so I stayed close to my room.)

What surprised me most of all was the fact that I was not hungry that whole day—nor was I hungry throughout the rest of the fourteen days. During these two weeks, the nurse brought me a cup of mint tea for breakfast, a cup of clear vegetable broth for lunch, and in the afternoon, at tea time, a cup of herb tea with honey. In the evening there was always a large glass of fruit juice. This is absolutely all I had for two weeks—and I repeat, I never was hungry. When I entered Dr. Buchinger's sanatorium, I weighed 205 pounds; after two weeks, I weighed 190 pounds and felt like a million dollars. Since I am six foot four inches, Dr. Buchinger decided that

I was about at my ideal weight and suggested that I stop the fast. He recommended a one-week transition diet, consisting of fresh salads, fruits, cottage cheese, and yogurt, which I carried out in my own home.

I speak of this personal experience only to show you that the body can get along on very little food. Actually the diets in this book are banquets, and you need not feel sorry for yourself ever when you restrict your food intake *temporarily*. Naturally, all such strict dieting and fasting should be supervised by a sympathetic doctor. I definitely do not recommend that you, my reader, go on such strict fare for more than one day. Fasting, if done for more than 24 hours, requires supervision by a physician specifically trained in this branch of the healing arts—and a physician who knows your physical background and present condition.

Dr. Buchinger and his son are both medical doctors, but they have specialized in scientific fasting for many years. So far, they have successfully supervised the fasting of more than thirty thousand men and women, and the results they are achieving in all sorts of so-called incurable conditions are absolutely amazing. I would not have believed it if I had not seen the results with my own eyes. Tired, overweight, toxic, rheumatic people, with all sorts of vague pains and aches, looked brighter and lighter and seemed to take a new lease on life after a few weeks of fasting.

People from all over the world go to these sanatoriums. While I was in Uberlingen, my friend John Ringling North was also taking the cure. (John is the head of the famous Ringling Circus family.) He is a yearly guest at the sanatorium. He is loud in his praise of this simple cure and what it does to keep him in top form.

So far there has been only one American guest in Uberlingen who "checked out," and the nurses are still laughing about *der kleine Amerikaner* who didn't have enough character to take the cure after he made the trip all the way to Uberlingen. It was Ludwig Bemmelmans who couldn't give up his beloved bockwurst and bockbier—even for two weeks!

If you or your doctor are interested in juice-fasting, I suggest you write directly to one of Dr. Buchinger's sanatoriums; both are equally modern and well staffed and the cost is extremely low for Americans:

Dr. Buchinger's Sanatorium, Bad Pyrmont, Germany, or

Dr. Buchinger's Sanatorium, Uberlingen-Bodensee, Germany Good news! As I wrote this I discovered that two American doctors seem to agree that fasting isn't a fad. (How could it—they fasted in Biblical times.) They are using it successfully, especially on hard-to-reduce and grossly overweight people. Dr. Walter Lyon Bloom, in Atlanta, Georgia, made his first experiments in 1958. He placed nine chronically obese men and women in the Piedmont Hospital and put them on short fasts, lasting from four to nine days, with excellent results. Dr. Bloom noticed especially that these patients were not depressed, and they were most enthusiastic about their weight losses. And, at the Pennsylvania Hospital in Philadelphia, another group of doctors, led by Dr. G. Duncan, is using fasting therapy with amazing success. One woman who had tried all sorts of low-calorie diets lost 25 pounds in 10 days and never felt hungry. Dr. Duncan, a specialist in weight reduction, has this to say about fasting: *"This may prove to be one of the most significant breakthroughs in obesity therapy in the last twenty-five years."*

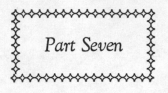

Part Seven

RECIPES AND FORMULAS

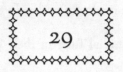

29

Proteins Build Better Bodies

THE MODERN WAY

Whenever and wherever I have met an unusually happy and good-looking family, there I also found a loving wife and mother who had learned to cook with her head, her heart, and her hands. Today there is a new movement among intelligent people for food that is honest, wholesome, and healthful. Homemakers everywhere are revolting against puffed-up white bread, foodless precooked cereals, ready cake mixes, artificially colored fruits, foodless white sugars and bleached flours, and all the highly tooted hydrogenated fats which settle on hips and in arteries. Millions of women have gone back into their kitchens to spend more time and thought on wholesome dishes such as they enjoyed as youngsters. Many even bake their own bread. Fortunate, indeed, is such a family where someone practices the fine art of tender loving cooking.

I believe any woman who cares about her own well-being and the health of the family can prepare delicious meals in the modern manner if she applies these five common-sense rules:

1. Undercook rather than overcook.
2. Learn to be more generous with the good proteins.
3. Be extravagant with fresh living foods, especially green growing things.

4. Use carbohydrates modestly and only the natural whole-grain whole-sugar variety.

5. Be a miser with animal fats; in their place, use golden vegetable oils and spreads.

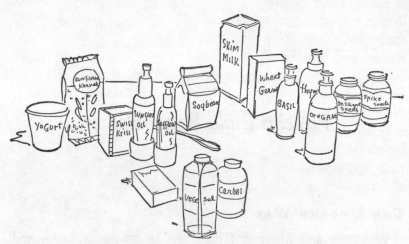

Herbs and spices add nonweighty delights

If you keep these five common-sense pointers in mind you can continue to cook your family's favorite dishes, with a tremendous increase of health and well-being. In the following pages you will find some old stand-bys, but you will also discover some new nutritious dishes which I hope will add to your eating pleasure.

Let us start with our most important group of foods, the important proteins, our valuable meats and fish. Any cut of beef, veal, lamb, or poultry can be used, provided always that you cook it lean. The only products of the pork family I can recommend with good conscience are the smoked ones: lean ham and lean bacon. Organ meats of all kinds, and especially liver, are super-proteins and should be used much more frequently. Also, fish and all foods coming from the sea should be enjoyed several times a week.

LEARN TO LOVE LIVER

I know that fresh raw liver is not particularly appetizing to the novice or squeamish cook. It has a consistency more like gelatin or aspic than like steaks or chops. But once it is properly cooked—

and that means very briefly—it takes on a delicate firmness that is quite pleasing to the eye and to the palate.

Liver contains first-class protein and is a treasure house of vitamins. Old-fashioned cookbooks still tell you to soak all the good out of the liver and then fry it like shoe leather. But, actually, the less liver is cooked the more beneficial it is. Modern chefs know that tender calf liver, chicken and turkey livers, should be quickly washed and quickly cooked—only until they change color. Beef liver, also an excellent food, is a little tougher, but it can now be tenderized. Lamb liver, the cheapest of all, is just as good nutritionally as the more expensive kinds. A fine old American custom is to have golden brown onions with all livers. For variety's sake, have some golden apple slices with your liver occasionally. To convince you of the amazing nutriments contained in the cheapest of all, lamb liver, let me give you a comparative analysis.

	Expensive		*Inexpensive*	
	Calf Liver (3 oz.)		Lamb Liver (3 oz.)	
Protein	16.2	gm.	17.8	gm.
Fat	4.2	gm.	3.3	gm.
Carbohydrates	3.4	gm.	2.5	gm.
Calcium	5.	mg.	7.	mg.
Phosphorous	292.	mg.	309.	mg.
Iron	9.	mg.	10.7	mg.
Vitamin A	19,130.	I.U.	42,930.	I.U.
Thiamine	.18	mg.	.34	mg.
Riboflavin	2.65	mg.	2.79	mg.
Niacin	13.7	mg.	14.3	mg.
Vitamin C	30.	mg.	28.	mg.
Vitamin D	45.	I.U.	20.	I.U.

Broiled Liver

If you can afford calf liver, you are lucky. If you use beef liver, sprinkle it on both sides with that easy-to-use tenderizer, and let it stand for 30 minutes at room temperature. Then take ½-inch thick slices and brush them lightly with a bit of golden oil. Place on broiler pan and broil 3 inches from the heat. This takes only 3 minutes on each side. Place on hot platter, season, and trim with parsley or watercress.

Enjoy Liver This Way

Take any fresh tender liver. Cut in noodle-like strips. If at all tough, sprinkle with tenderizer and let stand for 20 minutes at room temperature. Then put just 1 tablespoon of golden oil or margarine in heavy, heated skillet. Sauté one large sliced onion to a golden brown. Add the strips of liver and sauté for just 3 minutes. Sprinkle with a bit of vegetable salt and serve at once. This is my favorite liver recipe, and many liver-haters enjoy it when prepared this way.

Liver Loaf

1 lb. beef liver	1½ cups chopped carrots
3 tbsp. golden oil	1 tbsp. minced celery leaves
½ cup minced onion	2 tbsp. minced parsley
¼ cup diced celery	1 tbsp. wheat germ
4 tbsp. finely chopped green pepper	1 tsp. vegetable salt
	¼ tsp. paprika
1 lb. ground beef	2 fresh eggs

Have the liver cut in half-inch slices. Heat the golden oil in a heavy skillet and sauté the liver a few minutes. Remove the liver from the pan and put it through a food chopper, using the fine blade. Add the onion, celery, and green pepper to the hot skillet, adding more oil if necessary, and sauté for 3 minutes or until the onion is golden brown. Combine all ingredients and mix thoroughly. Place in a well-oiled dish or casserole, cover, and bake 30 minutes in a moderate oven (375° F.). Uncover and bake 15 minutes longer or until the top is brown. If your family leaves any of this delicious dish, your dog will gobble it up.

Chicken Livers

¾ lb. chicken livers	2 tbsp. sliced onions
1 tbsp. butter	½ tsp. vegetable salt
1 tbsp. golden oil	dash of rose paprika
2 cups sliced mushrooms	

Wash livers and cut into small pieces. Heat butter and oil in heavy skillet and sauté the livers, mushrooms, and onions over low heat for about 4 minutes, stirring occasionally. Add seasonings and serve.

Hi-Vi Liver-Heart-Kidney Tonic

The less you cook liver, the more potent a weapon against paleness and tiredness it is. However, up to now it has been impossible to eat raw liver; but with that clever invention, the liquidizer-blender, raw liver can be easily transformed into a palatable drink with the livery taste entirely eliminated. I highly recommend this Hi-Vi tonic to all who need nourishment quickly and in the most concentrated form. This liver tonic can win the *grand prix* every time for making rich red blood and rosy complexions within a few days' time.

Put half a cup of vegetable broth or chicken broth into the liquidizer-blender. To this add a tablespoon of fresh parsley and a slice of mild onion coarsely chopped. Spike with vegetable salt and a dash of soy sauce. Turn on liquidizer and, when the mixture is puréed, add one tablespoon of the freshest raw liver obtainable (chicken, calf, or very young beef). Continue until the mixture is smooth; then pour into a cup of hot tomato juice or chicken broth. Stir and drink at once.

P.S. Not only liver, but heart, kidney, and other inner organs can be prepared the same way; and they are also highly recommended by nutritionists. Raw organ meats are loaded with vitamins, hormones, and as yet undiscovered substances. Thousands of years ago, Chinese doctors ordered their patients to eat young hearts for strengthening the heart. Who knows? Scientists may yet discover that specific organ meats help to nourish specific organs.

Calf Liver with Avocado

1 lb. calf liver (¼ inch slices)
golden vegetable oil or
   margarine
1 large ripe avocado

¼ cup chicken or vegetable
   broth
lemon juice
vegetable salt to taste

Sauté the slices of liver slowly in the golden oil over medium heat. When browned on both sides, remove liver to serving platter and keep warm. Brown the sliced avocado in the same pan and put slices on top of the liver. Add hot vegetable or chicken broth to the pan and briskly boil down, stirring constantly. When reduced by half, pour over the liver and avocado. Sprinkle with lemon juice, add vegetable salt, and serve immediately.

BEEF—OUR FAVORITE PROTEIN

For Americans, particularly, beef has long been the favorite meat. Properly cooked, all cuts of beef offer flavor and high nutrition.

Broiled Steak

When you want a steak for broiling, ask the butcher for his best, the most tender cut, one and one-half inches thick, and have him cut off all visible fat.

Preheat the broiling oven 5 to 10 minutes, at 400° F. Brush the steak lightly with a little golden oil. Then brush the broiler rack with oil. Place the steak on the rack about 2 inches below the heat. Sear it on both sides, then reduce the heat and continue cooking. (Usually the door of the broiling oven is left open, unless directions for your range specify otherwise.)

For a rare steak, 1½ inches thick, broil 12 to 15 minutes; for a 2-inch steak, 15 to 18 minutes.

One of the most important steps in preparing a steak is to make sure it is seasoned delicately, yet adequately. Have a platter of the right size hot and ready. To season the underside of the cooked steak, add about one tablespoon of golden oil to the hot platter, one teaspoon of vegetable salt, and one teaspoon of chopped parsley. Stir. Place the hot steak on this seasoning. Season the top of the hot steak lightly and quickly, adding a little chopped parsley. Pour any lean juices from the broiling pan over the steak. Garnish the platter with parsley.

Fortified Beefburgers

1 lb. lean chopped beef	2 tbsp. chopped onions
2 tbsp. wheat germ	2 tbsp. chopped parsley
½ cup water	1 tbsp. chopped celery
1½ tbsp. nonfat dry milk	

Mix all ingredients and make into 4 flat patties. Put into a heavy pan which has its bottom covered with ½ tsp. salt, and brown quickly on both sides. Beefburgers may also be broiled on a slightly greased rack, but make patties ¾ inch thick for broiling.

Budapest Goulash

1 lb. lean beef cut in small cubes	1 tsp. rose paprika
1 lb. veal cut in small cubes	1 bay leaf
2 tbsp. golden oil	½ tsp. caraway seeds
4 large chopped onions	2 cups strained tomatoes
2 cloves chopped garlic	2 cups scrubbed, unpeeled,
1 tsp. vegetable salt	cubed potatoes

Sprinkle tenderizer over meat cubes; let stand for 30 minutes at room temperature. Then heat golden oil in heavy iron kettle or Dutch oven on top of the stove, and brown the meat with the chopped onions and garlic. Add salt, rose paprika, bay leaf, and caraway seeds. Heat tomatoes and pour over meat. Cover tightly and simmer about one hour and a half. If the mixture begins to dry, add more tomatoes or tomato juice. Add the potato cubes half an hour before meat is to be done. If desired, gravy can be thickened with a tablespoon of whole-wheat flour or a bit of vegetable thickener.

Beef Stroganoff

2 lb. lean beef cut into small cubes	2 tbsp. chopped parsley
	1 tbsp. soy sauce
2 tbsp. whole-wheat flour	½ pint thick yogurt
2 tbsp. golden oil	½ tsp. vegetable salt
1 medium or 2 small onions	rose paprika to taste
½ lb. sliced mushrooms	
2 cups vegetable or chicken broth	

Sprinkle tenderizer over meat cubes; let stand for 30 minutes at room temperature. Then dredge meat cubes in whole-wheat flour. Pour golden oil in heavy iron kettle or Dutch oven and heat. Brown the meat on all sides. Add the onions and mushrooms and cook until golden. Add the broth, cover the kettle, and let simmer over low flame for about one hour. Remove cover during the last half hour and let liquid cook down to half its quantity. Ten minutes before serving, add parsley, soy sauce, and yogurt. Season to taste with vegetable salt and rose paprika.

German Beefburger

1 cup ground raw carrots
1 cup ground unpeeled raw
  potatoes
2 tbsp. chopped onion
2 tbsp. chopped parsley
1 lb. ground lean beef

½ cup chopped celery
1 beaten egg
¼ cup milk
¼ cup wheat germ
2 tsp. vegetable salt

Mix all together, then form into patties and place them on lightly oiled shallow pan and bake in hot oven (400° F.) for 20 minutes.

Lean Beef and Black Olives

3 lbs. very lean top sirloin or
  round (1½ inches thick)
¼ cup golden oil
  whole-wheat flour
  vegetable salt
12 small white onions

1 clove garlic
1½ cups consomme
½ tsp. thyme
½ cup black olives (pitted)
¼ cup chopped parsley

Cut the beef into 1½ inch cubes and trim off any remaining fat. Coat cubes well with flour and salt. Heat the oil in a large heavy skillet and brown the meat quickly on all sides. Transfer the meat to a casserole. Brown the onions and crushed garlic lightly in the same skillet and add them to the casserole. Add the consomme and sprinkle with thyme. Cover the casserole and bake in pre-heated oven (300° F.) for about 1½ hours. Add the olives and parsley. Cover and continue to bake for 40 or 50 minutes, or until meat is completely tender.

VEAL

Sicilian Piccadillo—a Delightful Party Dish

2 lbs. ground veal
4 medium-sized onions
2 green peppers, diced
1 clove garlic, mashed
1 cup sliced olives
½ cup raisins
½ cup blanched sliced almonds

dash nutmeg
1 tbsp. chopped fresh basil (or
  1 tsp. dried)
1 tsp. honey
3 ripe tomatoes, quartered
  vegetable salt

Sauté the ground veal in a heavy skillet with just enough golden vegetable oil to cover bottom. Cook until all red disappears. Put veal into large pot or Dutch oven. In the same skillet sauté the onions, peppers, and garlic, adding a small amount of oil, until soft and golden but not brown. Add vegetables to veal in the pot. Add olives, raisins, almonds, nutmeg, basil, and honey. Combine well. Cover and simmer until all ingredients are blended. Remove from flame and hold until serving time. Just before serving, add quartered tomatoes and reheat. Salt to taste. Serve with fluffy rice. Fresh sliced bananas are often served on top of the piccadillo.

LAMB

Leg of Lamb Glazed with Golden Apricots

Leg of young lamb (6 or 7 pounds)	1 onion, sliced thin
	1 cup water
2 cloves of garlic, slivered	2 tbsp. golden oil
1 tsp. vegetable salt	½ lb. dried apricots

Remove skin and every bit of fat from lamb. Insert slivers of garlic in gashes made in leg of lamb with a sharp paring knife. Preheat oven to 275° F. Sprinkle lamb with salt and place on a rack in an uncovered shallow pan. Spoon the oil over the top of the lamb. Put water and sliced onions in the bottom of the pan. Bake about two hours.

While the lamb is baking, steam the apricots in enough water to cover, until soft (about 25 minutes). Pass through food mill and set aside.

Remove the lamb from the oven after two hours. Pour off the gravy and remove the fat. Mix the remaining gravy with the apricot purée and pour over the lamb. Return to the oven and continue to cook for one more hour, basting frequently with the apricot gravy. When the lamb is nicely glazed and golden brown, slice thin and serve on a warmed platter covered with the gravy. (Serves 8)

CHICKEN AT ITS BEST

Roast Chicken

For this delicate, wonderfully flavored low-fat dish of chicken, select a bird not less than 3½ pounds, or a capon of about 5 pounds. Rub the bird inside and out with a little golden oil and lemon juice. Place the chicken breast side up in an uncovered roaster. Roast in a hot oven, 450° F., about 20 minutes, or until brown. Reduce the heat to moderately slow, 325° F., and roast, allowing 18 to 25 minutes per pound. For a plump chicken roast a little longer, to be sure it is well cooked through and not red around the bones.

While the chicken roasts, baste it at 15-minute intervals with beautyfarm basting sauce (see below). When the chicken is nearly done, turn it breast side down and let the underside brown evenly. To test a chicken for doneness, insert a two-tined kitchen fork into the thickest part of the breast and the second joint. If the juices do not run red, the chicken is done.

Some prefer the moderate-temperature method of roasting. For this, heat the oven to 350° F. Roast the chicken at that temperature for 25 to 30 minutes per pound. (A 4-pound chicken requires 1 hour and 40 minutes to 2 hours.)

For a good poultry stuffing, mix about 3½ cups cooked brown or wild rice, add 4 chopped cooked prunes, and 1 chopped whole orange (seeds removed). Stuff and bake as described, allowing a few minutes more per pound.

For the added pleasure of eating herbed roast chicken, add 1 teaspoon each oregano and sweet basil to the stuffing; or add these herbs to the hot oil and water with which you baste the chicken, or to the beautyfarm basting sauce. A 3½-pound chicken serves four or more.

Beautyfarm Basting Sauces

You can prepare a delectable roast chicken, turkey, or duck without using any fat, even in the basting. Prepare the whole fowl, or separate pieces such as breast and legs, for roasting. Roast as usual, but baste every 20 minutes of roasting time with the following sauce:

2 chicken or vegetable bouillon cubes	1 cup orange juice
1 cup boiling water	¼ cup lemon juice
	½ tsp. vegetable salt

Dissolve the bouillon cubes in the boiling water. Combine with the fruit juices. Add salt and mix well. Use for basting with spoon or pastry brush.

For a roast *lamb*, skim the fat from the roaster continually during the cooking period. Baste the roast frequently with a warm mixture of white wine, bouillon, and a few chopped fresh mint leaves.

Blend tomato espresso (see page 509) with bouillon. Add a crumbled bay leaf and a dash of dried rosemary. Heat slightly, and use to baste *veal* as it cooks. Wonderful flavor in the roast when you carve it onto warmed dinner plates.

Baste roasting *chicken, turkey*, and other fowl with a warm mixture of orange juice, lemon juice, bouillon, flavored lightly with oregano and a little dried rosemary.

And, for superlative flavor in any roast, rub the meat thoroughly with vegetable salt before it goes into the oven. Basting washes some of the seasoning off, so add a light sprinkling of vegetable salt over the top of the roast after the last basting.

Modern Oven-Fried Chicken

2 1½-lb. broilers, quartered	1 clove garlic
½ cup golden oil	½ tsp. sweet paprika
1 tsp. vegetable salt	½ cup wheat germ

Mix the oil, vegetable salt, crushed garlic, and paprika. Apply to the chicken pieces with a pastry brush. Roll chicken in wheat germ and place, skin side down, in a shallow baking dish coated with remaining oil mixture. Bake for approximately 1½ hours in a 350° F. oven. Turn skin side up after 45 minutes.

Chicken with Curry

1 young chicken (about 3 lbs.)	1 large onion, chopped fine
2 cups water	1 tsp. vegetable salt
1 tsp. vegetable salt	½ tsp. allspice
2 stalks celery	1 tsp. curry powder
4 cups yogurt	1 tbsp. whole-wheat flour
2 fresh eggs, slightly beaten	½ cup margarine

Cut up chicken and put it in a pot with the water, salt, and celery. Cover and simmer for one hour or until tender. Cool and remove the chicken (save the broth for soup). Skin and bone the chicken, and cut the meat in strips. Put the yogurt in a double boiler and add the 2 eggs, onion, salt, allspice, and curry powder. Mix well.

Add the flour, little by little. Cook over a low flame, stirring constantly, until the yogurt thickens (about 10 minutes). Add the chicken and margarine and continue cooking and stirring for five minutes. (Taste. You may want to add more curry powder.)

A Note on Fats

Always remember that the younger the chicken, the less fat it contains. A spring broiler contains only about 10 percent fat, but an old stewing hen can contain as much as 40 percent fat. This is hard fat, remember. Don't you dare serve such a stew without skimming off the fat.

Turkey is another favorite and an excellent protein food. The fat content of turkey depends upon whether or not the turkey was fattened for the market, but most fowl contains only 10 or 15 percent fat. If you are lucky enough to go hunting for wild fowl, I envy you. All wild game is richer in nutrients and has much more muscle than fat, a good example of the shining effect of exercise. If you enjoy wild duck, pheasant, quail, or grouse, remember not to spoil these by serving greasy gravies.

Eat Fish and Live Longer

That's the new slogan the Fishery Council coined after it was discovered that the fats and oils in fish help to reduce cholesterol; and, of course, fish contains the same first-class protein that meat does. Fish is also richer in phosphorus, and has the added beauty-giving mineral: iodine. The fat content of our beloved steaks is as high as 40 percent, whereas the fat content of fish is only about 15 percent—and of the friendly unsaturated variety. Remember also that our oceans are still relatively uncorrupted and free from chemicals and additives. Do not use a lot of fat in fish cookery. Just a bit of one of the nonhydrogenated vegetable margarines or, still better, your favorite golden vegetable oil, will seal in the flavor and nutrients. In Sicily they prefer straight olive oil; sophisticated Romans cook with half oil and half butter; the French, with their clever thermos pan cover, can cook fish in a matter of moments with very little fat (or *no* fat, which is ideal). Here are a few unusual and delightful fish recipes, some from the sunny Mediterranean countries. Try them all.

Sesame Halibut Steaks

3 halibut steaks, 1 inch thick	1 tsp. vegetable salt
3 tsp. oil or margarine	3 tbsp. toasted sesame seeds
2 cups soft whole-wheat bread crumbs	½ tsp. thyme
	3 tbsp. melted margarine

Put steaks in an oiled baking pan; sprinkle with salt and pour 1 tsp. of margarine (or golden oil) on top of each steak. Combine bread crumbs, salt, sesame seeds, thyme, and remaining margarine, and spread on top of steaks. Place in oven preheated to 350° F. and bake uncovered for about 30 minutes, or until fish flakes easily.

Swordfish in Foil

1½ lbs. swordfish steak (four pieces)	2 tbsp. golden oil
1 cup sliced mushrooms	2 tbsp. lemon juice
1 onion, thinly sliced	½ tsp. dill seed
2 tbsp. chopped green pepper	½ tsp. vegetable salt
1 tbsp. chopped parsley	4 slices tomato
	4 small bay leaves

Line a baking pan with foil. Mix the mushrooms, onion, green pepper, parsley, oil, lemon juice, dill seed, and salt together. Put half the mixture on foil on bottom of pan. Add the swordfish. Sprinkle with salt. Top each piece with a slice of tomato and a small bay leaf, and cover with the remaining mixture. Cover pan with foil and place in oven preheated to 425° F. Bake about 40 minutes. Remove bay leaves. Serve from the baking dish, and use the pan juices and vegetables as a sauce.

Baked Bluefish

1 bluefish (approximately 4 lbs. cleaned)	chopped parsley
4 strips lean bacon	lemon wedges

Split the fish and place on an oiled baking sheet, skin side down. Top with bacon slices and bake in preheated oven (425° F.) for about 25 minutes, or until fish flakes when fork-tested. Sprinkle fish with parsley, and garnish with lemon wedges.

Grilled Salmon Steaks with Herbs

4 salmon steaks, ¾ inch thick
½ cup dry vermouth or white wine
½ cup golden vegetable oil
1 tbsp. lemon juice
generous pinch of thyme
generous pinch of marjoram
1 tbsp. minced parsley
small pinch of sage
½ tsp. vegetable salt

Put the steaks in shallow pan. Mix the other ingredients and pour over the steaks. Marinate for two hours, turning once. Lift steaks from marinade and place on preheated, oiled rack and place in hot broiler. While cooking, brush several times with the marinade. Turn once, after 7 or 8 minutes. Cook until tender (flakes easily with a fork), in all about 15 minutes.

Broiled Lobster Tails

If you use quick-frozen African lobster tails, follow directions on package. Usually one package makes two servings.

Oil broiler pan or grid with a bit of golden oil. Place lobster tails on broiler, flesh side up, and season with a bit of vegetable salt. Broil in moderate oven (325–50° F) for about 8 minutes (see directions on package). Baste twice during broiling period with a mixture of 1 tablespoon fresh lemon juice and 1 tablespoon of golden oil. Then turn lobster tails over, shell side up, and broil for 2 or 3 minutes more, basting once more with lemon and oil mixture. Remove from broiler. Serve lobster tails flesh side up, with membrane cut for easy eating, and sprinkle with a tablespoon of finely chopped watercress or dill. Serve at once.

Lobster tails can be served hot with a hot hollandaise sauce or chilled and served with cold hollandaise sauce.

DELICIOUS MEATLESS PROTEIN DISHES

When eggs, milk, brewers' yeast, wheat germ, nuts, or soy products are mixed with vegetable protein they become much more nutritious. Such combinations can be enjoyed, not only by vegetarians, but by all those wishing for more variety in their menus.

Walnut Loaf

2 cups walnuts, chopped
2 cups whole-wheat bread crumbs
2 tbsp. soy flour
2 eggs, beaten foamy

1 medium onion, chopped
½ green pepper, chopped
1 cup Hauser Broth

Put all ingredients into bowl, mix thoroughly, and put into a loaf pan. Place in a moderate oven and bake for about 40 minutes.

Georgia Pecan Loaf

1 cup pecans, chopped
½ cup cooked brown rice
½ cup whole-wheat bread crumbs

1 medium onion, chopped
1 tbsp. parsley, chopped
1 egg, beaten foamy

Put nuts, rice, crumbs, onion, and parsley into bowl. Add beaten egg. Mix all ingredients thoroughly. Put in loaf pan and bake in moderate oven for about 40 minutes.

Savory Nut Loaf

¾ cup finely chopped nut meats
1¼ cups cooked tomato
1 cup celery, chopped
⅓ cup parsley, chopped
½ cup onion, finely shredded
1 egg, slightly beaten

1 tsp. vegetable salt
½ tsp. savory
1 cup dry whole-wheat bread crumbs
2 tbsp. golden vegetable oil
2 tbsp. wheat germ

Combine first six ingredients and mix thoroughly. Add the remaining ingredients and mix again. Pack into a well-oiled loaf pan. Bake in a moderate oven about 40 minutes, or until firm. Serve with lemon wedges, parsley butter, or tomato sauce.

Golden Carrot Loaf

¾ cup raw carrot, grated
1 small onion, minced
2 tbsp. parsley, chopped
1 stalk celery (including some leaves) diced
½ cup chopped nuts
2 tbsp. dry whole-wheat bread crumbs

2 tbsp. cream
1 egg, slightly beaten
1½ tsp. vegetable salt
2 tbsp. golden oil whole-wheat bread crumbs
2 tsp. margarine

Mix thoroughly all ingredients but the last three. Coat the inside of a loaf pan with golden oil and dust oiled surfaces with remaining bread crumbs. Pack mixture into loaf pan, dot with margarine, cover pan, and bake in moderate oven about 35 minutes. Invert on serving platter. Serve with your favorite sauce.

Celery Loaf

½ cup celery, chopped
½ small onion, chopped
⅜ cup nut meats, chopped
¾ cup thick tomato juice
½ tbsp. grated cheese
1 tsp. vegetable salt

1 tbsp. margarine, melted
⅔ cup dry whole-wheat bread crumbs
1 egg, well beaten
2 tbsp. golden oil

Put celery, onion, and nut meats through food grinder, using medium blade. In a bowl, thoroughly mix celery, onion, nut meats, tomato juice, cheese, salt, margarine, and all but 2 tablespoons of the bread crumbs. Add egg and mix lightly. Coat inside of loaf pan with golden oil and dust with remaining bread crumbs. Pack the mixture in pan, and bake in moderate oven until firm, about 40 minutes. Loosen sides with knife and invert loaf onto serving platter. Sprinkle with chopped parsley and garnish with fresh tomato wedges.

Savory Stuffed Peppers

6 medium-sized green peppers
   vegetable salt
1½ tbsp. margarine, melted
¼ cup celery, chopped
1 medium-sized onion, chopped
¼ cup green pepper, chopped

½ cup nut meats, chopped
⅔ cup dry rye-bread crumbs
1 cup milk
½ tsp. vegetable salt
3 tbsp. wheat germ

Wash peppers, cut off stems, and remove seeds and veins. Sprinkle insides with vegetable salt. Combine all remaining ingredients (except wheat germ) and heat, in double boiler, stirring until well blended and hot. Fill green peppers with the hot mixture. Put filled peppers into baking dish just large enough for them to fit snugly, and pour about 1 inch of hot water around them. Cover, and bake in a moderate oven until peppers are done, about 35 minutes. Uncover and sprinkle wheat germ over tops of peppers. Return to the oven, uncovered, for 5 to 8 minutes, or until wheat germ is golden brown.

Oven Baked Beans

1 cup dried beans (kidney, lentil, navy, lima, pea)
5 tbsp. golden vegetable oil
4 tbsp. molasses (or honey, or 3 tbsp. brown sugar)

1 onion, cut into wedge-shaped pieces
1 tsp. vegetable salt
juice of ¼ lemon
2 tbsp. brewers' yeast

Rinse dry beans thoroughly, and soak 4 to 6 hours (or overnight). Pour into casserole, and add oil and seasonings. Add hot water *almost* to cover. Cover casserole, and bake in a slow oven (250° F.), stirring occasionally. Add more hot water as needed to keep beans almost covered until nearly done. Then add remaining ingredients, and return casserole to oven uncovered. Allow top to brown. Serve in casserole, garnished with parsley.

Special suggestions: Lima beans are delicious seasoned with garlic. Lima beans and lentils require no sweetening. Lentils are better with twice the above amount of lemon juice. Stewed tomatoes make a delicious vegetable accompaniment for any baked beans.

Quick Baked Beans—an Excellent Party Dish

There are many varieties of legumes, such as beans, peas, and lentils, that are canned in a wholesome manner. They can save you much time. But you may find them too bland for your taste. Here is an utterly simple and delicious way to make canned baked beans better:

2 one-pound cans of baked beans
1 tbsp. prepared mustard
1 tbsp. cider vinegar

2 tbsp. unsulphured molasses
1 sliced tomato
1 sliced onion

Mix mustard, vinegar, and molasses, and stir into beans. Pour in a pan or skillet. Top with tomato and onion slices. Heat slowly, stirring occasionally, until heated through (about 15 minutes).

These beans are especially delicious when served with Virginia bacon (the Duchess of Windsor's favorite). Place lean strips of bacon in a pan. Dribble two or three teaspoons of unsulphured molasses over the top. Place in moderate oven for 5 minutes or until molasses starts to bubble.

Wild Rice Nutburgers

2 cups cooked wild rice
1 egg, slightly beaten

½ cup coarse chopped nuts
   (pecans, hazelnuts, walnuts, or peanuts)

Combine ingredients. Form into patties, using one heaping serving spoon for each; or drop from the spoon directly into a well-oiled hot skillet or griddle. These are for special occasions—wild rice is expensive. However you can substitute whole brown rice, which is equally nutritious and also quite tasty.

Quick Wild Rice:

½ cup wild rice
1½ cups boiling water

½ tsp. vegetable salt
1½ tsp. margarine

Add rice to boiling salted water. Cover and cook over very low flame, without stirring, for 15 minutes. Remove cover and dot the margarine over the top. Let stand for a few minutes in a barely warm oven or on an asbestos mat over a very low flame to dry out the grains.

THE WONDER VEGETABLE THAT CAN TAKE THE PLACE OF MEAT

Soybeans—the meat without a bone. That's what millions of Orientals call this high-protein legume. Actually, this unassuming little bean is the only vegetable that contains a complete protein and can actually take the place of meat. So highly do Orientals regard this meat without a bone that wars were fought over the Manchurian fields where the finest soybeans grow to this day. Americans and Europeans so far have not profited by using soybeans, perhaps because they were once difficult to prepare. But now there are easy-to-cook soybeans grown in America and Europe, so no doubt more soy products will be used by people of the West.

Everybody knows that soybean oil is an excellent vegetable oil, with 53 percent of the valuable linoleic acid. Most people do not know that soy flour is as nutritious as egg yolks; and too many people have never tasted baked soybeans—a real stick-to-the-ribs protein dish costing pennies instead of dollars. Toasted soybeans are a delight; and they can take the place of expensive nutmeats. Soybean milk, on which millions of Oriental babies thrive, is a Godsend for our babies who are allergic to cow's milk.

With soy milk it is possible to make yogurt and a nutritious cheese called *Tofu*, but the real million dollar secret is that sprouted soybeans are a superfood, containing protein, vitamins A, B, and C, enzymes, and auxines (a type of vegetable hormone). Soybean sprouts are indeed a "living" food. Everybody should learn to grow them. Use them fresh in salads. Use a handful when making potent vegetable juices. Short-cook them as for chop suey. As emergency rations, a sack of soybeans could keep a person alive and chipper for weeks, so versatile and potent is the honorable little bean.

Grow Vitamins in Your Kitchen

Simply cover the bottom of a glass baking dish with a layer of soybeans—the small Mung variety are best. Cover with lukewarm water and let soak overnight. Next morning, pour off excess water, rinse, and add fresh water to cover. Cover glass dish with its lid or another dish of the same size and place where the beans will have even room temperature. Twice each day, pour off stale water, rinse, and add fresh water to barely cover. Young, tender vitamin sprouts will appear the second day, and they are usually ready to eat by the fourth day. The shells of the beans will rise to the top (or sink to the bottom) and are easily removed. These bean sprouts are an amazingly rich source of vitamin C. You derive greatest benefit from them when they are eaten raw in salads or sandwiches. They are also excellent sprinkled over cooked vegetables, and wonderful when mixed into chop suey. Bean sprouts are indeed a wonder food. After you have learned the secret of sprouting soybeans, you should also learn to sprout whole-wheat kernels and lentil and alfalfa seeds. In emergencies, when cut off from other fresh things, such a small vitamin garden can become a real lifesaver!

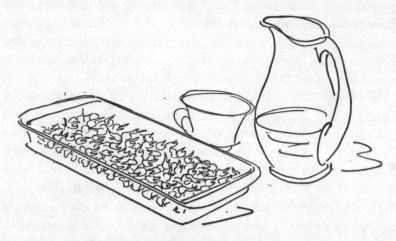

Grow your own bean sprouts—a Wonder Food

Baked Soybeans (oven baked)

Baked soybeans can provide a welcome change. They are a fine and inexpensive protein. (If you are too busy to cook soybeans, I recommend ready-cooked canned ones.)

1 cup dried large soybeans	1 onion, thinly sliced
3 cups water	1¼ tsp. vegetable salt
hot vegetable broth	juice of ¼ lemon
4 tbsp. golden oil	¼ lemon cut in thin slices
2 tbsp. unsulphured molasses	

Wash the soybeans and put them in a kettle in which you can boil them next day. Pour 3 cups of water over them and soak overnight. Next day, bring to a boil in the same water. Reduce heat and cook slowly, adding hot vegetable broth as needed to keep the beans almost covered. Simmer for 2 hours, or until the beans are a light tan. Transfer to a casserole, and add the oil and molasses. Cover casserole. Bake in moderate oven (325° F.) for 30 to 40 minutes. Stir occasionally. During the baking, keep the beans barely covered with liquid. Remove from oven, add the onion, salt, lemon juice, and lemon slices. Return to oven, uncovered, and bake another 30 minutes, or until the liquid is almost absorbed and the top is brown. Serve from casserole dish, garnished with chopped parsley or green onion tops. (4 servings)

Baked Soybeans (quick method)

You can save yourself time and work by buying canned soybeans. They are delicious and nutritious.

2 one-pound cans baked soybeans	1 tbsp. vinegar
¼ cup unsulphured molasses	1 tomato, chopped
1 tbsp. prepared mustard	1 onion, chopped

Pour two cans of baked soybeans into a deep, heavy pan. Add the remaining ingredients. Heat over low flame, stirring occasionally, until thoroughly hot and bubbly (about 15 minutes). Makes 6 delicious servings.

Soy Flour Adds Protein

This is one of the most nutritious foods of all. One tablespoon of soy flour has approximately the same food value as an egg. Soybean flour can be added to muffins, biscuits, waffles, and breads. Eating such soybean-enriched products for breakfast makes it easy to get sufficient proteins into this most important meal.

Soy Grits Save Money

These are made by breaking the soybean into 10–12 little pieces. In this way they cook much faster. Soy grits can be mixed with many other foods. They give a nutlike flavor to hamburgers and meat loaves. They can also be mixed with cereals. One tablespoon of soy grits gives an added 6 grams of protein to any dish. Actually, soy grits form the main part of the "meals for millions" which our government distributes to needy nations.

How to Make Soy Milk

This vegetable milk is used by millions of Orientals. When milk causes allergies, soybean milk makes an excellent substitute. It can now be bought in cans, but you can make it at home as follows:

Soak 1 cup of large soybeans in 3 cups of water for 24 to 48 hours. *Pour off water in which beans have been soaked.* Grind the beans through a meat chopper, or put them in a liquidizer until chopped very fine. Add 5 to 6 cups of warm water, and boil for 30 minutes. Strain through fine strainer; add a pinch of vegetable salt and 1 tablespoonful honey. This milk can be used exactly the same as cow's milk.

Tasty Soy Treats

Delicious and nutritious as toasted almonds are these easy-to-make soy treats. Simply cover ½ cup of big dry soybeans with 1½ cups warm water and let soak overnight. Next morning, dry the soaked beans with a towel. When dry, put beans into a heated heavy skillet and stir until beans are a golden brown. Just before removing from skillet, add 1 tablespoon of golden vegetable oil or sunbutter (see page 33) and sprinkle with ½ teaspoon of vegetable salt. A great success when served fresh and hot at cocktail parties!

Eggs, a Wonder Food

Fresh eggs are a complete food, so complete that they make a beautiful chick! More and more nutritionists feel that fertile eggs are preferable to eggs produced on the assembly line. Eggs contain all of the necessary amino acids, and they are a treasure house of vitamins A and B₂ and iron. However, raw eggs should not be used habitually. The raw egg white can cause all sorts of skin difficulties and allergies because the avidin in the white combines with the biotin, one of the B vitamins, and so prevents it from getting into the blood stream. Biotin deficiences can be responsible for many ugly skin conditions.

Eggs are nutritionally at their best hard-cooked, or at least cooked until the white is firm. Contrary to popular belief, hard-cooked eggs are not hard to digest. Each one contains seven or eight grams of first-class protein. It is wise to keep a few hard-cooked eggs in the refrigerator, for they have tremendous satiety value eaten with or between meals. They help to satisfy an overdemanding stomach. All healthy people should enjoy one or two eggs a day. *They are high in cholesterol, but they are also high in lecithin and the B vitamins which help to keep cholesterol on the move.* Unless your doctor has specifically forbidden you to eat eggs, I hope you will enjoy them daily. Eggs are also wonderful fortifiers of other foods.

Always get the freshest eggs available, preferably from a nearby farmer who has a rooster and lets his chickens walk on the fresh earth.

Eat Eggs in Every Form

Have eggs raw, soft-cooked, hard-cooked, poached, scrambled, even fried (but use the friendly golden oils, such as sesame oil which has a delightful flavor). Eggs fried hard in butter are definitely detrimental to good health and good looks.

Quick Pep Breakfast

Beat two fresh raw egg yolks into a glass of orange juice or any other unsweetened fruit juice. This makes an ideal breakfast or lunch for those poor souls who have to eat and run!

German Egg Tonic

Beat one fresh egg yolk into half a glass of sherry. Sip through straw. German doctors consider fresh egg yolk the richest source of lecithin, and prescribe this brain and nerve tonic for a quick pick-up.

French Omelet

½ cup fresh milk
4 eggs

2 tbsp. powdered milk
½ tsp. vegetable salt

Mix all ingredients until smooth. Pour in oiled heavy pan. With the French thermos cover you can make the fluffiest, lightest omelets in a matter of moments. If you use an ordinary frying pan, be sure to separate the eggs and beat the whites until fluffy. In France, when omelets are eaten for dessert, sweetened fruits or marmalades are added just before the omelet is folded.

Henrici's Egg Pancake

½ cup fresh milk
3 fresh eggs
½ cup whole-wheat flour

3 tbsp. powdered milk
2 tbsp. golden oil
½ tsp. vegetable salt

Mix all ingredients in a bowl, or preferably a blender; then pour into oiled pie tin (be sure it is cold). Bake at high heat for 10 minutes, then lower heat to about 350° F. Bake for 10 more minutes. Such a puffed-up pancake is a delight. It makes an ideal Sunday breakfast served with lean ham or bacon. The chef at Henrici's in Chicago kept this delightful recipe a deep, dark secret for many years. Now it is yours!

Protein Soups—a Meal in a Cup

When meats and eggs are expensive, it is quite a problem for the homemaker with a large family to get 20 to 30 grams of protein into each person at each meal. Here is where fresh and powdered skim milk can be most helpful. With them you can make many delightful soups. If you have a blender in your kitchen, there are dozens of cream soups you can make on a moment's notice. One cup of such a gourmet soup can give each member of the family 30 grams of good protein.

Potage au crème

The million dollar secret of a French chef's *potage au crème* is the gentle sautéing of finely cut-up or grated vegetables in mild butter or vegetable oil. Leek and onion soups are great favorites in France, but any vegetables—spinach, parsley, watercress, carrots, celery, mushrooms, young peas, and avocados—singly or in combination, make a meal in a cup in a matter of minutes. A level tablespoon of good-tasting brewers' yeast adds another 6 grams of good protein to each cup. Here is what you need for one serving:

½ cup shredded or grated raw vegetables (carrot, celery, spinach, parsley, etc.)
2 tsp. grated onion
1 tbsp. golden oil or margarine

1 cup fresh milk (8 grams of protein)
⅓ cup powdered skim milk (22 grams of protein)
1 tbsp. brewers' yeast (6 grams of protein)

Sauté the chopped or grated vegetables and the onion in the heated oil or margarine. Be sure to use low heat; do not allow the margarine to get brown. Stir constantly. Put the sautéed vegetables, the liquid milk, the dry milk, and the dry yeast into the blender. Blend for about 15 seconds. Pour into a double boiler and cook for 2 minutes; do not allow to boil. Season to taste before serving.

The onion improves the taste for most people, but it may be omitted. When using celery, remove the outside "strings."

Potage Hippocrates

If you are allergic to milk drinks of all kinds, learn to make nourishing soups and broths with meat stock, chicken broth, bouillon cubes, or dry brewers' yeast. The oldest of all vegetable broths was created five hundred years before Christ by Hippocrates, the wise Greek physician. He recommended that a rich mineral broth be made with carrots, celery root, parsley, and, especially, leek. Here is the ancient formula:

1 cup chopped or grated carrots	1 cup chopped leek
1 cup chopped or grated celery root	½ cup chopped parsley

Put all vegetables into 1½ quarts of water and simmer slowly for 30 minutes. This makes a rich combination of the water-soluble vitamins B and C. When Americans make Potage Hippocrates they add some onion, tomato, and other flavorsome vegetables, and season it with vegetable salt. On beautyfarms they add a tablespoon of celery-flavored brewers' yeast and call it their Complexion Broth.

Hi-Vi Mineral Broth

This is the most popular of all the "alkaline broths." When I created this in 1922, it was called Potassium Broth. This clear broth was based on the Hippocrates formula, which he recommended to all those who felt "under par." My broth is now used on many beautyfarms. It is also a part of my Seven-Day Elimination Diet (see page 415), which has become extremely popular as a one-week "housecleaning." Thousands of my students the world over take this diet in the spring, when all nature turns green and glad and when vegetables are at their best.

Here is the formula:

1 cup finely shredded celery, leaves and all	1 qt. water
1 cup finely shredded carrots	1 cup tomato juice
½ cup shredded spinach	1 tsp. vegetable salt
1 tbsp. shredded parsley	1 tsp. brown sugar or honey

Put all shredded vegetables into a quart of water. Cover and cook slowly for 30 minutes. Then add thick tomato juice (or tomatoes), vegetable salt, and honey or brown sugar. Let cook for 5 more minutes. Strain and serve. A sprinkle of chopped parsley or chives will add vitamins, minerals, and color. If you have no facilities for making this broth, you can get it in powder form at your diet and health shop.

California Soup

4 cups chicken broth (can be made   1 large or 2 small avocados
with cubes)

Heat the broth to boiling point. Transfer to blender and add the peeled and pitted avocado. Blend for 15 seconds. Serve immediately in heated bowls. A sprinkle of curry powder is a delightful addition.

Giuseppe's Nutritious Broth

Into each bowl of hot clear vegetable broth, stir one fresh egg yolk. Sprinkle with a bit of finely chopped basil or oregano. When unexpected guests arrive in my home, my clever chef fills them up with a cup of this delicious broth. It always makes a big hit.

Silemi Lemon Soup—Exciting and Delicious

When Mr. and Mrs. Joe Lambert, of Dallas, Texas, visited my new home, Casa Silemi, in Sicily recently, the lovely Mrs. Lambert kindly offered to make lunch for me and my guests, after she saw all the fresh things growing in profusion in my garden. (This delicious and unusual lemon soup was only the first course. It was followed by Sicilian Piccadillo (page 458) which makes a delightful party dish—guests always rave and want the recipe.

12 cups chicken stock   10 lemon wedges (including
8 medium cucumbers   rind)
                                  yogurt

Prepare chicken stock in advance, or use cubes or concentrate. Peel and remove all seeds from the cucumbers and cook them until soft in barely enough water to cover. Pass the cucumbers through mixer. Then add the cucumbers to the chicken stock and mix thoroughly. Pass the mixture through blender again, adding one lemon wedge for each cup of the mixture. Blend until lemon is thoroughly minced. Spike with vegetable salt and chill before serving. Just before serving, top each cup of soup with a teaspoon of yogurt. (Serves 10.)

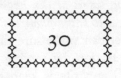

30

Sunlit Food

"Un giorno senza verdura é comme un giorno senza sole. A day without green things is like a day without sunshine." That's what they say in the sunny Mediterranean countries, and how right they are! It's the fresh green growing things that are loaded with sun energy. The sun makes them "living foods," which are of greatest importance in a high-vitality diet. American food scientists emphasize, and rightly so, the importance of more protein in our daily meals; but some of them neglect to stress the importance of the fresh green things. European food scientists insist that *frischkost* —fresh leaves, fruits, and seeds—contain the greatest health potential of any foods, and should be the mainstay of a healthy diet.

Forty years of research, teaching, and traveling all over the world has convinced me that the secret of any successful diet lies in its balance. And in balance there is strength. The ideal diet is one with good amounts of protein plus good amounts of fresh growing "living things"—our fresh vegetables and fruits.

Salads Are Protective Foods

Fresh tender salads should be eaten as a first course. In this way they protect us against overeating, against vitamin-mineral deficiencies, against constipation, against overweight; and they are the best insurance against excessive acidity. *If the alkaline-tablet slaves would eat a good salad at the beginning of the meal, they could say goodbye forever to their alkalizers!*

Any good homemaker can make sure that every member of her family gets health protection by serving the salad first. At the beginning of the meal, appetite is keenest; and the salad makes a good foundation for the meal to follow. Just make sure that salad vegetables are fresh and crisp. The green leaves, whether you use lettuce, escarole, or Bibb, should be washed *and dried*.

French and Italian chefs are masters in making delicious salads. They consider it an insult to their guests if the salad dressing does not adhere to the leaves. This is their secret: After the salad leaves are washed and broken (by hand) in small pieces, they *must* be dried. If you have traveled abroad you may have seen French peasants swinging wire baskets filled with lettuce, escarole, watercress, field salad, etc., shaking off every bit of water. (You now can buy such wire baskets in the United States.) Salad oils will cling to dry leaves, sealing in the chlorophyll, preventing the leaves from wilting, and keeping the salad fresh and crisp.

If you are lucky enough to have your own herb garden, cut some fresh mint leaves into half a cup of finely chopped chives, parsley, and young green onion tops. Put these in your wooden salad bowl with lettuce or romaine. Splash with your favorite golden oil and toss with a wooden spoon and fork until the salad shines like green gold.

Instead of always using the loud-mouthed garlic, spike your salad bowl with a tablespoon of minced fresh basil, watercress, chopped green pepper, or fragrant mint leaves.

Put the green leaves and other vegetables in the salad bowl, add the golden oil, and toss the greens until they are coated with oil. It is this tossing, lifting, and mixing of salad vegetables with the oil, which takes only a few seconds, that makes a salad a delight instead of a punishment. Then add the vinegar or lemon juice (the French use three parts oil to one part vinegar), and the salt, spices, and herbs. Toss lightly once more, and serve immediately.

Dress all salads well with golden oils. Season with vegetable salt and serve at once—while the herbs are still speaking to you.

Try These Delicious Salad-Bowl Combinations

Leaf lettuce, Bibb lettuce, watercress
Head lettuce, escarole, and Belgian endive
Tomatoes, green peppers, parsley, and avocado
Cucumber, artichokes, radishes, and watercress
Apples, cabbage, celery, and fresh mint
Carrots, celery root, and field salad
Chopped red cabbage and red apples
Chopped young beets, green peas, and onions
Chopped romaine lettuce, grated cauliflower, and radishes
Chopped carrots, green peppers, parsley, and celery
Chopped fresh or unsweetened pineapple, red cabbage, and parsley
Chopped Swiss chard, grated carrots, and onions
Young spinach, cabbage, and watercress
Thinly sliced Spanish onion, chicory, and spinach
Green apples, radishes, and watercress
Cucumbers, tomatoes, and avocados
Chopped endive, sliced beets, and watercress
Cabbage, carrots, celery, and fennuchi (anise)

These salad-bowl combinations are especially good when served with meat or other good proteins. Italians and many Californians and Floridians have discovered that salad bowls can be created with infinite variety.

Luncheons Fit for a King

Luncheon time should be salad time for many reasons. It gives us a chance to combine our two most important groups of foods: the proteins and the fresh, green, growing things. Such salad bowls are available at all good restaurants, but you will also want to make them at home. Always make a bed of greens, breaking them into bits by hand. Add vegetables, raw or cooked, and chopped fine. Then add any of your favorite proteins, depending on your taste and pocketbook—half a cup or more of tuna fish, salmon, lean ham,

Swiss cheese, chicken, hard-cooked eggs—all make delightful lunch-eon dishes. Or you can use any leftover meat or, still better, use cottage cheese or homemade cream cheese. The protein in these cheeses is just as valuable as that in meat. Mix your protein and salad greens with at least a tablespoon of golden oil dressing. All you need with such a salad is one slice of wholesome bread or toast—whole-wheat, gluten, soya, or rye. A glass of milk, butter-milk, yogurt, or Swiss coffee, and you have a nourishing luncheon, fit for a king!

Golden Vegetable Oils Galore

All diets or cookbooks that still recommend hydrogenated and animal fats, plus large quantities of butter, should be taken off the market. They do untold damage. One of my main concerns is to reduce the use of hard fats to a minimum and increase the use of our many golden vegetable oils. Research has proved that constant use of the hard saturated fats is conducive to high cholesterol levels, which can cause such serious conditions as heart trouble, strokes, gross overweight, and many other unfortunate problems. For cook-ing and baking purposes, the partially hardened vegetable-oil marga-rines may be used; but the fresh cold-pressed golden oils are much better for all purposes. Not only are they anticholesterol, they also help to avoid dry hair, dry skin, fat hips, and fat stomachs when used correctly. Years ago, a German chemist announced that a truly beautiful woman's fat content should be 11 percent of her total volume. He was referring to that most important fatty acid which we know today as linoleic acid. It is found in varying amounts in our golden vegetable oils. Take your choice.

Percentages of the important linoleic acid in oils:

Safflower	70	Sesame	41
Poppyseed	62	Avocado	39
Sunflower	57	Peanut	25
Soybean	53	Linseed	20
Corn	53	Sardine	15
Wheat germ	50	Olive	10
Cottonseed	50		

Use any of these oils singly, if you like. However, better results have been reported by my students when they combined several of the oils into a delightful golden oil dressing. Safflower oil is a great favorite, but it becomes rancid quickly. The other oils seem to be more stable. Sesame oil is mildest in flavor. Sunflower oil is probably the easiest to keep. In Germany, linseed oil, which is quite strong-flavored, is very popular; and in France, they prefer olive oil mixed with cold-pressed peanut oil. No matter what oil you use, be sure it is cold-pressed. These oils are worth looking for in your diet and health shops. Please make your dressings fresh and keep them refrigerated. Last, and very important, *the use of vegetable oils increases the need for vitamin E, so be sure to add a tablespoon of fresh wheat-germ oil whenever you make a batch of golden oil dressing or mayonnaise.*

Homemade Vinegar

If you can buy pure unadulterated apple cider, you can easily make your own full-strength vinegar. Simply go to your nearest Farmers' Market and buy a gallon jug of freshly pressed apple cider. Put the gallon jug in a warm place and remove the cork. In a few weeks time you will have a full-bodied wholesome vinegar. Taste it from time to time. When sourness is according to your taste, filter and put in quart bottles.

Swiss Herb Vinegar

Put your favorite herbs into pure apple or wine vinegar. The Swiss prefer a mixture of dill, mint, and tarragon. (Remove leaves from stems.) To get a full-bodied delightful *Krauter Essig,* just put 1 cup each of fresh dill, mint, and tarragon leaves, equal amounts, in a gallon of vinegar. Place bottles in a warm and sunny place and cork tightly. After 3 or 4 weeks, strain; put into clean bottles and cork tightly.

Golden Oil Salad Dressing

½ cup sunflower oil	1 tbsp. wheat-germ oil
½ cup peanut oil	2 tsp. honey
½ cup olive oil	2 tsp. vegetable salt
½ cup cider, wine, or herb vinegar	1 clove garlic

Place all ingredients in a covered jar and shake vigorously. You can give it a different flavor every time you make it by adding your choice of: 2 tablespoons of chopped fresh parsley, fresh chives, fresh mint, mild onion, or dried herbs; half a teaspoon of oregano or curry powder; 1 teaspoon dried mustard; 2 tablespoons of Roquefort cheese; 2 tablespoons chopped ripe olives. Use your imagination. There is absolutely no limit to the number of delightful salad dressing combinations you can enjoy. The million dollar secret of this dressing is that it contains *everything*—all the essential fatty acids, plus lecithin and vitamin E—and it tastes delicious. Should it be too rich for your taste or your pocketbook, do not hesitate to use some of the less expensive oils; but do be sure they are cold-pressed and fresh.

French 14-Carat Gold Mayonnaise

½ cup olive oil
½ cup peanut oil
 1 tbsp. wheat-germ oil

2 fresh dark egg yolks
1 tbsp. wine vinegar
½ tsp. vegetable salt

Mix oils in a measuring cup. Place fresh egg yolks in cold bowl and beat. Add a little oil very slowly and beat with rotary beater. Gradually add more oil. As mixture thickens, add vinegar and salt. Beat until thick and golden.

French Yogurt Dressing

Mix 4 tablespoons of yogurt with 4 tablespoons of French 14-Carat Gold Mayonnaise. Beat to consistency of heavy cream. Add a tablespoon of finely chopped carrots or parsley. This is particularly good with freshly chopped raw vegetables.

Avocado Dressing

1 cup avocado pulp
1 cup thick yogurt
1 tbsp. honey

1 tbsp. avocado oil
¼ tsp. vegetable salt
spike with favorite herbs

Place all ingredients in blender for one minute. This mixture is especially delicious with citrus and fruit salads.

Sunlit Appetizers

That is what they call their fresh young growing things along the balmy Mediterranean. You and your guests can eat these with good conscience. They are not only healthful, they are the most beautiful and sophisticated appetizers or hors d'oeuvres you can serve. A plateful of raw vegetable tidbits is served with a bowl containing a nutritious dip made from fresh yogurt, cream cheese, or cottage cheese, or a combination of all three, blended with fresh lemon juice, onion juice, chopped chives or dill, a tablespoon of golden vegetable oil, plus any of your favorite fresh or dry herbs. The dip should be stiff enough to cling to the vegetables without dripping. There are literally hundreds of recipes for dips. Just use your imagination. Add your seasonings a little at a time, and keep tasting until you have a delightful aromatic blend. For more fun and nutrition, try adding minced olives or clams or a mashed avocado.

You will be surprised at the number of vegetables that can be served: fresh raw carrots, cauliflower, sweet green or red peppers, celery, turnip, small zucchini, cucumber, young asparagus tips, tiny cherry tomatoes, red and white radishes, Belgian endive, mushrooms, Chinese cabbage, Italian fennuchi, and—for strictly family gatherings—green onions! The carrots, zucchinis, cucumbers, and peppers should be cut the long way into slim fingers. Cut the cauliflower into small knobs, always leaving a piece of the stem to serve as a handle. Put ice cubes over the vegetables to crisp them before serving and to preserve the vitamins.

Sunlit Food Needs Little Cooking

Fresh garden vegetables have the greatest health and beauty potential when served raw. A raw, fresh salad is a must with every big meal. Cooked vegetables, delicious as they are, should play a secondary role in a high-vitality diet. If the budget is limited, a good protein dish with a large salad makes an excellent meal. Of course, there is no reason why you should not also enjoy cooked vegetables. Just remember: The less you cook them, the richer they remain in vitamins and enzymes.

The Chinese, more than any other people, know the art of undercooking. For centuries they have cooked their vegetables in the quickest and most appetizing manner in a heavy, hot pan. No saturated fats are ever used; instead, they use such golden oils as soybean, sesame, or poppyseed. Everybody agrees that such short-cooked vegetables taste much better than the watersoaked, overcooked variety. The big secret in short-cooking is to cut the vegetables in small pieces or slices, and place them as quickly as possible in a very hot utensil; and, so the vegetable will not burn, put two or three tablespoons of chicken broth, vegetable water, or just plain water in the pan and drop the finely cut vegetables into this steaming liquid. Keep utensil covered for 2 or 3 minutes; let the steam tenderize the vegetable. When thoroughly tenderized, add a tablespoon of golden vegetable oil or sunbutter (see page 33) for each cup of vegetable. Spike with soy sauce, vegetable salt, and any herbs you desire.

LEAFY VEGETABLES

Pick over spinach, beet tops, turnip tops, and all green, leafy vegetables while dry. Then put the greens in a large pan and let the cold water run until greens are clean and crisp. Place them in a hot, heavy cooking utensil. Greens usually contain enough water of their own and do not require added water for short-cooking. Cook, keeping utensil covered for 2 or 3 minutes; then add golden vegetable oil, sunbutter, or nonhydrogenated margarine. Spike with vegetable salt and herbs.

Golden Carrots

Scrub them until they shine like gold. Then shred them medium (not too fine). Have 2 or 3 tablespoons of chicken broth steaming in hot utensil. Add shredded carrots. Cover for 3 minutes or until tenderized, but not soft and soggy. Add a tablespoon of golden oil for each cup of carrots, and sprinkle with vegetable salt. These carrots will still be a bit chewy and keep their golden color; and they are unbelievably delicious.

Rose Petal Beets

Select small young beets. Scrub, and shred on medium shredder. Heat a small heavy pan, and add 3 tablespoons of chicken or vegetable broth. When liquid is steaming, add shredded beets. Cover tightly and cook for about 5 minutes, depending on tenderness of beets. Then add sunbutter or golden oil, and sprinkle with vegetable salt. Short-cooked beets keep their rose-petal color and have a nutlike flavor all of their own.

Easy-to-Digest Cabbage

Shred young white or red cabbage on coarse shredder. Heat small heavy utensil and add 3 tablespoons of steaming broth. Place cabbage in pan and keep tightly covered. Young cabbage cooks in 3 to 5 minutes, and is easy to digest. All you add is a little vegetable salt and a bit of sunbutter or golden oil.

Delicious Cauliflower

Select a young white cauliflower. Shred on coarse blade. (Shred not only the flower but the whole stem.) Have heavy small utensil steaming with 3 tablespoons of vegetable or chicken broth. Drop in the white shreds and let cook, tightly covered, for about 4 to 6 minutes. They will cook tender but still chewy, and the shreds will keep their appetizing white color. Now add vegetable salt and a bit of sunbutter, and enjoy this new delicious flavor.

Young String Beans

Tender green or yellow beans can be finely shredded lengthwise and placed in small, heavy, hot utensil with 3 tablespoons of steaming broth. Cook tightly covered about 7 minutes. When tender, add golden oil or sunbutter and vegetable salt.

Elegant Beans Amandine

Short-cook the youngest and smallest green beans obtainable. In another iron skillet, toast coarsely chopped or slivered almonds to a golden brown. Sprinkle the toasted almonds over the very hot beans and serve at once. Any meal becomes a banquet with such a festive vegetable. I first ate these beans amandine at the Bel-Air home of that famous hostess Marian Mill Preminger, and I therefore dedicate this recipe to her.

Italian Zucchini

Select small zucchini; do not peel, only scrub with a brush. Slice thin or shred on coarse shredder. Put 3 tablespoons of vegetable or chicken broth in small heavy utensil; when broth steams, add shredded zucchini and cook, tightly covered, for only 3 to 5 minutes. Add golden oil or sunbutter and sprinkle with vegetable salt.

Easy Eggplant

Wash but do not peel young, tender eggplant. Shred on coarse shredder. Cook in heavy covered pot in 2 tablespoons of steaming hot vegetable or chicken broth for about 5 minutes. Then add golden oil and your favorite seasonings.

Eggplant Toast

Cut unpeeled eggplant into half-inch slices. Put under slow broiler and toast until golden brown. Spike with vegetable salt. Delicious under poached eggs. A favorite on sophisticated beauty-farms.

Onions Sauté

2 medium-sized mild onions, thinly sliced	2 tbsp. golden oil ¼ tsp. vegetable salt

Heat oil in heavy cooking utensil, add onions, and sauté. Cover pan, reduce heat, and let cook for about 5 minutes or until the onions are tender; then sprinkle with vegetable salt and serve.

Mushrooms Sauté

½ lb. fresh mushrooms 2 tbsp. golden oil	¼ tsp. vegetable salt

Heat oil in heavy utensil, add mushrooms, and stir in oil for 1 minute. Reduce the heat, cover, and cook for 5 more minutes. Add salt and serve hot.

DELIGHTFUL CHINESE DISHES

In recent years superior Chinese restaurants have sprung up like mushrooms in almost every city in America. Two famous ones are the Beachcomber's in Hollywood and Trader Vic's in San Francisco—a cuisine which is a combination of Cantonese, Hawaiian, and South Sea Island cookery. On a recent visit to the Hollywood Beachcomber I was invited to visit their kitchen, which is a marvel of modern efficiency. Chinese cookery requires a maximum of preparation and a minimum of cooking time and fuel. At the Beach-comber's there are bowls of neatly sliced and stacked vegetables (celery, bamboo shoots, water chestnuts, spinach, etc.), fresh and crisp, bowls full of sliced lean meats, all in refrigerators within easy reach of the chef. Upon receipt of an order, it takes him only a few seconds to select his ingredients, a skillful blending of meats and vegetables, and within ten or fifteen minutes a delicious meal is ready to serve. Only golden oils are used, never any hard fat. When necessary, a small amount of broth is added; seasonings such as soy sauce, vegetable salt, and monosodium glutamate are always added last.

Most Chinese recipes require too many special ingredients to make them popular. However, there is no reason why we should not include a few Chinese-type recipes to give spice and variety to our meals. Among my favorites (and the simplest to prepare) are Egg Foo Yong, Chicken with Vegetables, Lobster and Vegetables, Pepper Steak, and Chicken and Cucumber. Here are the recipes, which are easy to prepare:

Egg Foo Yong

2½ cups bean sprouts
3 green onions
6 water chestnuts
3 oz. mushrooms

1 cup finely chopped cooked chicken, shrimp, or lobster
5 eggs
peanut or soya oil

Toss drained bean sprouts in a small amount of flour; slice onions, water chestnuts, and mushrooms very thin; mix chopped meat and vegetables. Beat eggs lightly and stir in mixture of meat and vegetables. Heat oil in heavy skillet. Fry one ladleful of batter at a time, using medium heat. Fry each side about 3 or 4 minutes or until golden brown. Place in a warm oven until ready to serve. Add salt and seasoning to taste.

Dow-Jay-Gai (Chicken with Vegetables)

½ lb. string beans
2 tbsp. oil
1 lb. cooked chicken
⅛ lb. fresh mushrooms
1 cup celery

1 cup celery cabbage
1 cup chicken bouillon
2 tbsp. cornstarch
2 tsp. soy sauce
¼ cup water

Cut string beans into ½-inch pieces and short-cook until tender.

Preheat heavy pan containing 2 tablespoons of oil. Add chicken cut into thin slices. Slice and add mushrooms. Dice and add celery. Add celery cabbage, cut into ¼-inch pieces. Add chicken bouillon. Cover pan tightly and cook over moderate flame for 5 minutes. Add cooked string beans. Blend together and add 2 tablespoons cornstarch, 2 teaspoons soy sauce, and ¼ cup water. Cook for a few more minutes, stirring constantly, until the juice thickens. Add seasoning to taste.

Choy-Loong-Har (Lobster and Vegetables)

1 lb. green peas
1 cup diced carrots
2 tsp. oil
2 tbsp. onion, finely diced
1 clove garlic, diced
½ cup green pepper, diced
½ cup celery, diced
1 cup chicken bouillon
½ lb. lobster meat
2 tbsp. cornstarch
2 tsp. soy sauce
¼ cup water

Cook shelled peas and diced carrots separately. Preheat heavy pan containing 2 teaspoons of oil; add finely diced onions, garlic, green pepper, and celery. Add chicken bouillon. Cut lobster meat into small pieces and add. Cook over a moderate flame for 5 minutes, stirring constantly. Add cooked peas and carrots. Blend together and add 2 tablespoons cornstarch, 2 teaspoons soy sauce, and ¼ cup of water. Cook for a few more minutes, stirring constantly until juice thickens. Add seasoning to taste. Serve very hot with fluffy rice.

Pepper Steak

1 lb. round steak
1 tsp. brown sugar
3 tbsp. soy sauce
2 tsp. soy or peanut oil
1 medium onion, sliced
2 cloves garlic, minced
4 stalks celery, cut in slices
2 green peppers, cut in small squares
1 tbsp. cornstarch
2 tbsp. water

Cut meat into thin slices. Mix with brown sugar and soy sauce. Heat oil in a heavy pan. Add onion and garlic, and cook until onion is golden. Add meat. Cover and cook 8 minutes. Add vegetables; combine cornstarch with water, stir until smooth, and add. Cover and cook 10 minutes longer. Serve immediately over brown rice.

Chicken and Cucumber

1 double chicken breast
2½ tbsp. soy sauce
1 small onion, chopped
¾ tsp. powdered ginger
2 tsp. oil
½ lb. mushrooms, sliced

1 lb. fresh peas, shelled
½ cup consommé
½ cucumber, unpeeled
1 tbsp. cornstarch
2 tbsp. water

Cut chicken into thin slices. Mix with soy sauce, onion, and ginger. Heat oil in a pan. Add mushrooms and cook, covered, for 5 minutes. Remove and set aside. Place chicken mixture in pan with peas and consommé. Cover and cook 10 minutes. Cut cucumber in half, lengthwise, then in ¼ inch slices. Combine cornstarch and water and stir until smooth. Combine all ingredients and cook, covered, 5 minutes.

Chinese Rice

3 eggs
4 cups cold boiled rice (at least one
    day old)
4 chopped scallions

½ cup diced cooked chicken,
    turkey, veal, or lamb
1 cup chopped parsley
2 tbsp. soy sauce
1 tsp. vegetable salt

Beat eggs. Heat a little oil in skillet. Toss in rice and sauté until hot. Stir and gently press out all the lumps. Add chopped scallions and meat, and mix thoroughly. Stir a hollow in center of the mixture and pour in the eggs. When eggs are semicooked, resume stirring until rice and eggs are blended. Stir in parsley, soy sauce, and salt.

While on the subject of Oriental cooking, we should not overlook the Japanese, who have given the world at least one famous dish—Sukiyaki. I have dined at excellent Japanese restaurants in Los Angeles, San Francisco, Seattle, and New York. One of the best is Miyako, on West 56th Street in New York. But Sukiyaki is also easily made at home.

Sukiyaki—Japan's National Dish

Heat a heavy iron skillet. When the pan is hot, add 2 or 3 tablespoons of soy oil. Then add the meat and chopped vegetables. The meat should be very thinly sliced lean raw beef or chicken; the vegetables, onions, both Bermuda and green, celery, and spinach. Slice the Bermuda onions thin, and cut the green onions into 2-inch sections. Cut the celery into 2-inch sections and then cut them the long way into strips. Place all ingredients into the pan at the same time. The steam begins to rise immediately and in a few minutes you can see the meat change color and the vegetables begin to soften. At this time you add a small amount of broth and 2 tablespoons of soy sauce, and continue cooking for about 10 minutes. Covering the pan during cooking will speed up cooking time, preserve the color of the vegetables, and prevent loss of vitamin C. The Japanese usually add little squares of soybean curd cheese (Tofu) which resembles a thick salty custard; although it is a good source of protein, it is not essential when the Sukiyaki contains meat.

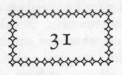

Wholesome Carbohydrates

When you load too much coal on a fire, you choke it. And when you load too many empty carbohydrates on your body fire—metabolism—you also choke it. The human body does not know what to do with an excess of foodless starches and sweets, and so it simply dumps them in the form of excess body fat. That's why over-refined empty carbohydrates are great trouble-makers. If the two chief offenders, the white-flour products and the white-sugar products, were to be taken out of our supermarkets, there would be a tremendous increase in the health and vitality of our people, and 80 percent of our overweighters would shed their blankets of fat.

However, this does not mean that healthy people should not enjoy the *wholesome* carbohydrates as nature prepares them in our *golden* grains and sugars. When man does not tamper with these, they are loaded with vitamins, minerals, and enzymes, and can be handled (burned) with ease by any healthy human body.

Here are some recipes prepared with the wholesome natural carbohydrates that you and your family can enjoy with good conscience.

A New Look at Bread

Nothing else can so quickly create a delightful homey atmosphere as the baking of wholesome bread. There was a time when life was less hectic, and most homemakers took pride in their own fragrant bread. You may remember, as I do, the aroma of freshly baked bread greeting you when you came home from school. In Sicily, where I am writing this, my cook is now making our own homemade bread, with all the goodness of the grain as it comes from the field. Let me give you a simple version of this delightful 100-percent natural bread. It's easy to make.

Hearty Whole-Wheat Bread (#1)

1 pkg. dry yeast (1 oz.)
1 qt. potato water or warm
  milk

1 tbsp. honey
3 lbs. fresh whole-wheat flour
1 tsp. vegetable salt

Place dry yeast with a bit of potato water and the honey in a warm cup. Put aside for 10 to 20 minutes. Place flour and salt in a large bowl and mix with a big spoon. Little by little, work in the yeast mixture and the rest of the potato water. When well blended, pour mixture into two or three well-oiled bread pans and place in a warm spot. When the dough mixture rises, close to the top of the bread pans, bake at 350° F. for one hour. This is a hearty, nutritious bread. The potato water helps to keep it firm and moist.

Hearty Whole-Wheat Bread (#2)

Here is another delightful bread you should bake for your family:

2½ cups whole-wheat flour
3 tbsp. fresh wheat germ
3 tbsp. soy flour
4 tbsp. powdered skim milk
2 tbsp. brown sugar

1 tsp. vegetable salt
½ cake yeast (½ oz.)
1 cup lukewarm water
1 tbsp. golden oil

Into a large bowl put whole-wheat flour (preferably stone-ground), fresh wheat germ, soy flour, powdered skim milk, brown sugar, and vegetable salt. Dissolve yeast in lukewarm water, and add this to the dry ingredients. Add golden oil. Mix thoroughly until you have a smooth dough; put it in an oiled bowl, and cover. Let rise in a warm place 1½ hours; punch down, and let rise 20 minutes more. Knead into a compact loaf and put into a large bread pan; cover, and let stand in a warm place. When dough has again risen to top of bread pan, bake for about 40 minutes at 400° F.

El Molino Bread—Fast and Delicious

If you are too busy or too lazy to follow the above recipes, I suggest you go to your nearest diet and health food shop and ask for the new El Molino Ready Mix. This is a delightful mixture containing stone-ground whole-wheat flour, unbleached flour, sesame flour, honey, skim milk, brown sugar, plus a fast-acting yeast, and even a bright, shiny bread pan. All you do is add water and bake.

This combination of ground fresh sesame seed and high-protein whole-wheat offers you an entirely new experience in bread eating. For real honest-to-goodness bread, I invite you to try this ready mix—nothing could be simpler! Most health and diet shops carry this exciting new product. If yours does not, drop a card to El Molino Mills, Alhambra, California. You might also ask about soy flour, quick-cooked soybeans, soy grits, and the delicious carob flour which this progressive firm introduced to America.

Famous Cornell Bread

1 pkg. dry granular yeast or 1 oz. compressed yeast	¼ cup sugar
	⅓ cup soy flour
¼ cup warm water (lukewarm for compressed yeast)	½ cup dry skim milk
	¼ cup fresh wheat germ
5 cups unbleached flour	1 tbsp. golden oil
1 tbsp. salt	1¾ cups water

Dissolve yeast in ¼ cup water. Combine dry ingredients in mixing bowl. Add dissolved yeast, oil, and water, mixing to blend well. Knead dough until smooth and satiny, then place in well-greased bowl. Cover, and allow to rise in a warm place for about 1½ hours. Punch down by plunging fist into center of dough, then fold over the edges of dough and turn the dough upside down. Cover and allow to rise again for 15 to 20 minutes. Shape into two loaves and place in oiled pans. Cover and allow to stand in warm place for about 55 to 60 minutes or until dough rises and fills pans. Bake at 400° F. for 45 minutes.

Grant Loaf from England—A New Idea

This bread needs no kneading and is a great time-saver. This popular English whole-wheat bread is from Doris Grant's fine book, *Your Bread and Your Life.*

3 lbs. whole-wheat flour	4 cups warm water
2 tsp. salt	2 tsp. dark molasses
1 oz. fresh yeast	

Mix flour with salt. Mix yeast in a small bowl with 1 cup of water. Let stand for 10 minutes or so, then pour this into the flour with the remaining 3 cups of water and the molasses. Mix well by hand for several minutes until dough feels elastic and leaves sides of bowl clean. Divide dough into three parts and place in three 1-quart bread pans which have been warmed and oiled. Cover pans with a cloth and leave in a warm place to rise by about one-third. Bake in a hot oven (about 450° F.) for 35 to 40 minutes.

Hi-Protein Gluten Bread—Easy to Make

1 cake yeast (1 oz.)	2 tsp. vegetable salt
2 cups lukewarm water	3 cups gluten flour
1 tbsp. golden oil	

Dissolve yeast in water and gradually add oil, salt, and gluten flour. Knead until mixture is smooth. Put in oiled bowl. Let rise until light, about 1½ hours. Then punch and knead again. Shape into small loaves and place in oiled pans. Cover, let rise until double in bulk (about 45 minutes). Bake at 400° F. for 40 minutes.

Milwaukee Rye Bread

2 cakes yeast	4 cups rye flour
2 cups lukewarm potato water	4 cups unbleached wheat flour
1 cup riced potatoes, solidly packed	1 tbsp. caraway seed
3 tsp. vegetable salt	

Dissolve yeast in ¼ cup lukewarm potato water. Add riced potatoes and salt to remaining 1¾ cups lukewarm potato water. Combine and blend the two mixtures. Combine both kinds of flour and caraway seed. Stir dry ingredients into liquid. When dough is no longer sticky to the touch, knead until smooth and elastic on a floured board. Then let rise, in oiled bowl, until doubled in bulk. Punch down, and divide dough into two parts. Knead each another minute or two, and form into loaves. Put into 2 oiled 4½ × 8½ × 2½ inch bread pans. When doubled in bulk, bake at 375° F. about 1 hour.

Sourdough Rye Bread

Place 1 cup of Milwaukee Rye Bread dough in a small stone crock. Cover, and let ferment. When baking a fresh batch of Milwaukee Rye Bread, set aside ½ cup of the fresh dough and replace it with ½ cup of sourdough. Then mix the ½ cup of fresh dough with the remaining ½ cup of sourdough to provide a starter for the next batch. Bake as above. This sourdough rye bread is a real stick-to-the-ribs bread, and it is most popular in Milwaukee.

Swedish Rye Crisps—A Delight for Dieters

2 cups sour milk
½ cup corn oil
½ cup honey
6 cups rye flour
2 tbsp. wheat germ
1 tsp. vegetable salt

Mix sour milk with oil and honey. Then add flour, wheat germ, and salt. Knead this stiff dough well. Roll out thin on floured board and cut into squares or triangles. Place on cookie sheets and bake at 400° F. for about 12 minutes.

Wheat Germ Sticks

2 cups whole-wheat flour
1¼ cups fresh milk
½ cup golden vegetable oil
2 cups fresh wheat germ
1 tbsp. honey
1 tsp. vegetable salt

Mix and knead all ingredients, then roll dough ¼ inch thick. Cut into sticks about ¼ inch wide and 5 inches long. Place on oiled cookie sheet. Sprinkle some of the sticks with caraway seeds and others with sesame seeds. Bake at 350° F. about 35 minutes, or until golden brown.

Hi-Protein Muffins

1½ cups soy flour
2 tsp. baking powder
1½ tsp. vegetable salt
2 fresh eggs
3 tbsp. brown sugar
1 tbsp. grated orange rind
1 cup milk
1 tbsp. golden oil
¼ cup floured raisins
¼ cup floured walnut meats

Sift together flour, baking powder, and salt. Separate eggs; beat yolks until very light and frothy. Beat sugar into the egg yolks, add orange rind, milk, and oil, and mix well. Pour the egg mixture into the dry ingredients and mix. Add raisins and nut meats, and mix thoroughly. Fold in whites, beaten stiff. Pour mixture into small muffin tins and bake in slow oven (300° F.) for about 30 minutes.

Important Note on Baking Powders: Whenever possible, use yeast as a leavening agent in your baking. Yeast adds nourishment. Whenever you must use baking powder, be sure you use one composed of tartaric acid (made from grapes) or phosphates. Get rid of any baking powder that contains aluminum derivatives. If you are unable to procure a wholesome baking powder, let your druggist combine the following:

Potassium bicarbonate	79.5 Grams
Cornstarch	56.0 Grams
Tartaric acid	15.0 Grams
Potassium bitartrate	112.25 Grams

Wheat Germ Muffins

2 fresh eggs
1 tsp. vegetable salt
1 tsp. brown sugar
½ cup golden oil

1½ cups milk
1½ cups whole-wheat flour
1 cup fresh wheat germ

Separate eggs. Beat yolks; add vegetable salt, brown sugar, and golden oil. Stir in milk, and add flour and fresh wheat germ. Fold in stiffly beaten egg whites. Bake in hot, oiled muffin tins at 350° F. for about 35 minutes.

Hi-Protein Popovers

¾ cup milk
2 eggs, beaten
¾ cup soy flour

¼ cup gluten flour
pinch vegetable salt
1 tbsp. wheat germ

Mix milk with eggs. Stir dry ingredients into the milk-egg mixture and mix thoroughly. Pour into well-oiled very hot popover pan. Bake at 450° F. for 30 minutes.

100-Percent Whole-wheat Rolls

½ cup milk, scalded
2 tbsp. golden oil
1 tbsp. honey
1 tsp. vegetable salt
½ cup warm water

1 cake compressed yeast
1 egg, beaten
3 cups whole-wheat flour
2 tbsp. fresh wheat germ

Make a mixture of scalded milk, golden oil, honey, and vegetable salt. Pour into this mixture ½ cup warm water. Then add in this order: crumbled yeast, beaten whole egg, whole-wheat flour (preferably stone-ground), and fresh wheat germ. Mix well, then let rise in warm place until bulk is doubled. Form into small rolls and place in oiled muffin pan. Bake at 400° F. for only 20 minutes.

Hi-Protein Beautyfarm Cake

2 eggs, beaten	½ tsp. vegetable salt
1 cup brown sugar	¾ tsp. cinnamon
⅓ cup whole-wheat flour	1 tbsp. cocoa
1⅓ cups soy flour	⅔ cup milk
1½ tsp. baking powder	⅓ cup golden oil

Beat the eggs, gradually adding the sugar; beat until very light. Sift the remaining dry ingredients together, and add to the egg mixture alternately with milk. Stir in oil. Pour into oiled shallow cake tin and bake in a moderate oven.

Nutritious Breakfast Puffs

1 yeast cake (1 oz.)	½ cup golden oil
¼ cup lukewarm water	2 eggs, well beaten
1 cup milk	3 cups whole-wheat flour
1 tsp. vegetable salt	2 tbsp. wheat germ
2 tbsp. brown sugar	2 tbsp. soy flour

Break yeast cake into lukewarm water. Scald milk, and add vegetable salt, brown sugar, and golden oil. Let cool until lukewarm, and add the yeast mixture. Stir in well-beaten eggs, add whole-wheat flour (sifted), wheat germ, and soy flour; and mix well. Set bowl in warm place and let rise for 1½ to 2 hours. Then drop by spoonfuls into oiled muffin pans, filling cups only half full.

¼ cup brown sugar	¼ cup chopped nutmeats
½ tsp. cinnamon	

Make a mixture of brown sugar, cinnamon, and chopped nuts, and sprinkle on tops of muffins. Let rise again until double in bulk, and bake in moderate oven (375° F.) for 25 minutes. Delicious for Sunday brunch.

Hi-Protein Waffles

1 yeast cake (1 oz.)	⅓ cup golden oil
2 cups buttermilk	1 tbsp. honey
3 eggs	⅓ cup dry skim milk
1 cup fresh wheat germ	1¼ cups whole-wheat flour
1 tsp. vegetable salt	

Put crumbled yeast into warm buttermilk. Separate egg yolks. To this mixture add egg yolks, wheat germ, vegetable salt, golden oil, and honey. Into these ingredients sift dry skim milk and whole-wheat flour. Mix well, then set bowl in a warm place and let rise for 1 to 2 hours. When bulk has doubled, stir with spoon. Then mix in stiffly-beaten egg whites and bake. Serve waffles hot, with honey or maple syrup. This recipe I dedicate to Virginia Fox Kennady, Director of Beautymasters, Detroit, Michigan.

CEREALS AND OTHER GRAINS

How to Cook Cereals While You Sleep

Before retiring, stir ½ cup of your favorite raw cereal—wheat, oats, rye, or buckwheat, preferably cracked—into 2 cups of salted boiling water. Stir for just 3 minutes, then pour into a wide-mouthed thermos bottle. Cork the bottle tightly. Next morning you will be greeted by a hot cereal, ready to be eaten with fresh milk and honey. For even more nourishment, cook cereal in milk instead of water. If fresh milk is not available, simply add ½ cup powdered skim milk to water. Serve with fresh milk and a sprinkle of honeyed wheat germ. (See below.)

Honeyed Wheat Germ

4 cups fresh wheat germ
½ cup honey

Pour wheat germ on large cookie tin and sprinkle with honey (also try maple sugar or molasses). Roast at 350° F. about 15 minutes or until golden brown. Store in a glass jar; and use it over hot or cold cereals. Many people who refuse to eat plain wheat germ love this toasted variety.

Kasha, a Special Grain

Kasha, or buckwheat groats, is an almost forgotten grain in America. In Russia it is one of the most important staple foods. It is high in energy and fairly high in protein; but most of all, it is a delicious and welcome change from rice and potatoes. Kasha is easy to cook. The whole kernel takes only about 20 minutes; the cracked ones take only 5 minutes. The Russian method is the simplest and leanest:

1 cup whole buckwheat groats (kasha)	2 cups water (if used for breakfast, otherwise chicken or beef broth)
½ tsp. vegetable salt	

Use heavy cooking utensil. Stir unwashed buckwheat groats into boiling liquid. Add salt, let boil for 1 or 2 minutes; then cover. Turn heat low and let simmer for 15 minutes, or until all liquid is absorbed. Every grain should be separate. Kasha must never be mushy!

My Favorite Method: Put 2 tablespoons of golden oil into heavy skillet. When oil is very hot, stir in 1 cup of buckwheat groats which have been mixed previously with a raw beaten egg. Add a teaspoon of vegetable salt. Finally add 2 cups of chicken broth, Hauser Broth, or vegetable water. Bring to a boil, then reduce heat; cover tightly and let cook until all liquid is absorbed, stirring occasionally.

Kashaburgers

These inexpensive and delicious kashaburgers make an excellent and different luncheon dish:

½ onion, finely chopped	1 egg, slightly beaten
1½ tsp. golden oil	1 tbsp. chopped nutmeats
2 cups cooked kasha (buckwheat groats)	

Sauté onion in oil to golden brown. Mix with kasha, egg, and nuts. Form into patties and sauté on hot oiled skillet, or drop heaping tablespoonfuls onto skillet. Sauté until golden brown.

Wholesome Boiled Rice

1 cup natural brown rice   1 tsp. vegetable salt
5 cups boiling water

Pick over rice and remove any husks and foreign particles. Put in a
wire strainer and rinse under cold running water to remove dust.
Bring water to boiling point, add rice, and boil briskly for 5 minutes. Turn heat low and simmer for 20 minutes. Turn off heat when
the rice is soft, add vegetable salt, and let stand over hot water until
any remaining water is absorbed, about an hour. The grains should
be whole and fluffy.

Swiss Rice Fondue

1 cup boiled brown rice   1 pimento, diced
½ cup grated Swiss cheese   2 eggs, separated
1 cup milk   ½ cup ground walnuts
1 tsp. vegetable salt

Mix together rice, cheese, milk, salt, and pimento. Beat egg yolks
until thick and lemon-colored, and combine with rice mixture. Beat
egg whites until stiff, but not dry, and fold lightly into rice mixture. Turn into a well-buttered baking dish. Sprinkle ground nuts
over the top and press them in a little so that they are moistened.
Bake in a moderate oven (350° F.) about 25 minutes, or until firm.
Serve garnished with parsley.

Golden Rice Pilaf

6 tbsp. golden oil   3 cups fat-free chicken broth
1½ cups brown rice   (or broth from chicken
½ tsp. saffron   bouillon cubes)
2 tsp. vegetable salt   ½ cup chopped sunflower
                                    seeds

Use a 2-quart heavy saucepan or flameproof casserole. Pour in
the oil. When it is hot, stir in the rice; cook, stirring, about 5 minutes. Sprinkle the saffron over the rice, stir well; add the seasonings, stirring continually. Add the broth and chopped seeds. Bring
to a boil. Cover, reduce heat, and cook until the rice is tender and
has absorbed the broth, about 15 to 20 minutes.

POTATOES CAN BE GOOD

Mashed versus "Smashed" Potatoes

When you peel, cut up, and boil perfectly good potatoes, and then pour off the water in which they have been cooked, and then mash the potatoes, you have what I call "smashed" potatoes, because all the good has been "smashed" out. To make nourishing, lean mashed potatoes, simply cook them in their jackets, in a small amount of unsalted water, until all the water is absorbed. Then pull off the thin peeling, sprinkle with 1 tablespoon dry skim milk, a bit of vegetable salt, and a handful of chopped parsley. Then mash, adding enough fluid skim milk to make them smooth and creamy. Yes, even on a reducing menu, you can occasionally have ½ cup of potatoes cooked this way.

Light-Hearted Baked Potatoes

Fragrant, delicate potatoes baked by this recipe need not add ounces to anyone's weight. Select medium-sized baking potatoes. Scrub them thoroughly and remove any blemishes. Wipe dry, then rub skin with a little golden oil.

Bake the potatoes on a rack in a moderately hot oven (425° F.) for 40 to 60 minutes, or until the potatoes feel soft when pressed with your towel-protected fingers. Remove the potatoes from the oven and break open the skin immediately to let the steam escape. Blend, for each potato, 1 tablespoon yogurt, ¼ teaspoon vegetable salt, 1 teaspoon finely cut chives. Scoop out the hot potato from the shells into a bowl, and blend quickly with the yogurt mixture. Return mixture to potato shells. Reheat for a few minutes in a slow oven and serve piping hot.

Potatoes à la Garbo

Scrub large baking potatoes; do not peel. Cut in half and scoop out most of the middle portion, until only about ½ inch of potato is left lining the skin. Rub with golden oil and bake in very hot oven until brown and crispy. Greta Garbo first served these potatoes to me and I dedicate this recipe to her. If you like a crisp baked-potato skin, you will love these.

Royal Hashed Potatoes

Heat 1 tablespoon golden oil in heavy iron skillet. Add 2 cups unpeeled potatoes, boiled and diced, and ¼ cup minced onion. Season with vegetable salt. Then add 3 tablespoons milk and let cook without stirring until browned on the bottom. Fold over like an omelet, and serve garnished with parsley. These are the favorite potatoes of Queen Alexandra of Yugoslavia. We ate them daily during Their Majesties' stay in America, so I respectfully dedicate this recipe to her.

Homemade Potato Chips

You can eat these with a clear conscience. Simply scrub potatoes until they shine. Do not peel, but slice very thin. Spread out thinly on a cookie sheet and sprinkle lightly with golden oil and vegetable salt. Place in moderate oven for about 40 minutes, or until potatoes turn into brown chips. Then turn off heat, but leave in for 15 minutes longer to make them extra crisp.

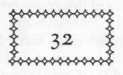

32

Make Delightful Vegetable Espressos

In Czechoslovakia there is a sanatorium where people with digestive difficulties flock by the thousands. There I learned about the
importance of fresh raw vegetable juices. Around this sanatorium
are acres and acres of vegetables, and they are grown on rich organic soil. The head gardener and his assistants collect golden carrots, baskets full of dark-green parsley, young tender spinach leaves,
celery and celery roots. From the orchard the men bring ripe red
apples, pears, and other fruits of the season. The head nurse,
Schwester Karoline, receives these vegetables and fruits with great
ceremony, and a buzz starts in the diet kitchen. The vegetables are
first picked clean, then put into a hydrochloric acid solution (see
page 100), and finally put into ice-cold water for exactly ten minutes to stop the loss of enzymes and vitamins. Carrots and other
roots are scrubbed till they shine, and the leaves are cleaned under
running spring water. Then, with handmills, they grind out the
juices of these very fresh vegetables. By ten o'clock every morning,
each patient in the Carlsbader Sanatorium has his 8-ounce glass
of fresh "live" vegetable juice.

I will never forget Schwester Karoline's expression when she
talked about vegetable juices. She called them the "blood of the
plant." The green magic of chlorophyll, she would say, is the quickest way of healing overfed and undernourished patients. Many
were English and Americans, with colitis, ulcers, liver and gall

bladder difficulties. It was in this sanatorium that, more than thirty years ago, I discovered the immense healing and invigorating power of freshly made raw juices. Since then, I have recommended a daily pint of fresh vegetable juice to every human being I have met. I am convinced, after all these years, that the addition of one pint of these vegetable espressos, as we call them today, to the daily diet is one of the best safeguards against tiredness and premature aging.

Needless to say, I was happy to see the excitement created all over America when Dr. Cheney, of California, announced that fresh cabbage juice cured ulcers in two weeks' time. His cure was based on giving his patients a quart of fresh cabbage juice or 75 percent cabbage and 25 percent celery juice. This is the first time that fresh vegetable juices were "officially recognized"—but why only cabbage juice or celery juice? *All* fresh juices have marvelous healing power, not only because of their vitamin and mineral content, but because of the *"matière vivante"* as Bircher-Benner calls it; and no chemist has yet been able to duplicate this energy. It takes the sun, soil, air, and water, Nature's mightiest forces, to produce young growing plants. No wonder the healing potential is so great in these fresh "live" juices.

If you have a specific health problem and are interested in the many health-giving and curative properties of fresh vegetable juice extractives, I suggest you read the book, *Vegetable Juices for Health,* by Dr. H. E. Kirschner, M.D., who has had years of experience in every phase of nutrition. In this book Dr. Kirschner gives many remarkable case reports of what fresh vegetable juices can accomplish in many so-called hopeless cases.

For people in the second part of life, these juices are doubly valuable because the chewing of raw vegetables may be a problem, or the raw bulk may be irritating. And, of course, much larger quantities of vegetables can be taken in espresso form. Not many people can eat five large carrots, yet a grandmother of 95 can easily drink the juice of five carrots. The vitamins and minerals have been extracted from the pulp and are more easily absorbed by the body, and there is no vitamin or mineral loss due to overcooking. Last, but not least, vegetable espressos are delicious and are therefore the easiest and laziest way to add vitamins, minerals, enzymes, and other as yet undiscovered factors, to the daily diet.

How to Make Fresh Vegetable Espresso

Wash all vegetables carefully. Do not soak any vegetables in water for any length of time—this will leach out vitamins B and C, which dissolve in water as salt does—but wash them under running cold water. Do not peel carrots and other root vegetables. Instead, scrub them with a stiff brush and cut them in pieces.

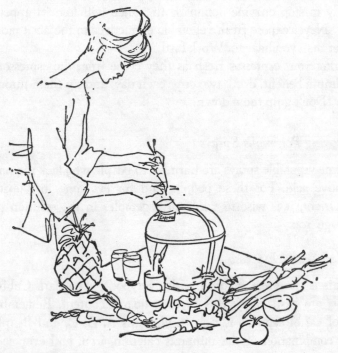

New electric espressor turns ordinary vegetables into potent cocktails

If you are buying a new vegetable juicer, buy the most modern one you can find, one that does not vibrate and get out of balance and one that gives you vegetable espresso with some of the vitamin-rich finely suspended microscopic pulp, not just the watery liquid. An efficient juicer is a good investment for the entire family. There are many on the market since I introduced the drinking of vegetable juices; some are made for bars and some for home use. The one I take with me all over the world weighs only about six pounds.

It is easy to operate because it has only four parts. Also, and this is important, if you buy a new device, the juice must not touch tin, lead, or aluminum; it must flow into a bowl of stainless steel which cannot possibly affect the color, taste, or chemistry of the vitamin-charged juices.

When you have scrubbed your vegetables sparkling clean, put them into the juicer and drink your first glass right from the spout. If you make extra juice, be sure to put it at once on ice and cover tightly to stop enzyme action or the juice will lose its appetizing color. Never expose fresh vegetable extractives to the air a moment longer than you have to. Work fast!

Drink your espressos fresh as they come from the espressor; for maximum benefit, drink two cups each day, and sip them through a straw. Don't gulp them down!

Removing Poisonous Sprays

Some vegetable sprays are harmful to people who lack the normal digestive acid. For these people, and for everyone in Mexico or the Orient, it is wise to wash all vegetables in the solution given on page 100.

Golden Carrot Espresso

This is the great favorite with everybody. The dark California carrots are best. Drink this to your heart's content. Remember, a cup of carrot espresso is rich in vitamins A, B, C, and B_2, plus a good combination of the minerals calcium, iron, and even iodine. Carrot espresso helps complexions to glow, helps the eyes, soothes the "inner man" with its vegetable mucilage. But more than anything else, it tastes so good, straight or mixed with practically any other juice.

Fresh Carrot Capucino

Half a cup of carrot espresso with half a cup of milk makes one of the finest "builder-uppers," rich in vitamins and double rich in calcium. It makes an ideal between-meal drink and is a favorite on beautyfarms. (Waistline watchers should use skim milk.)

Celery Espresso

This is a favorite in England. It is a natural digestive and one of the best appetizers. By all means use some of the dark-green outside stalks; they contain more chlorophyll. But do not use too many of the dark-green leaves; they make the juice too bitter, and they may have been sprayed heavily. Mixing a few drops of lemon or grapefruit juice adds to the flavor and prevents the juice from turning dark. Celery espresso contains vitamins A, B, C, and some E, also the minerals sodium, potassium, and chlorine. This makes it an ideal cocktail for reducers. Celery juice can be mixed with many other juices; try celery and carrot espresso, half and half.

Spinach Espresso

Fresh spinach juice alone has a sharp taste. It should be used sparingly and always blended with milder-tasting vegetables such as carrots and celery. Spinach juice is rich in pro-vitamin A, some vitamin B, and larger amounts of vitamins E and B2. There are also fair amounts of potassium and iodine, but the calcium in spinach is not assimilable. Try equal parts of carrot, celery, and spinach. For a supremely delicious spinach soup, heat a pint of milk, add a cup of spinach espresso, and spike with vegetable salt.

Fresh Parsley Espresso

Parsley espresso, made from the leaves and stems, has a beautiful dark-green color and is rich in chlorophyll; but, like spinach juice, it tastes much better when blended with other vegetable juices. Parsley is no mere table decoration, but a four-star vegetable. It is the richest source of vitamin A among the vegetables, contains some B vitamins, much vitamin C, and even a small amount of vitamin E. Parsley also contains many important minerals, especially iron. Make it a habit to add a bit of parsley to all your vegetable juice mixtures. Carrots, celery, and a bit of parsley make an ideal high-powered iron complexion cocktail.

Fresh Beet Espresso

Young beets, scrubbed and put through the espressor, make an extremely beautiful wine-red juice; but the taste is less agreeable, and only small amounts of beet juice should be mixed with other juices. Two-thirds pineapple juice and one-third fresh beet juice make a pleasant combination. Try "borsht" in the modern manner: Simply add half a cup of beet juice to a pint of milk, heat, and spike with vegetable salt.

Apple Espresso

Nothing can taste better than the juice from fresh ripe apples made by cutting the unpeeled apple into four parts and putting it through a juicer. The juice cannot be compared with ordinary apple juice or cider. It should be called "liquid apples" because it contains the whole aroma and goodness of the apple, including vitamins A and B in fair amounts, vitamins C and B_2 in good amounts, and minerals, including good amounts of sodium. Fresh apple juice has for years been recommended in gout and rheumatism; but in our program, it should be drunk for its deliciousness. Here's hoping that the apple growers of the Northwest install apple-juicing machines all over the land, the same as citrus growers have done. I am willing to bet that all their apples will be sold, once Americans have tasted these "liquid apples." Apple espresso is mentioned here because it also blends so well with vegetable juices, and apples are plentiful the year around.

P.S. Fresh apple espresso taken between meals while reducing is a welcome change, and the pectin of apples makes it especially soothing to the "inner man."

Fresh Cabbage Espresso

Pick tender young cabbage and cut in slices to fit vegetable juicer. This makes a sweet-tasting, light-green juice, but a few dark-green stalks of celery add flavor and character to cabbage juice. Fresh cabbage juice contains vitamins A, B, and C, which are important healing factors, as well as vitamin U, as Dr. Cheney calls the healing factor in cabbage juice. I see no reason why cabbage juice cannot be flavored with carrot juice or any other juice to help eliminate the monotony of just cabbage juice. In other words, 75 percent cabbage juice and 25 percent carrot juice (or tomato juice) can give the same results. Cabbage juice, as well as all other vegetable juices, must be made fresh daily and never kept from one day to the next.

Watercress Espresso

This dark-green liquid, like spinach and parsley juice, looks better than it tastes. You use both leaves and stems. Watercress juice contains practically all vitamins and minerals, including iodine. Therefore, a small amount fortifies other juices. Straight watercress juice, because of its sulphur content, can become an irritant; and it should therefore always be mixed with other juices.

Tomato Espresso

Like fresh apple juice, fresh tomato juice tastes delicious. Fresh tomato espresso, which is made by putting unpeeled ripe tomatoes into the espressor, bears no resemblance to watery canned tomato juice. You will be delighted with the flavor, the color, and above all the valuable contents of this fresh juice. There are plenty of vitamins A and C, some vitamin B. Flavored with a bit of lemon and a dash of vegetable salt, it makes one of the most delicious appetizers. Serve it well chilled.

Cucumber Espresso

Cut tender unpeeled cucumbers into strips and put through espressor. The juice in itself is flat-tasting and must be mixed with pineapple juice or carrot and celery juice. Cucumbers are believed to have a flushing action on the kidneys, and the juice is recommended in reducing and cleansing diets. Cucumbers also contain vitamins A, B, and C, plus chlorophyll and many minerals. When the divine Sarah Bernhardt was asked about the secret of her beautiful complexion, she said: "Cucumber juice is my favorite cosmetic—inside and out."

Gayelord Hauser Cocktail

Cut up equal amounts of dark-green celery, golden carrots, and red apples and put through your espressor. This contains an abundance of vitamins, minerals, enzymes, and chlorophyll. Three glasses a day of this pleasant combination is your best life and health insurance.

N.B. Always put the apples in *last*, because the pectin clogs up the strainer of your espressor.

Pineapple Espresso

Remove the tough outside skin from a ripe pineapple, and cut in slices to fit your electric juicer. The resulting foamy drink is one "fit for a duchess." Pineapple juice contains an excellent digestive called *bromelin* and is therefore most helpful before or after heavy foods are eaten. Besides bromelin, fresh pineapple juice contains the vitamins A, B, C, some B$_2$, plus nine necessary minerals including iodine. At your next dinner party, serve fresh pineapple juice flavored with a bit of watercress juice. This is the combination the Duchess of Windsor liked when I served it to her in Paris; I therefore dedicate this appetizer to her.

Grape Espresso

All fresh grapes contain the important vitamins A, B, and C, plus large amounts of minerals. And grapes have inert sugar that makes them an ideal food for elimination and reducing diets. Thousands of tired and overweight people take the "grape cure" in Meran, Italy, and other resorts. You eat grapes to your heart's content, but the peeling and seeds are not used. You can take your own "grape cure" right at home by drinking three large glasses of fresh grape juice while grapes are in season. (Be sure to wash off every trace of spray first.)

Rhubarb Juice Protects the Teeth

In tests with orange juice, grapefruit juice, and cranberry juice, it was proved that rhubarb juice contains a protective element for the teeth. Here is a million-dollar opportunity for some enterprising manufacturer to put up fruit juices combined with a small amount of rhubarb juice, so that those with sensitive enamel need not worry about the fruit acids ruining their teeth. (Until that time, it is a wise plan to rinse the mouth thoroughly with plain water after drinking acid fruit juices.)

LIQUID SALADS—IF CHEWING IS A PROBLEM

Liquid salads are an important part of the diet therapy used at the famous Bircher-Benner clinic in Switzerland. Old and young are given two glasses of vegetable juices a day. This "liquid salad" idea is an excellent one to adopt, since many people never completely chew their salads and raw vegetables to get all the food from them.

Let your imagination guide you. Put any combination of vegetables into the espressor. A combination of celery, carrots, and tomatoes tastes delicious, as does a combination of watercress, celery, and tomatoes. Another great favorite is a mixture of celery, apples, and a bit of parsley. You might even have a "liquid salad bowl" and put head lettuce, a bit of cabbage, celery, a small cucumber, tomatoes, and half a green pepper through the espressor. Spike with a bit of vegetable salt and a few drops of lemon. Such a liquid salad taken *before* a meal is a wonderful way of breaking yourself of overeating.

EAT, DRINK, AND BE BEAUTIFUL!

Distinguished hostesses all over the world now serve at least one cocktail without alcohol for guests who do not wish martinis and for those who watch their waistlines. One of the most elegant parties I ever attended was at the French Embassy in Constantinople on the Bosporus. Madame de Saint Hardouin, the Ambassadress, served cool carrot and celery espresso and chilled peach and mint cocktails in high-stemmed champagne glasses, side by side with the other cocktails. A king and his queen, many princesses, and diplomats from many lands enjoyed these refreshing drinks and asked for seconds. It is no wonder that Madame de Saint Hardouin is one of the most beautiful women of our time. Her blond hair and skin have long been the envy of every diplomat's wife. Ily de Saint Hardouin, I am happy to say, is a long-time friend and student; and because of her, the entire French Embassy had the benefit of beauty-full eating.

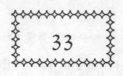

33

Desserts You Deserve

There is no dessert in the whole wide world that can compare with fresh, ripe fruit. Traveling the world over, I am happy to notice that more and more homes and smart restaurants serve fresh fruits at the end of a good meal. In France and Italy, they serve their fruits with the proper flourish. The waiter brings a whole box of beautiful peaches, pears, or grapes to your table. Very often each piece of fruit is carefully nested on its own bed of cotton to prevent bruising. You pick the ripest and juiciest fruit, and then proceed to eat it with the proper fork and knife.

I wish more people would acquire the good habit of eating ripe fruits. It is a fine way to train the palate away from gooey desserts. All fruits are excellent; select the ones you like most. For waistline watchers, ripe melon is especially recommended. To make it more flavorsome, squeeze over it lemon or lime juice. Ripe berries of all types—eat them in as natural a state as possible; or do as South Americans do: sprinkle them with orange or pineapple juice, then they won't need any further sweetening.

One of the favorite desserts at my home is a big crystal bowl full of every kind of fresh fruit. You start the bottom layer with ripe strawberries; on top of that you place a layer of sliced, ripe peaches, then a layer of blueberries, and still another layer of red raspberries, and so on. When the fruits are ripe, they need no sweetening; however, some sweet, fresh orange juice sprinkled over each layer gives added flavor. If the fruits are not sweet enough, sprinkle them with a bit of mild honey. But never sweeten fruits so much that you drown the natural taste.

Lady Mendl's Honey Compote

I learned this secret from the fabulous Lady Mendl's chef, Monsieur Fraise, who has made this compote for kings and queens, dukes and duchesses. I also have seen Sir Winston Churchill eat the compote with delight.

Select ripe fruit or berries, such as peaches, pears, apricots, strawberries, raspberries, blackberries. Use them singly, or in combination when a variety are on the market. If the fruits are cut into wedges they will "cook" more readily. Small ripe peaches or apricots can be used whole or cut in half.

Make a syrup of 1 part honey and 1 part water. When it boils up, pour it over the fresh fruit, cover, and allow to stand until cool; then put compote in refrigerator until serving time. Make just enough syrup to coat the fruit. For variety, add a few slices of lemon or orange and perhaps a bit of cinnamon.

Lady Mendl's Cherries Flambé

No.-2 can large black pitted cherries	¼ cup cognac
	1 tbsp. grated orange peel
1 cup cherry juice	¼ cup kirsch

Drain cherries, saving their juice. Heat cherries in 1 cup of juice in chafing dish. With a large, deep ladle, dip up some of the hot juice, add cognac to the ladle and ignite with a match. When the flames die down, add orange peel and kirsch, and pour at once into the chafing dish. Serve hot as a winter dessert. This flaming dessert was another favorite at Lady Mendl's Petit Trianon in Versailles. It is delectable and colorful, and impresses rich relatives no end. Don't worry about the alcohol; it vanishes into the air, and only the elegant flavor remains.

Broiled Grapefruit Caribbean

Half a fresh, ripe grapefruit is always a welcome dessert, but occasionally you might like it broiled. Simply cut ripe grapefruit in half, remove seeds, and cut the sections; but do not cut out the center. Place 1 teaspoon of brown sugar in center, also 1 teaspoon of sherry. Place in broiler pan under a low flame and broil for about 10 minutes. Be sure to put a little water on bottom of pan to prevent burning.

Jamaican Bananas

This picturesque dessert is no more fattening than baked apples. Peel 6 large, ripe bananas, split in half, and place in a shallow baking dish, cut side down. Mix 1 tablespoon sesame oil, ⅓ cup brown sugar, and 2 tablespoons lemon or lime juice, and pour over bananas. Bake 20 minutes in a slow oven (300° F.), basting several times. Sprinkle with shredded coconut and serve hot.

Pineapple au Kirsch

At Maxim's in Paris, fresh pineapple is served with pomp and circumstance. The headwaiter slices a very ripe peeled pineapple with a long sharp knife. On two paper-thin slices he pours a spoonful of kirsch, and serves it with a low bow. We lucky people in the land of plenty can eat pineapple without cutting it so thin, and with or without kirsch (but, of course, no extra sugar).

Pineapple de Luxe

1 ripe pineapple	1 qt. orange sherbet
honey	2 small tangerines

Pare the pineapple, slice, and cut in small cubes. Pour a little honey over the cubes; mix until all of the pineapple is coated lightly with honey. Put in a glass dish or china bowl, and chill.

To serve, spoon pineapple cubes and a little of the honey liquid from the bowl into a tall, flared dessert glass, or into a large wine glass. Fill glass with orange sherbet. Garnish with peeled sections of tangerine. Makes 8 or more servings—and always wins compliments.

French Yogurt Desserts

Fresh yogurt takes the place of cream or whipped cream for people who value their waistlines. You can make many attractive dessert combinations. Place ripe sliced peaches in your finest crystal goblets, cover them with a tablespoon or two of yogurt, and sprinkle the top with just a bit of honey and some finely grated lemon peel.

Raspberries and strawberries look beautiful in crystal glasses and become more delicious when you add fresh yogurt. People who love the taste of thick cream over strawberries or raspberries, as they make them in Paris, say that these yogurt fruit desserts are tops.

Light-Hearted Pie Crust

The most tasty and flaky crusts can be made with the light golden oils, fragrant whole-wheat flour, and sesame, poppy, or chopped sunflower seeds. Fresh and honeyed fruits of all kinds can be piled high into these tender pie shells. Small individual pie shells also make welcome and elegant desserts without insulting the waistline. To add more nutrition and glamour to fruit pies, before baking the crust sprinkle a tablespoon of your favorite seeds over pie shell and press in.

½ cup sesame oil (or sunflower oil)   1 tsp. vegetable salt
⅓ cup cold water   1 tbsp. sesame seeds
2 cups whole-wheat or
   unbleached flour

Mix sesame oil with the water and quickly add flour and salt. Mix as quickly as possible with a fork. Form into a ball and place mixture between two sheets of waxed paper and roll thin. Line pie plate with the crust, sprinkle with seeds, and bake to a light golden brown. Fill crust with your favorite fruit, and top with yogurt if you wish.

Quick Viennese Pie Shell

1 cup whole-wheat flour   1 hard-cooked egg yolk,
½ cup golden oil or sunbutter   finely mashed
1 tbsp. honey   ½ tsp. vegetable salt
                                    ½ tsp. grated lemon peel

Mix ingredients well. Press on pie plate and chill in refrigerator. Then bake to a golden brown. Let cool. Fill with fresh honeyed fruit. Also makes delightful individual tart shells. So easy to make, and delicious.

Honeyed Wheat Germ Pie Crust

1 cup sifted whole-wheat flour	¼ cup golden oil
⅛ tsp. grated nutmeg	2 tbsp. milk
¾ tsp. vegetable salt	¼ cup honeyed wheat germ

Sift flour, nutmeg, and vegetable salt together into a mixing bowl. Pour over, all at once, without combining, the oil and milk. Stir all ingredients lightly together. Add honeyed wheat germ, and continue stirring until blended. Form mixture into a ball. Place on a large sheet of waxed paper, flatten slightly, cover with another sheet of waxed paper, and roll out the dough. Remove the top paper. Invert the rolled dough and its bottom paper into a pie pan. Remove the paper. Shape the dough into the pan as usual, trim the edge, and make a decorative rim with thumb and forefinger or by pressing with a fork. Prick bottom of crust well with a fork. Bake in a hot oven (475° F.) 10 minutes or until golden and crisp.

Let crust cool. Pile high with sliced ruby-red strawberries. Or pour honey custard (page 520) in to half-fill the crust, and chill; then fill with fresh fruit slices, raspberries, or blueberries. This is also wonderful with fresh plums prepared this way: Cut them in half, do not peel; remove stones. Simmer halves in a mixture of equal parts water and honey, to cover, about 7 minutes. Let cool in honey mixture. Then spoon the fruit carefully on the custard filling. I dedicate this delightful dessert to my adorable sister-in-law Mrs. O. R. Hauser, who first served it to me.

Eighteen-Carat Orange Cookies

Here's an excellent "orange diamond" that contains real nourishment and is delicious:

½ cup sunbutter or margarine	1 cup shredded coconut
2 cups brown sugar	1 cup chopped nuts
2 unbeaten eggs	1½ tsp. baking powder
1 tsp. vanilla	¼ tsp. salt
1½ cups unbleached flour	1 cup orange juice
½ cup wheat germ	

Cook butter and sugar together over low flame until mixture bubbles. Cool. Add unbeaten eggs and beat thoroughly. Add vanilla, mix, and add dry ingredients alternately with orange juice. The mixture should be quite thin. If necessary, add more orange juice. Pour onto lightly oiled cookie-sheet and bake at 350 degrees for about 20 minutes. Cut diagonally into diamonds while still warm.

You Can Make Gelatin Doubly Nutritious

Since gelatin lacks many of the important amino acids and is an incomplete protein, many nutritionists do not recommend it. However, when gelatin is eaten with a meal containing a complete protein—as in meat, milk, eggs, or cheese—the inferior gelatin protein becomes a valuable and nutritious first-class protein. Therefore, gelatin desserts, when served with a balanced meal, are valuable. Naturally, we use only the pure white unsweetened gelatin, which you can buy by the pound. The highly colored sweet gelatins are mostly sugar and should not be used by intelligent homemakers. For color and flavor, we add pure unsweetened fresh or frozen fruit and vegetable juices. Follow directions on package.

Unsweetened Grape Juice makes a delightful dish, a doubly nutritious and decorative gelatin dessert. When it is partially set, remove it from the refrigerator and beat it until it is light and foamy. Then pour into a mold which has been rinsed in cold water. Chill. Serve with fresh milk or a spoonful of honey custard (see page 520).

Orange Juice, flavored with a little sherry, makes a golden jelly. For variety's sake, try this orange-sherry gelatin. Whip it as described above; pour it into a mold and chill. Serve this garnished with thin sections of fresh orange, and sprinkle with a bit of coconut. Or pour it into a square pan and chill; when firm, cut in small cubes. Pile the sparkling golden squares into dessert glasses. Garnish with fresh cherries, if available.

Wine Jelly—A Fine Party Dessert

There is an elegant aura about wine jelly. The color captures the sparkle of dinner table candles, the flavor reminds one of summer and the vineyards of France. Incidentally, it is a nutritious and easy-to-make dessert, and a favorite of weight-watchers.

4 tbsp. unflavored gelatin
1 cup cold water
3 cups boiling water
2 tbsp. honey

juice of 1 orange
grated peel and juice of 1 lemon
2½ cups sherry, Madeira, or port wine

Soften gelatin in cold water about 5 minutes. Then add boiling water and honey and stir until gelatin dissolves. Stir in fruit juices and peel, and let cool. (Some cooks strain out the peel after a few minutes.) When the gelatin mixture has cooled, add the wine. Pour into a 2-quart mold which has been rinsed with cold water. Chill until firm. Unmold onto a chilled serving dish. Garnish with grape leaves and small clusters of grapes. Makes 8 to 12 servings.

French Sherbet

1 cup thick yogurt
½ cup fresh or frozen fruit juice
¼ cup honey

1 tbsp. lemon juice
vegetable salt
2 fresh egg whites

Mix yogurt with fresh or frozen fruit juice. Add honey, fresh lemon juice, a pinch of vegetable salt; and mix thoroughly. Place mixture in freezing tray and freeze until quite firm. Then remove to a bowl and stir until smooth. Now fold the fresh egg whites, beaten stiff, into the mixture. Return to freezing tray. Dozens of smooth French yogurt sherbets can be made with the fresh or frozen fruit juices in your market.

Raspberry Sherbet—A Great Favorite

2 tsp. unflavored gelatin
¼ cup cold water
1 qt. fresh or quick-frozen red raspberries
¼ cup lemon juice
1¾ cups water

¾ cup honey
2 egg whites
⅛ tsp. salt
few reserved whole berries and fresh mint leaves

Soften gelatin in the ¼ cup cold water. Press the berries through a sieve or ricer, or use a blender. Add lemon juice to the berries, and mix. Combine the 1¾ cups water and honey in a saucepan and boil 10 minutes. Remove from heat and stir the soaked gelatin into this hot syrup to dissolve. Let syrup cool. Add sieved berries and mix to combine smoothly. Pour into refrigerator tray; chill about 30 minutes. Whip egg whites with salt until they are stiff and stand in peaks when beater is withdrawn. Fold egg whites into the chilled berry mixture. Pour back into refrigerator tray. Freeze for 30 minutes, then beat well. Freeze 3 hours or more, beating the sherbet at half-hour intervals. Beat once again before serving. Makes 5 or 6 servings. To serve this fragrant frozen dessert, heap it in large wine glasses instead of the usual dessert dishes. Place a geranium or grape leaf under each stemmed glass on dessert plate. Garnish sherbet with a few whole berries and a mint leaf.

Golden Carrot Sherbet

1 quart fresh carrot juice	3 med. size bananas
1 can (6 oz.) of frozen orange juice	3 tbsp. honey

Place all ingredients in electric blender and mix until very smooth. Pour mixture into refrigerator tray and freeze. Stir several times before serving.

Golden Papaya Ice

1 cup water	⅓ cup lemon juice
1¾ cups honey	2 cups sieved fresh ripe or
1 tbsp. grated lemon peel	cooked papaya

Combine water, honey, and lemon peel in a saucepan. Cook over low heat and stir until blended. Then bring to boiling, and boil gently 5 minutes without stirring. Let cool. Add the lemon juice and papaya, and mix well. Pour papaya mixture into a freezing tray. Freeze until firm. Then remove from tray and break up the mixture with a wooden spoon into a large bowl. Beat with electric mixer or hand rotary beater until it is free of lumps, but still of a thick consistency. Return it to freezing tray, and let freeze again. Beat once more before serving; then serve at once. Garnish as desired.

Honey Ice Cream—For Skinnies

2 cups whole milk
¾ cup honey
¼ tsp. salt

2 eggs
1 cup cream

Scald milk in top of double boiler. Add honey and salt. Beat eggs. Pour scalded milk into egg mixture, and stir until well blended. Return to top of double boiler and cook over hot water for 3 or 4 minutes. Let the mixture cool. Beat cream and fold it into custard mixture. Pour into refrigerator tray and freeze. Stir once or twice during the freezing period.

Golden Honey Custard

4 eggs
½ cup golden honey

3 cups whole milk
⅛ tsp. vegetable salt

Separate egg yolks. Beat yolks until lemon colored, adding honey gradually as you beat. Then add milk gradually, beating the mixture smooth. Whip egg whites, with the salt, until they are stiff and stand in peaks when the beater is withdrawn. Fold yolk mixture into egg whites. Pour into 6 or 8 individual custard cups. Place the cups in a shallow pan, and add about 1 inch hot water to the pan around the cups. Bake in moderate oven (325° F.) until the custard is firm. This should be about 1 hour. To test, insert a silver knife blade; if custard does not adhere to the blade, it is ready to be removed from the oven. Let cups cool a little, then chill in refrigerator.

California Apricot Soufflé

¾ lb. dried California apricots
5 egg whites

5 tbsp. brown sugar
vegetable salt

Soak apricots in warm water overnight. Press through sieve, or put in mixer and purée. Beat egg whites until stiff, and beat into them the brown sugar and a pinch of vegetable salt. Fold into apricot purée. Pile lightly into a buttered baking dish, and bake in slow oven (300° F.) until center is firm, about 45 minutes. Served with vanilla or fruit sauce, it makes a festive dessert. I dedicate this recipe to my friend Dagmar Godowsky, who loves all the good things in life.

Quick Apricot Whip

1½ cups of slightly cooked dried apricots are folded into 1 cup chilled yogurt, and sprinkled with honey and grated orange peel. Prune whip can be made the same way. Both prune and apricot whip make delicious fillings for individual pie shells.

Molasses Meringue

Beat 2 egg whites until foamy. Then add ⅓ cup molasses to the egg whites and beat until it stands up in peaks. Pile gently on top of pie, and place under broiler until delicately brown.

Plump Juicy Prunes, Apricots, and Raisins without Cooking

Simply wash dried prunes, apricots, or raisins, and place in quart jar. Cover with warm water, 1 tablespoon honey, and 1 tablespoon lemon juice. Cover jar, let stand 24 hours; then enjoy the juiciest, plumpest fruits you ever tasted. Excellent for breakfast or dessert.

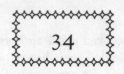

34

Coffee or Tea?

COFFEE FOR CONNOISSEURS

We in the Americas have the best coffee beans in the world; but we do not always use them wisely. What was once an aromatic lean beverage has become a sugar-and-cream-laden concoction with which millions of Americans wash down their food. Yes, many thousands of Americans, who otherwise do not overeat, carry twenty or more pounds of excess weight around because of this sugar-and-cream habit. If you are one of these sugar-and-cream coffee drinkers, here's hoping I can help you break the habit.

Café au Lait

Why not acquire the *café au lait* habit? Thus you get the mild stimulation of fresh coffee plus the nourishment of hot milk; and it requires no sugar at all. Or learn to enjoy a cup of hot freshly brewed coffee as is; you will be surprised at how soon you will enjoy your cup of coffee clear. I find that more and more smart people the world over would not think of spoiling the aroma of coffee with cream and sugar.

Café Espresso

The fight against the cream-and-sugar habit is also sweeping Europe. Café espresso is the strong black coffee the Italians have

enjoyed for many years; even the small restaurants have their espresso machines and serve very small cups of flavorsome black coffee. I was delighted to see this coffee served not only in Italy,
but also in Germany, the home of the fattening *Schlag,* and in
France, the home of sugared chicory coffee. In New York and
Chicago you find espresso coffee being served, and the way people
stand in line for it is a sign that they like this new coffee treat. It is
quite strong, but there is so little of it in a serving. Italians claim
that its bitters aid digestion. The first time you drink espresso, try
a little honey with it, if you wish; then use less and less until you
can enjoy the fragrant brew just as it comes out of the steaming
machine.

Mint Coffee—A New Delight for Sophisticates

As you enter the new and beautiful Hotel Phoenicia in Beirut,
an attendant wearing a fez welcomes you with a steaming-hot cup
of mint-flavored coffee. The Sheik of Kuwait was so impressed
with this gesture of hospitality that he now plans to build an elaborate hotel on the Persian Gulf and serve mint coffee to his royal
guests. Here is the recipe for this delightful and new coffee treat:
Simply add a teaspoon of dried peppermint leaves to finely ground
drip coffee. Put in a drip coffee maker and pour on boiling water.
(You can increase or decrease the amount of peppermint leaves.)
Serve very hot in small cups with honey or brown sugar.

American Coffee

It can be made in many different ways, but I believe that the
most flavorsome is drip coffee, made in one of those wonderful
porcelain pots. There is no tin or aluminum to change the delicate
flavor of freshly ground coffee. My morning cup of coffee is brought
to me in one of these porcelain pots, and it is always fragrant and
never bitter. The next-best method for making coffee is in the
glass vacuum-type of coffee-maker, where the freshly boiled water
goes just once through the freshly ground coffee and extracts only
its aromatic flavor and none of the bitter-tasting acids. Clear, fragrant coffee is the dieter's delight, and it can be taken several times
a day. Whenever coffee tastes bitter, it has been cooked too long;

and that's why millions of people have acquired the fattening sugar-and-cream habit.

Swiss Coffee

Thousands enjoy this lean and delicious beverage. You simply fill a large cup half full of freshly made coffee, then fill the rest of the cup with hot fortified milk. In Zurich, Switzerland, they pour coffee and milk at the same time; the coffee pot is in one hand and the milk pot in the other. Both streams meet in the cup, and the result is a frothy cup of delicious brew which needs no sweetening. (If you must, add just a bit of honey.) The extra milk provides added protein, which is so important, especially for breakfast.

Instant Swiss Coffee

If you are in a hurry, you can simplify the whole procedure and make instant Swiss coffee. Simply put 2 to 3 teaspoonfuls of instant dry lean milk and one teaspoon of your favorite instant coffee into a cup. Fill the cup with hot water and stir. This is a most pleasant and easy-to-make drink. Nervous and sleepless people should use the decaffeined coffee.

Italian Capuccino Coffee

Fresh hot milk is put in blender for 30 seconds to make it fluffy and foamy. When this is added to coffee, it makes it look like *schlag,* or whipped cream. Just a bit of cocoa sprinkled on top makes it different and delightful. It was my pleasure to serve this coffee to Mr. and Mrs. Ridder when they visited me in my home in Taormina, and I dedicate this recipe to the charming Agnes Kennedy Ridder.

New Orleans Cup

If even decaffeined coffee keeps you awake, stir 2 teaspoons of unsulphured molasses into a cup of very hot milk, add a pinch of salt, stir, and drink immediately.

Tea for Connoisseurs

Tea drinkers talk about themselves, and coffee drinkers talk about others—so goes a saying. I don't know if that is so, but I do know that there are two distinct camps—coffee-lovers and tea-lovers. There are many ways to make good coffee, but there is only one way to make good tea. The water should be fresh—it should be "singing," not boiled flat. The pot should be earthenware or porcelain. Metal pots change the flavor, say the real tea connoisseurs. The hot water and tea should steep in the pot for exactly 5 minutes, and no more, to get all the flavor but not the tannic acid from the tea leaves. Such tea is delicious. It can be drunk, hot or iced, to your heart's content. Drink it clear or with lemon; and if you must use a sweetener, try a little honey. *A cup of tea with a teaspoonful of honey taken 30 minutes before dinner is another way to curb a ravenous appetite.*

Tea Variations

With *minted tea,* you can combine the "lift" of regular tea with the fragrance of mint. You simply use ⅔ of your favorite tea leaves and ⅓ of dried peppermint leaves. This makes a delicious between-meal or five-o'clock pick-up. My friend the lovely Ann Astaire, who lived for many years in England and Ireland, has long enjoyed this tea; she now serves it to her guests. I must say it is a wonderful drink.

Papaya tea, a century-old after-dinner digestive, is becoming more and more popular. The dried papaya leaves contain a digestive enzyme; a mixture of half papaya and half mint tea makes a delicious after-dinner drink to help digestion.

Rose-hip tea is an old standby in the Bircher-Benner Sanatorium in Switzerland. Rose hips are rich in vitamin C, and when steeped for 4 minutes they make a beautiful and flavorsome pink drink.

Strawberry tea, made from the dried leaves of wild strawberries, makes an excellent brew, and tastes very much like regular tea. A teaspoon of dried leaves is simmered in boiling water for 3 minutes. Delicious served with milk and honey.

If you are a chronic tea drinker, may I suggest that you acquire the excellent habit of mixing your tea leaves with any one of the above fragrant and healthful herbs—all free of tannic acid.

Maté Tea

This delightful beverage was a new taste thrill for me. It was served to me for the first time during my tour in Argentina. There they love it, and drink it every morning as an eye-opener. They drink it from elegant silver cups and through solid silver straws. Real connoisseurs drink it without sugar; others spoil the beverage by sugaring it too much. Maté tea is inexpensive and obtainable everywhere. I recommend that you add it to your list of beverages. A cup of maté tea with a teaspoon of honey is wonderfully refreshing and can give you a real lift.

Tranquillitea

Instead of synthetic tranquilizers and dangerous sleeping tablets, try this century-old recipe. Mix 1 ounce of dry peppermint leaves (nature's digestive), 1 tablespoon rosemary leaves (nature's tranquilizer), and 1 teaspoon sage leaves (nature's sleep producer). Mix and keep in tightly closed jar. Use 1 heaping teaspoon of mixture to a cup of boiling water. Let steep for one minute, strain, sweeten with honey, and sip! Amazing tranquilizing effect—without a hangover.

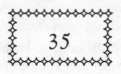

35

Milk and Milk Foods

Milk, like eggs, contains first-class tissue-building protein. It would be ideal if we could get fresh milk directly from healthy, well-fed cows. There now are some certified herds, and the milk from such a dairy is well worth the price. The milk you buy in your market is pasteurized, and often homogenized, and many important elements are lost; but all milk still contains its valuable protein. One quart contains about 35 grams. Therefore, if an adult drinks a pint of milk a day, he gets 17½ grams of protein, plus the important calcium.

Milk is an ideal food for fortifying other foods. In some parts of Italy people have learned to cook their spaghetti in milk, thus increasing the low protein value of their spaghetti; and in the Scandinavian countries, cereals are often cooked in milk instead of water. Millions of homemakers here have learned the secret of increasing the protein value of many dishes by using the inexpensive dry powdered skim milk. Dry milk should never take the place of fresh milk, but it is ideal for fortifying the watery skim milk; simply add 1 to 1½ cups of dry skim milk to a quart of fresh skim milk. This doubles its protein value and gives you 70 grams of protein, plus calcium, riboflavin, and other needed B vitamins.

Hi-Vi Milk

I recommend Hi-Vi Milk as sheer kitchen magic, especially for families who have to economize. Use this good-tasting milk in your coffee, over cereals, and in cream gravies. Always have a bottle in your refrigerator. (Check up on your protein intake before retiring—60 grams for ladies and 70 grams for gentlemen—and make up any deficiency with a glass of Hi-Vi Milk.)

Hi-Vi Milk Formula

Combine 1 quart of fresh skim milk, 1 to 1½ cups dry skim milk, and 2 tablespoons of golden vegetable oil. Thoroughly mix in blender or with egg beater. Use this formula not only as a beverage but also for cooking purposes and for pouring over cereals.

You may add any healthful flavor to your Hi-Vi Milk—one or two tablespoons of dark molasses (rich in iron), one or two tablespoons of caruba powder to give a chocolaty flavor, or a tablespoon of instant coffee.

Coffee Cream—If You Must!

1 cup fresh skim milk   ½ cup dry skim milk
1 tbsp. golden vegetable oil

Combine all ingredients and mix at high speed in blender. Serve at once.

Fortified Milk for Reducers

Most of the calories are in the cream of milk, but removing the cream from whole milk still leaves too much fat. It is therefore wise to buy skim milk and fortify it with dry skim milk. In this manner you receive double the amount of protein, calcium, riboflavin, and other vitamins of the B family, in one quart of milk. Such fortified skim milk prevents hunger pains and gives that satisfied feeling when taken with or between meals. I recommend this fortified milk drink to everyone—and for overweighters, it is their best friend. Here is how to make this superfood so that you won't even know it is skimmed milk:

Put a little less than a quart of fresh skim milk into a Mason jar or electric mixer and add ½ cup of dried skim milk. Then add 2 tablespoons dried brewers' yeast and 1 tablespoon molasses or honey. Shake well or mix until frothy. Keep on ice and drink to your heart's content during the day. Heat a cup to the simmering point (do not boil) and take as a nightcap for deep, sound sleep. A cup of this fortified milk provides 13.7 grams of protein, and a total of 145 calories. Of that total, 75 calories are derived from lactose. Many adults do not absorb lactose completely, and what they fail to absorb fails to add weight.

Famous Milk Lassie

Beat 2 level tablespoons powdered skim milk and 2 teaspoons unsulphured molasses into 1 cup fresh milk. Add 1 teaspoon powdered brewers' yeast. Beat until smooth. Serve cold between meals or hot (but do not boil) before retiring.

Honey Lass

Put 1 teaspoon honey into 1 cup hot vitamin D milk. Stir with fork until smooth. Excellent for weight-*gaining* when taken between meals or before retiring.

Chocolaty Caruba Milk

Unfortunately, the widespread habit of drinking "chocolate milk" is a bad one, especially for youngsters. Recent tests show that the important calcium in chocolate milk is not nearly so well absorbed as it is in plain milk. Therefore, since so many adults and children are already woefully short of calcium, chocolate milk cannot be recommended.

Carob powder, made from the dried fruit of the locust tree (St. John's Bread of Biblical times), has a delightful chocolate-like flavor. One tablespoon of carob powder, beaten into a cup of fortified fresh milk, makes a delightful and nourishing milk drink. It can be served hot or cold. Most diet and health shops now have delightful carob powder to make chocolaty drinks instantly.

Vanilla Milk Shake

Simply put 2 tablespoons dry skim milk powder into 1 pint of fluid skim milk, add a few drops of vanilla, and stir or shake the mixture. This milk shake is a wonderful bracer between meals. It helps to keep your energy up and spirits high. You can also use this double-protein-rich milk in your coffee. For festive occasions, put milk in the blender or whip until foamy.

Cinnamon Milk Shake

Blend 2 tablespoons skim milk powder into 1 pint of fluid skim milk and add ¼ teaspoon powdered cinnamon. Shake well and put in refrigerator. Shake again before using.

Nutmeg Milk Shake

To 1 pint fresh skim milk, add 2 tablespoons skim milk powder and ¼ teaspoon powdered nutmeg. Shake. Keep in refrigerator; shake again before using.

Ginger Milk Shake

For a spicy combination, put 2 tablespoons dry skim milk powder into 1 pint fluid skim milk; add ¼ teaspoon powdered ginger. Shake. Place in refrigerator; shake again before using.

Instant Coffee Milk Shake

Mix 1 teaspoon instant coffee with 1 pint fluid skim milk and 2 tablespoons dry skim milk powder. Shake and refrigerate. Shake again before using.

Orange-Lemon Milk Shake

This is a refreshing combination. Add ½ teaspoon grated orange and lemon peel to 1 pint fresh skim milk, plus 2 tablespoons dry skim milk powder. Shake and refrigerate. Shake again before using.

Licorice Milk Shake

Here's a new and interesting combination from Paris. Put 2 tablespoons dry skim milk powder and 1 teaspoon real licorice into 1 pint fluid skim milk; shake. This can also be served hot as a delicious good nite cap.

Molasses Milk Shake

Into 1 pint fluid skim milk, mix 2 teaspoons unsulphured molasses and 2 tablespoons dry skim milk powder. Shake and refrigerate. Shake again before using. This also makes a delicious hot coffee substitute.

Milk Shakes Unlimited

With a little practice, you can make a different mixture for practically every day of the year. Always use the same base: 2 tablespoons dry skim milk powder and 1 pint fluid skim milk. Remember that this gives you 25 grams of good protein. And it has been found that taking milk drinks between meals is the best and surest way to keep the stomach contented and happy.

Hi-Vi Fruit Drinks

Many who are allergic to fresh milk—or just plain don't like it—enjoy the following nutritious mixtures. The addition of dried skim milk, brewers' yeast, wheat germ, and natural fruit sugars make Lucullan drinks. These are rich not only in vitamin C, but also in vitamins of the B family, vitamin E, many minerals, and the ever-necessary amino acids. Most of these drinks can be made in a cocktail shaker; but for superb results, you should invest in one of those electric mixers that blends everything into smooth, easier-to-digest liquids. Be inquisitive; try each of the various drinks. Then experiment and create new combinations. But don't overdo, as some health faddists do, and make combinations that taste like hay. There must be pleasure in eating. *We also eat with our eyes, so make everything as attractive and appetizing as possible.* Drink these concentrated mixtures through a straw—and slowly, please. Here are some of my favorite combinations:

Orange Milk Shake

Shake or mix 1 glass orange juice with 2 tablespoons powdered skim milk and 1 tablespoon honey. Mix until smooth and frothy. Drink at once for quick energy. I dedicate this drink to Jessica Dragonette, beloved singing star, who passed this secret formula on to me.

Pineapple Shake

Put ¼ cup powdered skim milk and 1 teaspoon honey into a large glass of unsweetened pineapple juice. Beat until frothy. For better nourishment, also add 1 teaspoon brewers' yeast; gradually increase to 1 heaping tablespoon as you become accustomed to the flavor. You can also try this combination with grape juice, loganberry juice, apricot juice, or apple juice.

All-in-One Cocktail—A Meal in a Glass

Pour a glass of pineapple juice or apple juice into your mixer. Add 1 tablespoon dry skim milk, 1 tablespoon nut kernels, 1 teaspoon wheat germ, 1 teaspoon powdered brewers' yeast, and 1 teaspoon honey. For extra flavor, add 1 tablespoon of berries and a few slices of banana. Mix thoroughly. In one minute you will have a most delicious "building drink"—a meal in a glass! This combination I dedicate to the dynamic Leopold Stokowski, whose energy seems to increase with each year.

Curvaceous Cocktail

Into 1 cup milk (or 1 cup orange juice) beat 1 egg yolk, 2 teaspoons peanut oil, 1 tablespoon wheat germ, and 1 teaspoon honey. Excellent for weight *gaining*.

Pineapple Delight

Pour 1 cup unsweetened pineapple juice into an electric mixer. Add 2 tablespoons wheat germ, 1 tablespoon powdered skim milk, and 1 teaspoon honey or molasses. Mix until smooth and creamy; serve at once.

Special Banana Milk for Skinnies

Mix in an electric mixer 1 very ripe, almost black, banana, 2 tablespoons powdered skim milk, 1 teaspoon honey, and 1 glass of vitamin-D milk. This combination, taken with meals, has helped many people to *put on* healthy pounds.

Special Formulas for Reducers

Mix 4 tablespoons dried brewers' yeast (celery flavor) with 1 quart canned tomato juice. For additional flavor, add ½ teaspoon vegetable salt, 1 tablespoon lemon juice, and your choice of 1 tablespoon parsley or chives or green onion, or 1 teaspoon caraway seeds. Shake in Mason jar, or whip in electric blender, until frothy. Keep in refrigerator. Taken 30 minutes before meals, it prevents overeating.

Mix 1 pint tomato juice, 1 pint sauerkraut juice, 4 tablespoons dried brewers' yeast, and a pinch of caraway seeds if you like. Keep in refrigerator. Excellent as a first course or between-meal snack.

Mix 1 pint tomato juice, 1 pint yogurt, dash of vegetable salt, and 2 tablespoons dried brewers' yeast. Shake in Mason jar or in electric mixer until smooth. Keep in refrigerator.

Mix 1 teaspoon dried brewers' yeast into a glass of unsweetened grapefruit juice.

Note: Since dried brewers' yeast is such a wonder food, try to increase the amount to a tablespoonful. In France they take brewers' yeast before meals to help satisfy enormous appetites.

Make Your Own Buttermilk

A newly discovered secret about buttermilk is that it is an anticholesterol drink. It is rich in protein, calcium, and vitamin B₂. Cool buttermilk is a tasty between-meal drink. Here's how to make your own:

Pour half a cup of buttermilk from your dairy into a quart bottle of warm (not hot) fresh milk from which ½ cup has been removed, and let stand in a nondrafty place overnight. When milk has thickened, shake bottle and place in refrigerator. (Save half a cup for the next batch.)

Homemade Kefir

This cultured milk drink is enjoyed by millions who do not possess refrigerators. You can find Kefir at health and diet shops. Simply place some Kefir grains in a quart of fresh milk. Let stand overnight. The next day you will have a delightful milk drink. Many who do not like sweet milk enjoy this tart Kefir milk. Be sure to strain out the Kefir grains and save them for next batch.

Protein Whipped Cream

With ordinary skim milk you can make a delectable and protein-rich whipped cream to be used over your favorite desserts. Try it on berries and apricots and over fruit pies:

1 cup skim milk	½ tsp. vanilla
1 tbsp. pure gelatin	pinch salt
1 tbsp. honey	

Warm milk, and dissolve gelatin in it. Add honey, vanilla, and salt. Whip to consistency of whipped cream. Use at once.

For Milk Haters

Where there is a real dislike for milk, or an allergy to it, use Dr. Irvine McGuarrie's formula:

½ cup stewing beef	2 tbsp. honey
½ tsp. veal bone ash (very fine bone flour)	1 tbsp. rice (heaping)
1 tbsp. soya oil	enough water to make 1 pint

Put all ingredients in blender and liquidize. According to Dr. McGuarrie, this combination has nourishment equal to that of a pint of fresh milk.

Make Your Own Cottage Cheese

Heat 1 quart of milk in a heavy utensil or double boiler. When warm, add 1 tablespoon lemon juice. Stir and keep heat low. When milk curdles, remove from stove. Pour entire quart into muslin bag or cheesecloth and drain. This makes a delicious cottage cheese. (Be sure to save the water, which contains the valuable whey—rich in minerals and a most valuable food for troubled intestines. Mix whey with apple juice and drink once a day.)

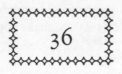

36

Yogurt Means Long Life

Through the ages, yogurt has played an important part in the diets of many people. The Armenians call yogurt *matzoon*. The Yugoslavs call it *kisselo mleko*, and King Peter assured me that there are hundreds of centenarians in his country who thrive on it. The Russians love their yogurt with black bread; they call it *varenetz*. The French eat quantities of yogurt with *fraises de bois*, and call it *yoghourt*. In Sardinia, they call it *gioddu*; in India, *dadhi*; in Egypt, *lebenraib*. But in any language, yogurt always means *long life*.

Whether there are so many one-hundred-year-olds in the Balkans because they love yogurt is debatable. But what interests us most is that although milk in itself is a good food, in the form of yogurt it becomes nutritionally superior in many respects. The important protein in yogurt is partially predigested by the yogurt bacteria, and the calcium in the mild lactic acid is easier to digest. The valuable bacteria in yogurt, living in the intestines, help break down milk sugar into lactic acid; and many of the bacteria which cause gas and fermentation are destroyed. These are some of the reasons why many people who are allergic to sweet milk can enjoy yogurt without difficulties. Even more important, according to the Warner Laboratories who have done so much yogurt research, the bacteria in yogurt synthesize or manufacture valuable B vitamins; so the person who daily uses yogurt has a built-in vitamin B factory in his intestines. For this reason, many doctors now recommend yogurt after antibiotic treatments have destroyed many friendly and valuable bacteria. You can also make your own.

How to Make Real Yogurt

The easiest way to make yogurt is to heat one quart of fresh skim milk. Heat this mixture carefully until it is hot, but do not boil. This is important, boiling kills the *bacillus bulgaricus*. Into this hot, but *not* boiling milk, you stir one cup of powdered skim milk, plus three tablespoonfuls of ready-made yogurt. Pour this mixture into a wide-mouthed thermos jar, cover and let it stand over night. It takes from four to six hours for yogurt to become solid. The next morning, remove top of thermos and place the yogurt in refrigerator.

If you are unable to buy ready-made yogurt in your city, write or go to your nearest health food store and purchase some real yogurt culture. With such culture you can make yogurt for a whole month. After your first initial batch, made with this culture, always save a half cup to make the next batch. If you make yogurt for a whole family, I suggest that you invest in a professional yogurt maker which costs less than ten dollars and turns ordinary milk into creamy yogurt while you sleep.

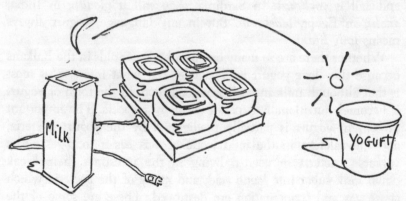

Automatic yogurt maker

French Yogurt

Ever since Elie Metchnikoff wrote in his book, *The Prolongation of Life,* that the good health and long life of the Balkans was due to their custardy milk food, the use of yogurt has steadily increased.

Ordinary yogurt is made by simply heating ordinary milk, adding yogurt culture, then placing the mixture into a bowl of hot water, keeping it covered until the mixture thickens. But the best yogurt to be found anywhere today is the way they make it in France. French yogurt is firmer, more like custard. It is low in fat and highest in protein. Instead of ordinary or homogenized milk, use a quart of fresh skim milk; add one cup of powdered skim milk, and mix well. Into this mixture pour the yogurt culture or 2 tablespoons from your last batch. Pour into clean jars and place in yogurt maker. Preparing this yogurt takes only a few minutes. In a few hours you will have the most delicious and nutritious yogurt you ever ate. This method never fails—and it is a tremendous money saver.

Yogurt Cocktail

Put 1 cup yogurt and 2 cups tomato juice in a shaker. Spike with a pinch of caraway seeds, a teaspoonful of finely chopped onion, a pinch of vegetable salt. Add two pieces of ice, and shake well. This is excellent for nondrinkers at cocktail parties.

Morning-After Yogurt

Mix ½ cup yogurt with ½ cup thick tomato juice; spike with pinch of vegetable salt and a few drops of fresh lemon juice. This is an excellent pick-up for the morning-after, and does much more good than a Bloody Mary. It is also a delicious appetizer and between-meal lift.

Cholly Breakfast Yogurt

For a delicious and nutritious drink, mix equal amounts of tomato juice and fortified yogurt. Add a bit of vegetable salt and paprika, or a pinch of your favorite herb. Blend well and serve chilled. This delicious mixture keeps well when refrigerated. It is excellent for Sunday breakfast or as an appetizer before dinner. I recommend this combination highly and dedicate it to Count Cassini, our Cholly Knickerbocker of New York, a yogurt enthusiast who frequently eats it for breakfast.

Orange Yogurt

Mix 1 tablespoon frozen orange juice concentrate with 1 cup fresh yogurt.

Pineapple Yogurt

Mix 1 tablespoon fresh frozen pineapple concentrate with 1 cup fresh yogurt.

Blue Grape Yogurt

Mix 1 tablespoon fresh frozen Concord grape concentrate with 1 cup fresh yogurt.

These make delightful and nutritious breakfast or between-meal drinks, each one giving about 10 grams of first-class protein. Any frozen fruit concentrate can be used, provided it is unsweetened.

Yogurt Avocado Soup

2 ripe avocados
1 quart stock (chicken or
    vegetable)
2 cups yogurt
pinch vegetable salt

Peel and pit the avocados and add them to the stock and yogurt in blender. Add vegetable salt to taste. Blend until very smooth, and chill before serving. Garnish with chopped fresh dill or parsley. A delightful summer night surprise!

Cold Yogurt Soup from Armenia

2½ cups yogurt
  1 chopped cucumber
  1 chopped hard-cooked egg
½ cup whole milk
¼ cup chopped green onions
  2 tsp. vegetable salt
6 ice cubes
½ cup raisins
1 cup cold water
1 tbsp. chopped parsley
1 tbsp. chopped fresh dill or
  1 tsp. dill seed

Place the yogurt, cucumber, hard-cooked egg, milk, green onions, salt, and the ice cubes in a large salad bowl. Add the raisins (previously soaked in cold water for 5 minutes). Add one cup of cold water and stir well. Chill in refrigerator for several hours. Garnish with parsley and dill when serving.

The Easy Way. A simpler version of cold yogurt soup, which makes a wonderful outdoor party dish on a warm summer evening, can be made by combining cold yogurt with chilled chopped vegetables, such as cucumber, onion, watercress, parsley, chives, onion tops, mint leaves, radishes. Put the yogurt in a bowl and arrange the chopped vegetables in small dishes around the bowl. Put two ice cubes into each chilled soup plate and invite your guests to help themselves, first to the yogurt and then to spoon into the yogurt the vegetables of their choice. Garnish with a slice of red tomato, a bit of grated lemon peel, a spoonful of chopped olives or chives. Season with vegetable salt and paprika. Delicious with dark rye or pumpernickel bread, or Armenian flat bread—the kind that is covered with sesame or poppy seeds.

Hot Yogurt Soup with Meatballs

4 cups yogurt	1 tsp. whole-wheat flour
¼ cup rice	1½ tsp. vegetable salt
1 egg	4½ cups water

Combine all ingredients, except water, in a 3-quart pot and beat well. Stir in the water. Cook over a very low flame until the mixture thickens (about 20 minutes). Stir constantly while cooking. Next, add meatballs, and simmer for another 10 minutes.

Meatballs: ½ lb. ground beef   ½ tsp. vegetable salt
                 1 onion chopped fine   ¼ tsp. white pepper

Mix all ingredients and form into walnut-sized meatballs.

Now Add: ½ cup chopped   ½ cup cooked
                  parsley   garbanzo beans
               ½ cup chopped green
                  onions

Continue to simmer for 15 more minutes, still stirring. Sauté one or two cloves of garlic in butter. Add 1 tablespoon dried powdered mint. Ladle a teaspoon of this sauce into each plate of soup when serving.

Delightful Cucumber Relish

1 cucumber	1 tbsp. fresh chopped dill
1½ cups yogurt	or 1 tsp. dried dill
	vegetable salt

Chop the cucumber fine and add it to the yogurt. Add the chopped dill and vegetable salt, and stir. Chill before serving. Makes an excellent appetizer, relish, or salad.

Green Yogurt Dressing

Add a handful of chopped greens—parsley, chives, fresh mint, green onion tops, watercress, or green peppers—to a cup of yogurt. Use the greens singly or in any combination that appeals to you.

Yogurt Spring Salad

1 cup yogurt	2 cucumbers (sliced thin)
1 tbsp. chopped fresh mint	vegetable salt
1 clove garlic	3 red radishes (sliced thin)

Add the mint and garlic (put through a press) to the yogurt. Stir well. Add cucumber slices and vegetable salt. Garnish with radish slices.

Yogurt Cream Pie—for Skinnies

1 cup yogurt	1 tbsp. honey
1 large package cream cheese	½ tsp. vanilla extract
(9 oz.)	

Combine all ingredients and whip to the consistency of whipped cream. Pour into a baked pie shell and put in refrigerator until it sets. Sprinkle with honeyed wheat germ and/or grated lemon peel before serving.

French Cream Cheese

This creamy cheese is a protein food. You will find many uses for it because it is made from yogurt. It also is friendly to the "inner man." Here is how to make your own:

Simply dump a cup of yogurt (bought or homemade) into a piece of muslin or thick cheesecloth and let it hang above your sink overnight. Next morning you will find a white ball of the tenderest, creamiest cheese you ever ate. To give the cheese more savor and flavor, add a pinch of vegetable salt or a pinch of brown sugar to the yogurt before placing it in the muslin bag. For sandwiches, salads, and dips, add Roquefort cheese to taste.

Index

Guide to Recipes